14.50

P9-CRI-847

GERRIT BEVELANDER
*Formerly, the University of Texas, Dental Branch,
and the Graduate School of Biomedical Sciences,
Houston, Texas*

JUDITH A. RAMALEY
*University of Nebraska Medical Center,
Omaha, Nebraska*

Essentials of
HISTOLOGY

Seventh edition

With 322 figures and 4 color plates

The C. V. Mosby Company

Saint Louis   1974

Seventh edition

Copyright © 1974 by The C. V. Mosby Company

All rights reserved. No part of this book may be reproduced
in any manner without written permission of the publisher.

Previous editions copyrighted 1945, 1952, 1956, 1961, 1965, 1970

Printed in the United States of America

Distributed in Great Britain by Henry Kimpton, London

Library of Congress Cataloging in Publication Data

Bevelander, Gerrit, 1905-
  Essentials of histology.

First-3d ed. by M. M. Hoskins and G. Bevelander.
1. Histology. I. Ramaley, Judith, joint author.
II. Hoskins, Margaret Morris, 1886-   Essentials
of histology.   III. Title.
QM551.B43 1974   611'.018   73-12625
ISBN 0-8016-0677-2

CB/CB/B 9 8 7 6 5 4 3 2 1

Preface

The continuing purpose of this textbook is to provide a clear and concise introduction to the principles of histology—the microanatomy of tissues and organs. The material presented is appropriate for an understanding of basic structure. Such understanding is a prerequisite for the effective study of function as well as the basis for the study and recognition of differences that exist between normal and diseased tissues (pathology). Before one can understand changes in tissue and cellular structure, it is necessary to develop a clear idea of what normal tissue is like. That is what this book is all about.

The major changes in this edition have been made in the chapters on the male reproductive system, the female reproductive system, and endocrine organs. Other chapters have been updated and revised in part.

Several new figures have been added where it was felt that a transition from gross structure to fine structure might help in understanding the microanatomy of a tissue or organ. As in the past, the relation between structure and function has been emphasized and enlarged upon in this edition. This treatment of the material, we believe, will make the text more meaningful and readily understood, especially in relation to the other basic sciences.

Thanks go to those several colleagues whose micrographs appear in the text and also the many instructors who have offered suggestions over the years for improving the presentation of material.

Gerrit Bevelander

Judith A. Ramaley

Contents

COLOR PLATES

Essentials of
HISTOLOGY

1

Introduction

Histology is the science that deals with the detailed structure of animals and plants and in its broader aspects correlates structural features with function. Vital functional units are called cells. Not only do different kinds of cells exhibit variations in form and structural content, but the same cell may vary in these respects with changes in its physiologic status. Our knowledge about cells and cell products has been obtained by a study of "fixed" or dead cells and by a variety of ingenious methods developed to study living cells. Each of these methods has advantages and disadvantages, but they are mutually complementary and we may conclude that all normal cells have certain attributes in common.

Cell structures and cell products are made visible by fixing these structures with suitable chemicals, followed by sectioning and staining with certain dyes. The traditional stains are hematoxylin and eosin (H & E). The basic dyes, like hematoxylin, stain the chromatin of the nucleus (basophilia), whereas the acid dyes, such as eosin, tend to stain the cytoplasm (acidophilia, oxyphilia). Although many other dyes are used, most slides utilized in routine histologic and pathologic studies are hematoxylin and eosin preparations. These dyes have the great advantage of relative stability, universal use, and reproducible results.

In addition to the use of stained preparations, several other methods have been and are currently used to study cells. Histochemical techniques, for example, are currently being used and developed to aid in the localization of specific chemical substances within the cell. By means of these methods, it is possible to localize substances such as enzymes, lipids, nucleic acids, and glycogen. Modifications of ordinary light microscopy are also employed. Some of these are phase microscopy, which enhances contrast and is especially useful for observing living cells, and dark-field microscopy, which utilizes a special condenser producing a dark field. The latter method permits observation at a higher resolution than is possible with the usual light microscope. Ultraviolet rays, x-rays, and polarized light are also utilized for observing specimens to enhance resolution, density, or birefringence, respectively.

The most recently developed instrument used in microscopy is the electron microscope, which employs a system analogous to that of the optic microscope. It differs from the optic system, however, in that the illuminating source consists of a beam of electrons accelerated to a high velocity in a vacuum. The electron beam is projected through a specimen and focused on a fluorescent screen or photographic plate by means of electromagnetic fields that serve as lenses. Although the electron microscope permits visualization of specimens at much greater magnification than is possible by optic methods, the important advantage of this instrument is the great increase in resolution over that afforded by other methods. Whereas the optimum resolution possible with the light microscope is of the order of 0.5μ, the electron microscope can resolve cell structure at approximately 10 Å and thus permits visualization

1

Cell wall   Mitochondrion

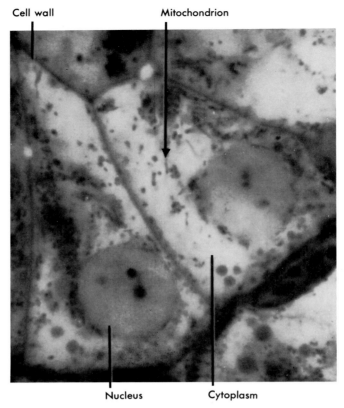

Nucleus   Cytoplasm

Fig. 1-1. Liver cells of turtle showing mitochondria and other cytoplasmic inclusions. (Iron hematoxylin; ×1,000.)

of structures that have the dimension of macromolecules.

THE CELL

Most cells are composed of a single nucleus embedded in cytoplasm (Fig. 1-1). The term *protoplasm* is used to designate the living substance of both the nucleus and the cytoplasm. Protoplasm is a grayish viscous liquid (hydrosol) enclosed at all interfaces by a membrane (cell membrane). The cell membrane selectively regulates the interchange of materials between the cell and surrounding environment and upon death becomes completely permeable, or nonselective.

Cytoplasm

Cytoplasm (protoplasm) is usually considered to be a colloid and consists of ap-

proximately 60% to 75% water, part of which is free, the other part protein-bound (Fig. 1-2). Cationic salts are present as potassium, magnesium, and traces of several others; anions occur as bicarbonate and phosphate. Cytoplasmic components that are particularly concerned with the organization and structure of the cell consist of the following macromolecules: carbohydrates, proteins, and nucleic acid.

Carbohydrates of biologic interest are glycogen and mucopolysaccharides. Glycogen is a storage product from which glucose is released on demand for a variety of metabolic activities. Mucopolysaccharides are frequently present as hyaluronic acid and chondroitin sulfates, components of the ground substance of connective tissue and cartilage, respectively.

Proteins responsible for the characteristic

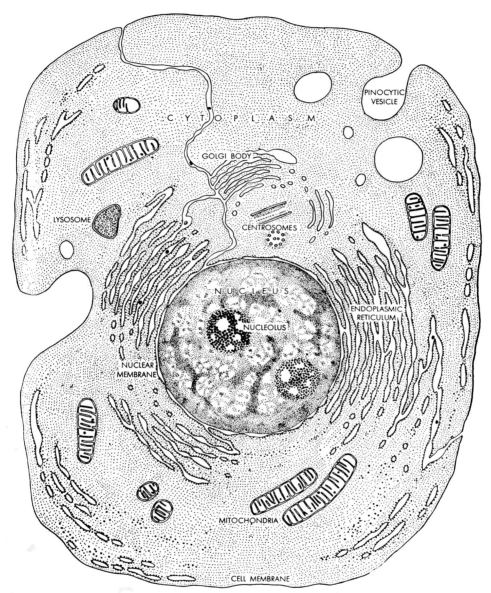

Fig. 1-2. Diagram of typical cell based on what is seen in electron photomicrographs. Mitocondria are sites of oxidative reactions that provide the cell with energy. Dots that line the endoplasmic reticulum are ribosomes, the sites of protein synthesis. In cell division the pair of centrosomes, one shown in longitudinal section (rods) and the other in cross section (circles), part to form poles of apparatus that separate two duplicate sets of chromosomes. (From Brachet: Sci. Am. **205**:51, 1961. Reprinted with permission.)

structure of the cell are molecules of high molecular weight and consist of many amino acid monomers linked in sequence by peptide bonds. They occur as structural proteins such as glycoproteins and keratin or as nonstructural proteins such as enzymes, contractile proteins, and some hormones.

Nucleic acids are polymers of nucleotides concerned with protein synthesis. They are remarkable in that they can exist in infinite varieties because the variation in the base pairs of the nucleic acids and the variation of the sequence of amino acids of the protein elaborated provide a code with limitless combinations.

The most important constituents of the nucleus are the nucleic acids. Two general types of nucleic acids are present—deoxyribonucleic acid (DNA) and ribonucleic acid (RNA). There is more DNA than RNA in the nucleus. DNA is a constituent of chromatin, the material in the nucleus that becomes differentiated during cell division to form discrete structures called chromosomes. Each chromosome contains a number of smaller units, called genes, consisting of DNA and some associated protein. There is excellent evidence that the DNA associated with a specific gene can transfer its information to govern the exact sequence of amino acids in specific proteins. The nuclear DNA is the molecule of heredity, and the sequence of the base pairs is the genetic code providing information and direction regarding the specific function of the cell. This information is transferred to a class of molecules known as messenger RNA, complementary to nuclear DNA, which carry genetic information from the DNA of the gene to the ribosomes, where specific protein synthesis takes place. DNA is found in every living cell and issues the orders of cell pattern and tissue organization to determine the uniqueness of a cell and its ability to duplicate itself; each type of cell contains the duplicating stencil of itself in its own DNA molecules.

CELL (PLASMA) MEMBRANE

The cell (plasma) membrane is visible with the light microscope in some cells as a delicate structure separating one cell from another. Actually what is seen at this magnification is not the plasma membrane itself, whose dimensions are smaller than the resolution of the light microscope, but rather cellular secretions that coat the cell surface. In places, the cell boundaries become visible because of elaborate folding of the cell membrane (brush borders). The plasma membrane serves in both an active and a passive manner to regulate the interchange of metabolites and other substances from the cell and its environment. At the electron microscope's level of resolution the plasma membrane, also known as a "unit" membrane, consists of a three-layered, polarized structure comprised of two dark layers separated by a light interval. Chemically, it is considered to be a bimolecular leaflet made up of a chain of lipid molecules located between two protein layers. In addition to this complex, there is an outer layer of proteoglycan known as the *glycocalyx*, or "fuzz," the latter being composed of N-acetylglucosamine, mannose, and sialic acid. This surface coat is illustrated in Fig. 1-3.

Cell surfaces are frequently specialized. Cells specialized for absorption exhibit fingerlike projections on the free surface, called *microvilli*, which greatly increase the surface area (Fig. 1-3). Absorption or ingestion also occurs in other cells by a process known as *pinocytosis*, which is effected by the formation of small vesicles at the cell surface that ingest materials and transport them to other parts of the cell. *Phagocytosis* is another method of cellular ingestion and is similar in some respects to pinocytosis.

The space between the unit membranes separating adjacent cells is approximately 100 to 200 Å. The membranes separating the cells are often parallel to one another but vary considerably in arrangement. Some, for example, exhibit a serrated or interlocking arrangement (Fig. 1-4). Toward the distal surface of certain cells the lateral cell interfaces are often specialized in the form of thickened membranes known as *terminal bars*. At the base of some cells, for example, of the kidney, prominent infoldings of the basal surface occur. This is

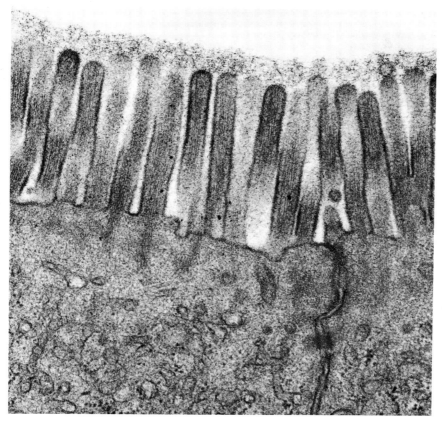

Fig. 1-3. Electron micrograph of microvilli forming striated border of small intestine of mouse and showing surface coat at periphery of microvilli. (×60,000.) (Courtesy Dr. Caramia, University of Rome.)

another modification to increase surface area for transport of materials.

In addition to the situations just described, it has also been observed that there is probably a continuity between the plasma membrane and the endoplasmic reticulum and also indirectly with the Golgi apparatus and other organelles.

ENDOPLASMIC RETICULUM (ERGASTOPLASM)

The cytoplasm of many cells such as nerve cells, salivary gland cells, and the acinar cells of the pancreas exhibits diffuse or discrete masses of material that stains with the same basic dye as does the chromatin material of the nucleus. This material, formerly known as chromophil substance, contains ribonucleoprotein and

changes markedly during cellular activity.

With the electron microscope, regions of the cell exhibiting chromophil substance have been shown to consist of accumulations of osmiophilic granules approximately 150 Å in diameter. These granules, known as ribosomes, are made up of ribonucleoprotein and are believed to be the site of protein synthesis (Fig. 1-5).

The endoplasmic reticulum consists of a complex of cisternae and tubules, which often extend throughout the cytoplasm. It is enclosed by a membrane approximately 75 Å thick. Two varieties of reticulum have been identified: (1) agranular (smooth), in which the cisternae and vesicles do not exhibit osmiophilic granules on the surface of the membranes, and (2) granular (rough), in which the surface of the mem-

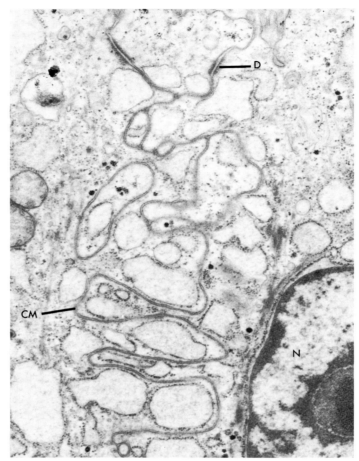

Fig. 1-4. Electron micrograph of part of an epithelial cell of mollusc mantle showing marked folding and interdigitation of adjacent, lateral surface cell membranes. *D,* Desmosome; *CM,* cell membrane; *N,* nucleus. (×27,000.)

branes are studded with granules (ribosomes). The lumen of the reticulum may contain material that has a greater density than the surrounding cytoplasm, and it is apparently in this region that synthesis of some cell products occurs.

GOLGI APPARATUS

The Golgi apparatus (complex) consists of an irregular network usually located in a supranuclear position, that is, between the nucleus and the free surface of the cell. The network may be fairly discrete and localized in one part of the cell, or it may be diffuse and localized in several areas within the cytoplasm.

Electron microscopy shows that the Golgi apparatus consists of a series of parallel arrays of smooth-surfaced membranes. The contoured membranes circumscribe flattened sacs piled one upon another (Fig. 1-6). In some instances, the sacs appear dilated and are then known as Golgi vacuoles. The Golgi apparatus has been associated with secretory activities for some time. Recent studies have confirmed this concept, although many details regarding this mechanism await further clarification.

CENTROSOME (CYTOCENTRUM)

With the light microscope one may observe a small dark body, usually located

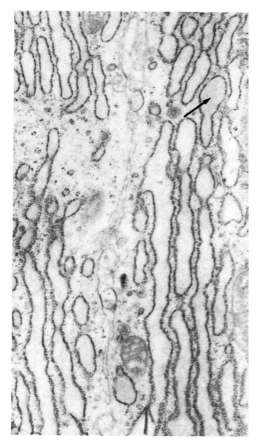

Fig. 1-5. Electron micrograph of the granular or rough endoplasmic reticulum of a young odontoblast. The lumina of the cisternae contain a dense material (arrow), and the external surfaces are studded with granules (ribosomes). (×28,000.)

near the nucleus, called the *centrosome.* The centrosome contains two or more small granules known as centrioles. In many instances the centrosphere (centrosome) is surrounded by a group of delicate, radially arranged fibrils called the *aster.* During the nuclear phase of cell division the centrioles separate and migrate to opposite sides of the nucleus. With the aid of the electron microscope the centriole appears to be a short hollow cylinder having a dense wall in which are embedded nine, longitudinally arranged, tubular elements. In transverse section, the centriole

appears as a dense ring. It is usually located close to the Golgi apparatus.

MITOCHONDRIA

Mitochondria are present in all living cells and require special techniques for visualization at the level of the light microscope. They vary in number from a few to several hundred per cell. They appear as spheres and also as rods and filaments. When observed with the electron microscope, they all have basically a similar structure. They are bounded by two unit membranes. The outer membrane is smooth and the inner membrane is thrown into infoldings, usually in a transverse direction (Fig. 1-7). These infoldings are known as *cristae.* Minute granules, the elementary particles, believed to be the source of several enzymes, are attached to the inner membrane. The core of the mitochondrion is filled with an amorphous fluid known as the *matrix.* A variable number of particles containing calcium, magnesium, and RNA have been observed in the matrix. It has been postulated that the RNA in the particles serves to hold the calcium phosphate in an amorphous form rather than the crystalline form (hydroxyapatite). The mitochondria contain enzymes concerned with oxidative phosphorylation, as well as electron and ion transport mechanisms. They are also involved in cellular respiration and in the storage and transference of energy.

FIBRILS AND FILAMENTS

Fibrils occur in many cells. They are especially prominent in nerve (neurofibrils) (Fig. 8-1) and muscle cells (myofibrils) (Fig. 7-8). In epithelial cells of the skin, they are known as *tonofibrils.* Structures formerly described as fibers at the optic level have been shown to consist of subunits of much smaller dimension that can only be observed with the aid of the electron microscope. For example striated muscle cells contain many myofibrils that can be seen upon further magnification to be made up of smaller filaments. This is true also for collagen fibers in the extracellular matrix.

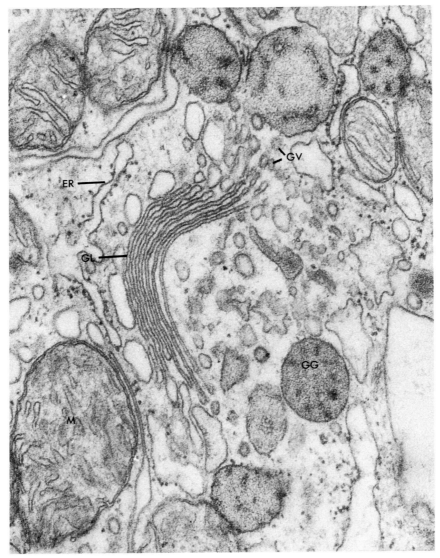

Fig. 1-6. Electron micrograph of part of calciferous gland of *Lumbricus terrestris* showing Golgi apparatus. Note proximity of rough endoplasmic reticulum, *ER*, to the stacks of Golgi lamellae, *GL*, which transmit and modify protein derived from the *ER*. The material is then conveyed to Golgi vesicles, *GV*, which undergo further changes in the cytoplasm as represented by the Golgi granules, *GG*, which are eventually extruded at the free surface of the cell. *M*, Mitochondria. (×77,000.)

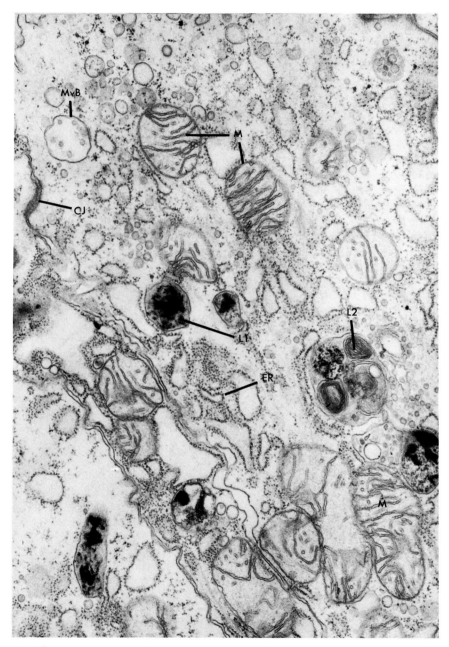

Fig. 1-7. Electron micrograph showing several organelles in the mantle epithelium. *CJ,* Cell junction; *ER,* endoplasmic reticulum; *L1, L2,* phagocytic vesicles (lysosomes); *M,* mitochondria; *MvB,* multivesicular body. (×29,000.)

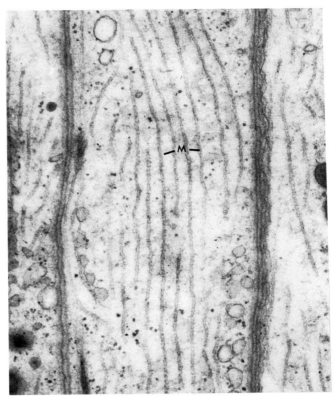

Fig. 1-8. Electron micrograph of longitudinal section of several microtubules, *M*, from marginal gland of Littorina. (×46,000.)

MICROTUBULES

In addition to the microfilaments previously mentioned, cytoplasm frequently exhibits straight *microtubules* having a diameter of approximately 200 Å (Fig. 1-8). The wall of the microtubule is composed of several filamentous subunits. Microtubules are numerous during mitosis and on other occasions when the cell alters considerably in size or shape. The exact function of these structures is not known for certain. It has been suggested that they may function as cytoskeletal elements or that they may be contractile and function in changes in cell shape or movement.

Nucleus

The nucleus of the cell at the interphase exhibits several morphologic characteristics that can be observed with the optic microscope. The nucleus usually appears as a spherical or ovoid body bounded by a nuclear membrane. The nucleus contains a fluid (nucleoplasm) in which is found one or more dark-staining, eccentrically placed spheres (nucleolus) and, in addition, a delicate lacy network upon which dark-staining *chromatin granules* or flakes appear to be lodged (Fig. 1-9). Although the nucleoplasm is rarely stained, both the nucleolus and chromatin granules are strongly basophilic and stain a deep purple or blue with hematoxylin. When stained with toluidine blue, the two may be distinguished. The chromatin stains blue (orthochromasia), whereas the nucleolus, containing RNA, stains purple (metachromasia). In some cells such as white blood cells and megakaryocytes, the nuclei appear to be lobed and connected by fine

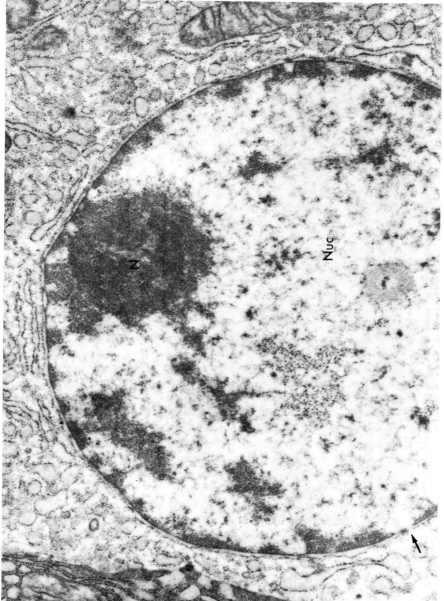

Fig. 1-9. Electron micrograph of a nucleus of a pancreatic acinar cell. The prominent nucleolus, *N*, is made up of granules arranged in irregular strands (nucleolonema). The nuclear envelope is made up of two membranes bonding a narrow perinuclear cisterna. At frequent intervals the nuclear membrane appears to be interrupted (arrow) by pores. Chromatin granules are scattered throughout the nucleus, *Nuc.* (×18,000.)

strands. In others, such as liver cells, osteo-clasts, and skeletal muscle fibers, two, three, or more nuclei may be present. In the red blood cell the nucleus is extruded, rendering these cells incapable of cell division.

The nuclear envelope consists of a double-layered structure interrupted at frequent intervals by openings or pores (Fig. 1-9). The membranes are separated by an interval known as the perinuclear space. The outer membrane is continuous at several sites with the cisternae of the endoplasmic reticulum and, like the latter, often bears ribonucleoprotein granules on the cytoplasmic surface. It is believed that a transference of large molecules such as RNA occurs in the region of the pores.

Nuclear sap (karyoplasm), which appears structureless at the optic level, has been shown at the electron microscope level to contain dispersed particles and delicate filaments. These dispersed materials are believed to condense at mitosis to form the chromosomes.

Chromatin particles previously mentioned represent portions of the chromosomes that were not dispersed during reconstruction following mitosis. There is a marked variation in the amount of chromatin present in the cells of various species.

NUCLEOLUS

Each nucleus may contain one or more nucleoli, since they sometimes fuse and at times new nucleoli arise. They consist in part of acidic and basic proteins, RNA, and at times DNA. They are especially large in neurons. It has been shown that there is a correlation between nucleoli size, number, cell growth, and protein synthesis. In actively growing or dividing cells and those actively synthesizing protein, the nucleoli are large and multiple, which is probably correlated with the fact that they are the site of RNA production. At the optic level one may observe in favorable preparations that the nucleolus is made up of two components: a structureless *pars amorpha* and a threadlike portion, the *nucleolonema*.

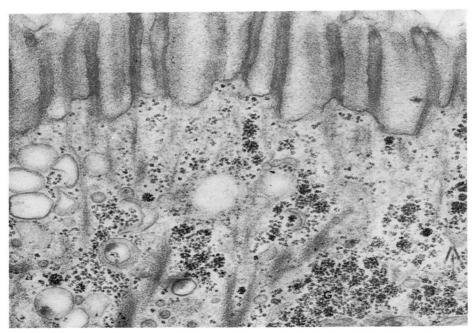

Fig. 1-10. Electron micrograph of part of epithelial cell showing clusters of dark granules, *G*, glycogen, arranged in form of rosettes. (×45,000.)

NUCLEOLONEMA

At the electron microscope level, the nucleolonema has been shown to consist of a mass of granular material that is arranged in irregular strands embedded in an amorphous material (Fig. 1-9). The structure of the nucleolonema is further subdivided into a fibrillar component and a granular component. The latter is believed to consist of ribosomes.

INCLUSIONS

Inclusions are structures in the cytoplasm that vary in number and size during different physiologic states of the cell. They consist of lipids, carbohydrates, proteins, and occasionally crystalline material. In routine histologic preparations these structures are usually not well demonstrated. Lipids can be demonstrated after osmium fixation as dark brown or black granules or masses of material. Carbohydrate in the form of glycogen is readily demonstrated at the light level by the use of the periodic acid–Schiff reaction. When observed with the aid of the electron microscope, glycogen appears as particulate material, either as single granules or in the form of rosettes (Fig. 1-10).

SECRETION GRANULES

Secretion granules occur in a variety of cells, especially in epithelium. The appearance of these granules is cyclic in nature, depending upon the activity of the cell. In many instances the granules contain enzymes or precursors of enzymes and are periodically discharged at the free surface of the cell.

PIGMENT GRANULES

Pigment granules occur in diverse tissues and are prominent in the skin and eye. They are either endogenous in nature—for example, hemosiderin, an iron-containing pigment, or melanin, a dark pigment responsible for skin color—or are exogenous pigments, those formed outside the organism.

LYSOSOMES

Lysosomes occur in a wide variety of cells and appear as scattered granules at the light level. Observed with the electron microscope, they appear as granules of varying size, being characterized by the presence of a membrane (Fig. 1-7). Lysosomes are pleomorphic; that is, they occur in diverse forms inasmuch as the appearance of the material enclosed by the membrane is concerned. They may arise by different methods, for example, as the result of the coalescence of pinocytotic vesicles, by the fusion of vacuoles, and possibly by other means. Their content may consist of a dense lipid or osmiophilic substance, myelin bodies, parts of organelles, and, in some instances, precursors of hormones. They contain hydrolytic enzymes such as acid phosphatase and aryl sulfatases and are concerned with intracellular digestion.

Table 1 summarizes the staining reactions of cell constituents most frequently mentioned in modern texts.

STUDY OF TISSUES AND ORGANS

One's view of the organization of cells and tissues is dependent upon the degree of detail (smallest size visible) that he can see through the microscope. The maximum magnification possible with a light microscope is about 1,000× and the smallest detail visible with ordinary student microscopes is about 1 μ. The latter will vary according to the properties of the optic system and the wavelength used to illuminate the tissue specimen. The limit of resolution depends directly upon the minimum contrast detectable by the human eye and the wavelength of the light used, and it varies inversely with the *numerical aperture* of the lens system. The term *numerical aperture* (NA) is a measure of the light-gathering properties of the lens system and depends upon both the light-bending (refractive) properties of the medium used to embed the specimen and the angle at which light enters the field (controlled by the condensor). It follows, then, that the resolution of the field will depend on how well the slide was prepared and how well the microscope is adjusted, as well as on several other considerations.

The best theoretical numerical aperture

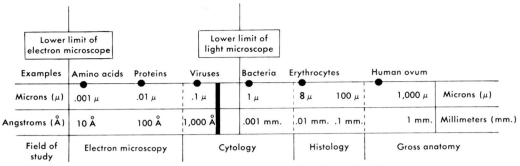

Lower limit of electron microscope			Lower limit of light microscope				
Examples	Amino acids	Proteins	Viruses	Bacteria	Erythrocytes	Human ovum	
Microns (μ)	.001 μ	.01 μ	.1 μ	1 μ	8 μ 100 μ	1,000 μ	Microns (μ)
Angstroms (Å)	10 Å	100 Å	1,000 Å	.001 mm.	.01 mm. .1 mm.	1 mm.	Millimeters (mm.)
Field of study	Electron microscopy		Cytology		Histology	Gross anatomy	

Fig. 1-11. The size of objects encountered in the study of anatomy.

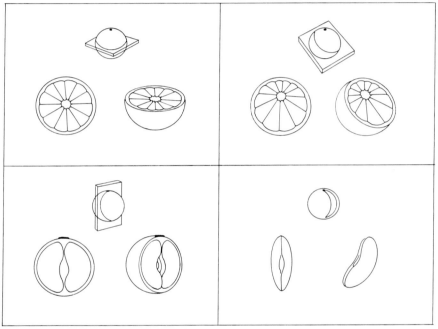

Fig. 1-12. Effects of plane of section on appearance of an object. Upper left, Orange cut perpendicular to long axis segments (cross section); lower left, orange cut parallel to long axis of segments (longitudinal section); upper right, orange cut obliquely to axis of segments; lower right, appearance of segments in space (three dimensional). (Drawing by Emily Craig.)

obtainable with the light microscope is 1.4× for oil immersion and 1.0× for high dry (40× objective). This limits resolution to a theoretical maximum of about 0.2 μ using short wavelength (blue) light. The electron microscope employs beams of electrons having properties very much like light but of ultrashort wavelength. However, since the electrons in the short wavelengths of the beam can be captured by air particles in their path, the beam and the specimen must be placed in a vacuum. The electron beam is focused by magnets that serve the same function as lenses in an optic system using visible light.

Fig. 1-11 gives an idea of the sizes of objects normally studied in anatomy. The usual range encountered in histology varies from the limit of resolution of most student microscopes ($1.0\ \mu$) to the limit of resolution of the unaided human eye (0.1 mm. to $100\ \mu$). Cells range in size from $8\ \mu$ (red blood cells) to $150\ \mu$ (ripe ova). The size of most cells falls between these two values. A useful standard for approximating cell size in a tissue section is to use the red blood cell as a standard. It measures approximately $8\ \mu$ in diameter and is usually present in the vasculature of most tissue. However, it must be remembered that processing tissues almost always causes some variation in the cell size.

One of the main objectives should be to develop an ability to visualize and construct a three-dimensional image of the cell or tissue from the flat, roughly two-dimensional object found on the microscope slide. To demonstrate how an objective can apparently change in shape depending upon how it is cut, one should consider the appearance of a simple spherical object such as an orange that has been cut in several planes (Fig. 1-12). The segments of the orange vary in shape depending on the *plane* of the section. The same kinds of variation will arise in connection with the study of structures.

Cellular detail visible with the light microscope even when special stains are used is somewhat limited, since most organelles are smaller than the resolution of the light microscope. For this reason it is essential to learn to recognize cells and tissues on the basis of several simple criteria. For example, one clue useful in identifying cell types is the appearance of the nucleus. In examining a slide of loose connective tissue (Fig. 3-10, for example), one can readily observe that the nuclei differ from each other in size, shape, staining intensity, presence or absence of nucleoli, degree of clumping of chromatin, and distinctness of the nuclear envelope (visible at the light microscope level only because of a rim of chromatin attached to it). Usually little if any cytoplasm is visible, and in addition the boundaries between cells may be very indistinct. When cytoplasm *is* visible, the presence of variations in its staining properties (regions of basophilia, for instance)

or the presence of visible inclusions (glycogen, pigment granules, vacuoles left by dissolved fats) should be noted. The identification of cells or tissues on the basis of color alone is not feasible because of the diverse coloration that stained specimens may exhibit.

Another aspect of prepared specimens used in the study of histology both clinically and experimentally is the presence of *artifacts*. Poor tissue preservation or too long a delay before fixation results in autolysis (self-digestion) of the tissue and disruption and shrinkage or swelling of the cells. As slides age the stain fades, reducing color contrast. Such distortions in the appearance of normal tissues may be present in the slides available for study.

Cellular activities

Tissues are made up of communities of cells in various functional states. Cells may be vegetative, growing, reproducing, differentiating, or performing specialized functions. Each of these stages in the life cycle of a cell will be reflected in its organelle composition and its appearance at the light microscope level. Changes in nuclear appearance, in the cytoplasm, and in the relative size of nucleus and cytoplasm can be expected. The result of these changes will be to produce a diversity of overall appearance in groups of cells of the same kind. The *matrix* (structural frame) of a tissue may also be altered in different functional states.

VEGETATIVE ACTIVITIES

Vegetative activities are concerned with minimum activity for maintenance of the cell, such as resorption, assimilation, and excretion of waste products. These cells, capable of further division, are called *intermitotics*.

GROWTH AND REPRODUCTION

Growth involves the elaboration of additional structural materials. Reproduction is a complex series of events involving division of the cells into two genetically equal daughter cells in the usual method of cell division (mitosis). Prominent roles are

Table 1. Staining characteristics of cell components

Cell constituent		Chemical constituent	Characteristics
Nucleus	Chromatin	DNA	Purple, blue, or black with hematoxylin—basophilia
			Blue with toluidine blue—orthochromasia
			Blue-green with methyl green—pyronin
	Nucleolus	RNA	Purple, blue, or black with hematoxylin—basophilia
			Purple with toluidine blue—metachromasia
			Red with methyl green—pyronin
		Ribose	Red-purple with Feulgen reaction
Cytoplasm			
Organoids	Ground substance	Protein	Pink-red with eosin—acidophilia, eosinophilia
	Mitochondria	Complex	Blue with Janus green B supravital, black with iron hematoxylin, red with acid fuchsin
	Centrioles	Protein	Rarely seen in hematoxylin and eosin, black with iron hematoxylin
	Chromophil substance	RNA	Same as nucleolus
	Fibrils	Protein	Special methods, argyrophil in nerve cells
Inclusions	Lipids	Fats	Blackened by osmic acid—osmiophilia
			Negative image in hematoxylin and eosin removed by solvents
	Zymogen	Protein	Red with eosin—acidophilia
	Mucigen glycogen	Carbohydrate	Unstained in routine hematoxylin and eosin negative image; red to purple with PAS

played by the centriole and nucleus in this process.

SPECIAL ACTIVITIES

In addition to the usual vegetative activities common to all cells, certain cells in multicellular animals have become differentiated, which means that certain cell activities become more prominent, whereas others become less prominent or may even be lost. Thus muscle cells exhibit the property of contractility; epithelial cells, of secretion and absorption; nerve cells, of hyperirritability, which permits reception, integration, and transmission of impulses. At the same time, however, such highly differentiated cells may lose the properties of mobility and reproduction. Those that lose the ability to reproduce are called *postmitotics*. Macrophages and certain white blood cells retain the property of mobility and also have the ability to phagocytize particulate matter, including bacteria.

The several changes in form and function occurring during the life of the cell are referred to as *cytomorphosis*. Distinct enlargement or growth of cells is called *hypertrophy*. Most of the lifespan of the cell is spent in the vegetative state, which represents a dynamic equilibrium between the cell and environment. With the passage of time the cells undergo regression or *atrophy*, until finally death *(necrosis)* and cell loss occur. In the latter phase the nucleus shrinks and the chromatin forms a deeply staining mass, a process known as *pyknosis*.

TISSUES AND ORGANS

It has already been indicated that living cells carry on several physiologic processes, such as response to stimuli, contraction, metabolism, and reproduction, in connection with their own maintenance and perpetuation. In multicellular organisms, moreover, groups of cells have the ability to perform one or another of these functions beyond their own needs for the benefit of the organism as a whole. Such specialized collections of similar cells are called *fundamental tissues* and are divided into groups as follows: (1) epithelia, (2) connective and supporting tissues, (3) blood and lymph, (4) muscle, and (5) nervous tissue. Some authors include reproductive tissue as a separate group because of certain special characteristics.

The fundamental tissues are not evenly distributed throughout the body but are gathered together to form organs, and the locations of these organs are studied in gross dissection. Further analysis of organs is accorded by microscopic study from which we may learn what kind or kinds of tissue are present in each and estimate the activity the organ performs. We shall find in such examination that many organs consist of an arrangement of epithelium, con-

nective tissue, and muscle, with a supply of nerves and blood vessels. Some, however, may lack epithelium, muscle, or both of these tissues.

It will be our object in the study of organs to analyze each organ and relate this analysis to the results of histochemical and physiologic studies. Before undertaking the study of organs, however, it will be necessary to acquire a full knowledge of the fundamental tissues. Each of the groups already mentioned has subdivisions, and these subdivisions have morphologic and physiologic pecularities that must be recognized and understood to make organology intelligible. The first chapters of this book are accordingly devoted to the subject of the fundamental tissues, whereas the remaining chapters present the various combinations of such tissues forming the different organs.

2
Epithelia

Epithelial tissues have two types of arrangement and two functions. First, they are arranged in sheets, one or more layers in thickness, covering the surface or lining the cavities of the body to form a protective sheath or limiting membrane. Second, they are grouped in solid cords, tubules, or follicles, which have developed as outgrowths from an epithelial sheet and are specialized for secretion, absorption, or excretion. The separation of function is not complete, however, since cells are present in many lining epithelia that have a secretory function.

GENERAL FEATURES OF EPITHELIAL TISSUES

Covering and lining layers of epithelium, regardless of thickness or function, have several features in common.

1. The cells are somewhat regular in shape and without extensive protoplasmic processes; they generally fit tightly together and are held in this position by specialized portions of their cell surfaces known in general as *junctional complexes.*

2. Between the cells there is very little structural framework (extracellular material or *matrix*). The matrix material present consists of *ground substance* composed of acid mucopolysaccharides (glycosaminoglycans) such as hyaluronic acid and the chondroitin sulfates. Calcium bound to the matrix is important in cell adhesion. Less is known about the composition of this matrix than is known about connective tissue matrices (see Chapter 3).

3. Epithelial tissues lack a vascular supply and must be nourished by diffusion from underlying capillary beds.

4. Epithelial tissues are firmly bound to underlying connective tissue by a thin membrane called a *basal lamina* or *basement membrane* (Fig. 2-3) and are produced jointly by the epithelium, which elaborates the ground substance, and the underlying connective tissue, which provides the fibrous elements of the matrix.

5. Numerous mitotic figures may be observed in epithelia and, when present, are an indication of cell renewal. Estimates for the complete renewal of the cells of epithelial membranes range from a few days for the intestinal mucosa to a few weeks for parts of the lining of the respiratory tract.

EPITHELIAL CELLS AND INTERCELLULAR SUBSTANCE

Many epithelial tissues perform the function of maintaining a concentration difference between the fluid on one side of the cell sheet and that on the other side. Cellular attachments, the cell base, and the free cell surface of cells making up such a sheet are specialized for supporting fluid transport, absorption, and secretion.

Cell attachments. A modification of cell membranes, known as desmosomes, occurs in most epithelial cells. They are made up of two plaques that consist of thickened parallel cell membranes separated by an intercellular space approximately 200 Å wide (Fig. 2-2). Attached to the cytoplasmic surfaces of the thickened membranes or plaques are numerous delicate

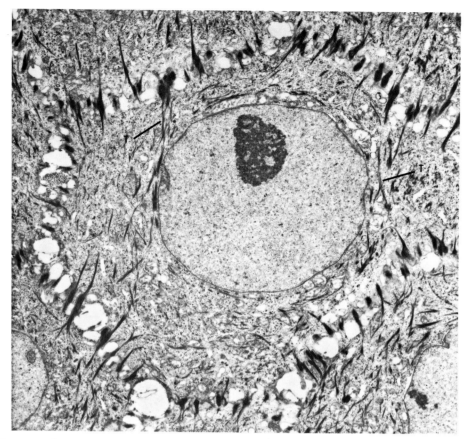

Fig. 2-1. Electron micrograph of cell from stratum germinativum of the gingiva. These cells exhibit many tonofibrils, *T* (the intercellular bridges of light microscopy). The fibrils terminate in desmosomes on the cell surface and do not, as was formerly supposed, extend to adjacent cells. (×6,000.)

tonofilaments. *Hemidesmosomes* occur in regions such as the basal layer of stratified epithelium of the skin adjacent to the basement membrane. As their name implies, they consist of one half a desmosome. They serve to attach the cells to the underlying matrix.

A more complicated cell junction occurring in many epithelial cells is the so-called *junctional complex.* It consists of three parts: (1) *zona occludens,* also known as the tight junction, occupies the most distal position and lacks an intercellular space between the membranes; (2) *zonula adherens,* located below the zona occludens, exhibits an intercellular space of approxi-

mately 200 Å, as well as bands of filaments in the adjacent cytoplasm; and (3) *macula adherens* or desmosome was described above.

Cell base. The epithelia, which are arranged as coverings and linings, rest upon a *basement membrane,* or lamina. At the optic level the basement membrane may appear to be hyaline and structureless or composed of a band of tightly or loosely packed (reticular) fibers. The hyaline material stains with the PAS method, whereas the fibers require special silver techniques for visualization. The basement membrane is often so fine that it is imperceptible in routine preparations. Some epithelia exhibit

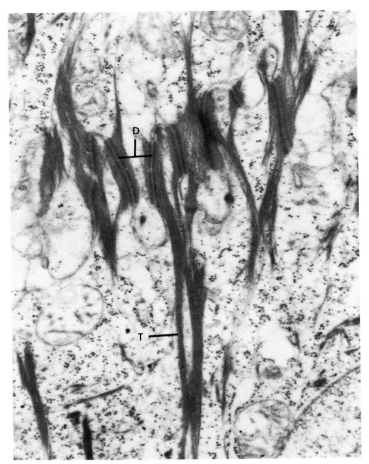

Fig. 2-2. Electron micrograph showing termination of tonofibrils, *T*, in desmosomes, *D*. The opposing plasma membranes of the desmosomes appear thickened, and a fibrillar material lies between the membranes. (×24,000.)

a well-marked membrane (pseudostratified of the trachea). Epithelial tissues are avascular, and blood capillaries are found only below the basement membrane.

Electron microscopy has shown that the basal lamina is separated from the basal epithelial cells by a light zone about 400 Å in width. The lamina exhibits a texture because of the presence of fine filaments embedded in the amorphous mucopolysaccharide (Fig. 2-3). The basal lamina is concerned with cell permeability and certain immunologic reactions.

Cell surface. Epithelial cells lining moistened membranes or tubules exhibit either free smooth surfaces or protoplasmic projections known as *cilia*. Cilia of the motile variety are prominent structures in well-preserved material. They appear as slender elongated processes exhibiting an axial filament and a refractile basal body. The electron microscope has shown that cilia contain nine longitudinal filaments on the periphery and two centrally placed filaments. In transverse section the outer filaments appear double. The basal bodies appear similar to a centriole. They are hollow and contain nine peripherally located filaments (Figs. 2-4 and 2-5). Motile cilia are associated with the respira-

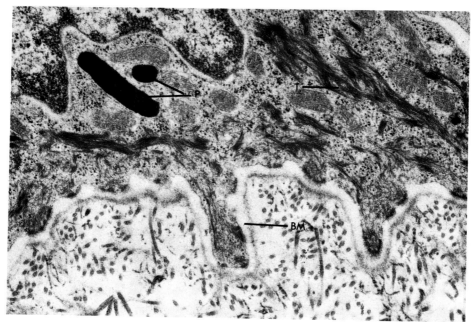

Fig. 2-3. Electron micrograph of the basal region of the epithelium of the monkey lip, showing the basal lamina, or membrane, *BM*, pigment granules, *P*, and tonofibrils, *T*. (×34,000.)

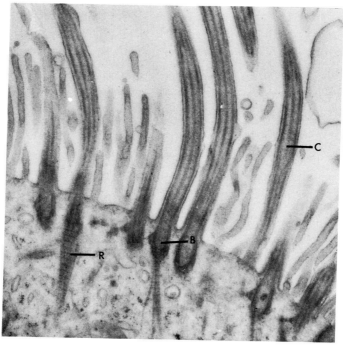

Fig. 2-4. Electron micrograph of longitudinal section of cilia, *C*, of epithelial lining of cat bronchiole; *R*, rootlet. The internal longitudinal filaments form a junction with the basal bodies, *B*. (×25,000.)

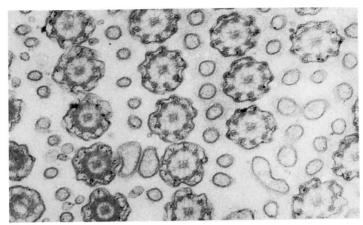

Fig. 2-5. Transverse section of cilia. (×45,000.)

tory passages and the female reproductive tract. Stereocilia are elongate and non-motile. Formerly described as cilia, they are now known to be attenuated microvilli. They occur in portions of the male reproductive tract.

When viewed with the electron microscope, striated borders are shown to be composed of many extremely thin, short, uniform, and closely packed protoplasmic projections known as microvilli. They are found in locations where absorption and secretion are the primary activities of the cell. In the small intestine the striated border is covered by a thin layer of mucoprotein secretion, and in poorly stained or preserved material an ill-defined layer is observable on the surface of the cell. This layer is sometimes referred to as a cuticle, or cuticular border.

Cell surfaces beset with protoplasmic projections of an irregular arrangement are said to have a *brush border*. The projections known as brush borders are somewhat longer than those occurring as striated borders and appear at the electron microscope level as fingerlike projections on the distal surface of the cell. They, too, as known as *microvilli*. (See Fig. 1-3.) They consist of a solid core enclosed by extensions of the plasma membrane. The heights of microvilli vary in diverse cells. They are numerous and relatively tall in the digestive tract. In some cells a fibrillar

condensation of the apical part of the cytoplasm extends into the core of the microvillus, which is also continuous with fibrillar material in the region of the terminal bars. This fibrillar material is often referred to as the terminal web.

VARIETIES OF EPITHELIA

The epithelia are divided into groups on the basis of *cell shape* and *thickness* and number of *cellular layers* in the sheet. The two main groups are simple epithelia and stratified epithelia. Simple epithelia consist of a single layer of cells, all of which are in contact with the basement membrane. Stratified epithelia consist of cell layers superimposed one upon the other, and only the basal cell layer is in contact with the basement membrane. The two main groups are further subdivided according to the shapes of the component cells, as shown in the following classification outline.

Simple epithelia	*Stratified epithelia*
Squamous	Stratified columnar
Cuboidal	Stratified cuboidal
Columnar	Transitional
Pseudostratified	Stratified squamous

Simple epithelia

Squamous epithelium. The cells of simple squamous epithelium are extremely flattened. Viewed from the surface they appear as fairly large cells with clear cyto-

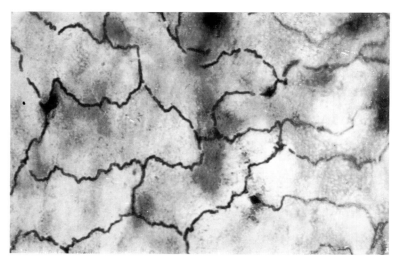

Fig. 2-6. Surface view of mesothelium. (Silver nitrate preparation.)

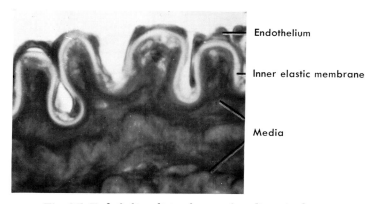

Endothelium

Inner elastic membrane

Media

Fig. 2-7. Endothelium lining lumen of medium-sized artery.

plasm. The nucleus of each is round or oval and eccentrically placed. Cell outlines are not ordinarily visible but may be demonstrated by the reaction of silver nitrate on intercellular substance. In such preparations the polygonal cell boundary may be somewhat wavy, serrated, or sometimes smooth (Fig. 2-6). In section, the cytoplasm is barely visible but may be seen in the region of the nucleus, where the cytoplasm appears to bulge (Fig. 2-7). The boundaries between adjacent cells are not visible in routine preparations.

Simple squamous epithelium is not found in exposed regions or in sites where ab-

sorption and secretion are the primary activities. Generally it forms barriers in regions where diffusion or filtration rather than protection is the basic requirement. This is the case in Bowman's capsule of the kidney and in lung alveoli, which are used as examples of this tissue type. It forms the barriers of the blood–tissue fluid, tissue fluid–lymph, and tissue fluid–gas interfaces. *Endothelium* is the type of simple squamous epithelium found lining blood vessels, heart, lymphatic ducts, and bone marrow. It forms the entire thickness of the walls of blood and lymph capillaries. *Mesothelium* is the same type of tissue found on the so-called serous membranes lining the peritoneal, pleural, and pericardial cavities of the body. Endothelium and mesothelium are not, however, morphologically distinguishable other than by location. They arise from mesoderm and mesenchyme and are said to be related to primitive connective tissue. In repair of mesothelial tissues, new cells are derived from cells of adjacent connective tissues; in repair of other types of epithelia, cells are replaced by mitosis of similar cells. For these and other reasons, mesothelium is often considered to be an epithelium with special properties or potencies. The mesothelium-like layer found lining the anterior chamber of the eye, the inner ear, and the cerebrospinal spaces is known as mesenchymal epithelium. The flattened cells lining joint cavities are said to be fibroblasts derived from the dense connective tissue in those regions and are not considered to be epithelial at all.

Cuboidal epithelium. In surface view the cells of cuboidal epithelium are smaller and more regular than simple squamous cells and appear roughly hexagonal in outline (Fig. 2-8). The cell boundaries are often clearly visible because of the presence of terminal bars. In vertical section (Fig. 2-9) the cell appears square with a rounded nucleus in the center of each, and in specially stained preparations the terminal bars are visible. The square shape is modified to that of a trapezoid when the cells are grouped around the lumen of a small duct. When they are closely packed around the lumen of some glands, the cells resemble a truncated pyramid and are accordingly called pyramidal cells. The cytoplasm of these cells may appear clear or granular, and in the latter case the cell boundaries are often indistinct in sectioned material. Examples of simple cuboidal epithelium may be found in certain kidney tubules (Fig. 2-9) and in the partly distended cells of the thyroid gland. In the thyroid the cells elaborate secretions, although this function is more commonly associated with columnar cells.

Columnar epithelium. In surface view, columnar epithelium fits the description given for cuboidal epithelium, including the terminal bars as well. In sections, however, the cells are seen to be taller than they are broad, that is, they have the form of rectangles with the long axis perpendicular to the free surface. The nucleus is characteristically close to the base of the cell, except when the cells are extremely

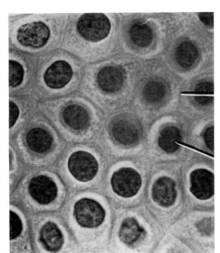

Intercellular cement

Nucleus

Fig. 2-8. Transverse section of cuboidal epithelium from kidney.

compressed. The free surface may be composed of a smooth plasma membrane covered by a thin or thick mucous secretion, or it may have microvilli or cilia of the varieties described in the introduction to this chapter. The cytoplasm may be clear or may contain granules, secretion droplets, or a large clump of secretion droplets in a vacuole near the surface of the cell (Fig. 2-10, *A*). (See discussion on goblet cells, Chapter 14.)

Mucous cells occur in varying numbers in the mucosa of the intestine and respiratory tract. They are modified columnar cells in which secretory droplets (mucinogen, the precursor of mucus) accumulate distally, resulting in a goblet-shaped cell. Eventually the cell surface ruptures, the secretion is discharged, and the cell repeats its secretory cycle.

The difference between cuboidal and columnar cells is not sharply marked. It depends on the height of the cells as seen in vertical section. An organ may be said by one author to be lined with cuboidal epithelium, whereas another will use the term *low columnar* in describing the tissue.

An example of low columnar epithelium is shown in the illustration of the kidney (Fig. 2-9). Tall columnar epithelium is illustrated in Fig. 2-10, drawn from a section of the small intestine.

In studying columnar epithelium, it is important to select a region in which the section passes through the tissue in a plane perpendicular to its surface. When a slanting, or tangential, section is studied, the appearance is that of two or more layers of cells, and the tissue may be erroneously classified as stratified or pseudostratified epithelium (Fig. 2-10, *B*). Columnar cells are found in regions where the epithelial lining of an organ combines the function of secretion with that of a limiting membrane (for example, digestive tract).

Pseudostratified epithelium. Pseudostratified epithelium consists essentially of columnar cells, which are crowded very closely together. Because of this, the rectangular form is distorted and not all of the cells reach the free surface of the epithelium. Those that do reach the surface have an upper part like a columnar cell and a much-constricted base. Some have a

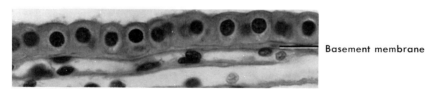

Basement membrane

Fig. 2-9. Vertical section of cuboidal epithelium from kidney.

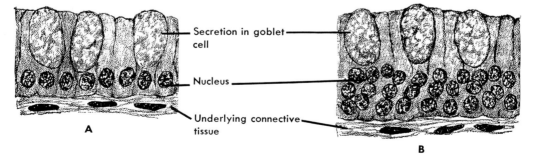

Secretion in goblet cell

Nucleus

Underlying connective tissue

A

B

Fig. 2-10. Tall columnar epithelium from intestine. **A**, Vertical section; **B**, tangential section.

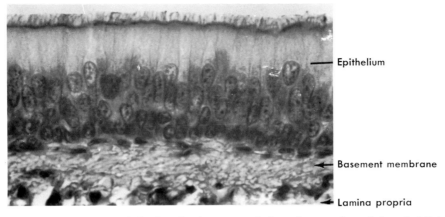

Epithelium

Basement membrane

Lamina propria

Fig. 2-11. Pseudostratified ciliated columnar epithelium from trachea of dog. (×640.)

wide base and an irregular spindle shape, and still others are short and rounded. The nucleus of each lies at its widest portion, and this gives the tissue the appearance of a stratified epithelium with nuclei at several levels. Only in the best preparations can it be demonstrated that, whereas approximately only one cell in three touches the free surface, all have a portion touching the basement membrane. In all preparations there seems, at the first glance, to be little difference between a vertical section of pseudostratified epithelium and the tangenital section of simple columnar epithelium described. The nuclei of the two kinds of tissue offer the best means of distinguishing between the two. In pseudostratified epithelium these are of several types—those at the base of the tissue being small and dark, those nearer the surface being larger and paler. In the tangenital section of columnar epithelium, on the other hand, only one type of nucleus is present. The cytoplasm of the cells of pseudostratified epithelium is sometimes clear, sometimes granular. It may contain drops of secretions, and the surface cells are ciliated. The nuclei are round or oval according to the shape of the cells in which they lie. The usual appearance of this type of epithelium is illustrated in Fig. 2-11 (trachea). It is functionally adapted to serve as a fairly resistant limiting membrane.

Stratified epithelia

In all stratified epithelia a complete layer of small modified cuboidal or columnar cells lies next to the basement membrane. These cells are called *basal cells.* Above this, except with a two-layered epithelium, are one or more layers of polygonal cells. At the free surface lies a layer of cells that have a different shape in each subdivision of the group. The shape of the cells at the free surface of a stratified epithelium determines its classification into one of the four subdivisions.

Stratified columnar epithelium. Stratified columnar epithelium differs from the pseudostratified type in having a continuous layer of small rounded cells next to the basement membrane. The columnar cells at the surface of the epithelium are thus entirely cut off from the basement membrane, and the epithelium is truly stratified. This type is of rare occurrence. (See Fig. 21-15.)

Stratified cuboidal epithelium. Stratified cuboidal epithelium is extremely rare, the best example occurring in the ducts of the sweat glands. A definite basement membrane is present, whereas the free surface bears a distinct border. Certain cell layers in the testis and ovary are also included in this group by some authors.

Transitional epithelium. Transitional epithelium is a stratified epithelium whose

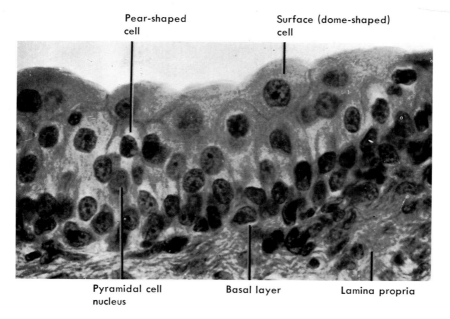

Pear-shaped cell   Surface (dome-shaped) cell

Pyramidal cell nucleus   Basal layer   Lamina propria

Fig. 2-12. Section of mucosa of urinary bladder showing transitional epithelium. (×640.)

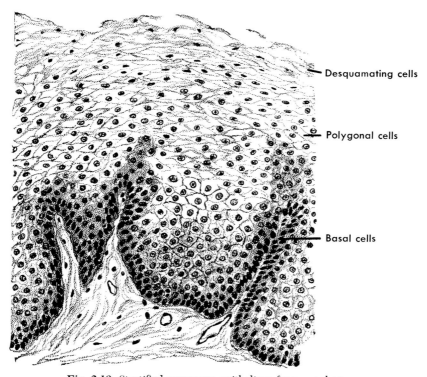

Desquamating cells

Polygonal cells

Basal cells

Fig. 2-13. Stratified squamous epithelium from esophagus.

surface cells do not fall into the truly squamous, cuboidal, or columnar categories. The basal cells are like those of stratified columnar epithelium. Above them is a varying number of polygonal cells of which those immediately below the surface layer tend to have an elongated, pearlike (piriform) shape. The layer at the surface is composed of large, somewhat flattened cells, generally described as dome shaped. One of these cells often covers three underlying pear-shaped cells, with indentations to receive the latter. The dome cells are so large that in sectioned material many of the nuclei are not visible because they are not in the plane of the section, although dome cells are known to have as many as two or three nuclei each. The cytoplasm just under the free surface of the dome cell appears to be more condensed and deeply staining, which is an aid in the identification of this tissue at the optic level. Basement membrane, terminal bars, and cilia are not found in this nonsecretory tissue (Fig. 2-12).

The cells of this epithelium possess to an unusual degree the ability to change their position by sliding over each other, so that if the viscus they line (for example, the urinary bladder) is distended, the epithelium is reduced to three or four layers. When the viscus is empty, the cells heap up, forming several layers between the basal and surface cells. This tissue changes in appearance not only with the state of distention of the lined structure but also from place to place along the urinary tract to which it is confined. It is accordingly advantageous to examine this tissue from different regions of the urinary tract.

Stratified squamous epithelium. In stratified squamous epithelium the thickness and number of cells vary in different parts of the body; the shape and arrangement of component cells, however, follow the same general plan. In this epithelium the basal cells are covered by several layers of polygonal cells. Near the base the polygonal cells are quite small, but they gradually increase in size toward the middle of the tissue (hypertrophy); beyond this point they begin to flatten out and become smaller. As they approach the surface, they may become flattened, shriveled (atrophy), and scalelike with pyknotic nuclei, which is the situation existing in the mucous membranes of the mouth and esophagus (Fig. 2-13). In more exposed, dry epithelia, such as the skin, the cells may incorporate a tough resilient material (keratin). When this condition exists, the epithelium is said to be *cornified* or *keratinized*. This tissue is particularly well adapted to perform its protective function because of (1) its great thickness and keratinization, (2) its ability to slough off surface cells under the impetus of abrasion, and (3) the replacement of these cells from below. Whereas surface cells are typically flattened, as on the surface of the cornea of the eye, or scalelike, as described before, they differ from simple squamous cells in that the flattened nuclei do not generally produce an enlargement of the cell. The addition of hair also increases the protective function of this epithelium.

The cells that make up the basal and polyhedral layers of this tissue, the so-called *stratum germinativum*, are characteristically basophilic, suggesting their great metabolic activity. In addition, shrinkage of this region produced during preservation (fixation) reveals prominent intercellular bridges containing tonofibrils, a characteristic that has earned for them the name "prickle cells." Since none of the epithelia described is penetrated by blood vessels, their nutrition apparently depends on transmission through interstitial cellular fluids. This would create a serious nutritional problem for epithelia as thick as stratified squamous epithelia. At any rate, it has been suggested that the death of surface cells and possibly keratinization may be the result of lack of nutrients. The thicker stratified squamous epithelia have fingerlike projections of connective tissue, known as *papillae*, penetrating quite deeply into the stratum germinativum, thereby increasing the surface area available for the diffusion of nutrients. In summary, then, we have surface cells that may be flattened or scalelike, keratinized or nonkeratinized. The epithelia appear papillate or nonpapillate.

3
Connective tissue proper

In the connecting and supporting tissues the arrangement of cells and intercellular substance is quite different from that seen in the epithelia. Rather than being closely applied to each other in the form of a sheet or a cord, the cells lie more or less scattered, sometimes not in contact, sometimes touching only at the ends of long protoplasmic processes. The intercellular substance is much more prominent than among the epithelia and becomes the most important part of the majority of the tissues in the group.

The type of cell most frequently found in these tissues is of an irregular branching form, sometimes called stellate. Its nucleus is vesicular and its cytoplasm is somewhat granular and prolonged in the form of processes. Cells of this type make up the mesenchyme (Fig. 3-1), the embryonic tissue from which all the members of the group are derived. The original shape of the cell is retained in some of the connecting and supporting tissues after they have been fully differentiated. In others it is modified. The intercellular components of the connective tissues consist of (1) fibers, (2) ground substances, and (3) tissue fluid.

FIBERS

The fibers are of three kinds and are distinguishable by their appearance and chemical reactions: collagenous or white, reticular, and elastic.

Collagenous or white fibers. Collagenous fibers are the most common. They possess little elasticity, are dissolved by weak acids, and yield gelatin when boiled. Collagenous fibers consist of bundles of fine fibrils, known as fibrillae, which lie parallel to each other and give the fiber its longitudinally striated appearance. The fibrillae are held together by a cementing substance. The fibrillae do not branch. The bundles or fibers, however, branch and anastomose and appear in section sometimes straight, but usually wavy. They stain fairly readily with eosin, giving a pink color to tissues containing many of them.

Studies made with the electron microscope have shown that the diameter of the collagen fibrils varies considerably, averaging about 1,000 Å. The fibrils reveal characteristic periodic cross bandings with an

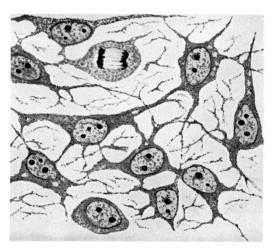

Fig. 3-1. Mesenchyme in a 60-mm. dog fetus. (Silver stain; ×1,200.) (From Nonidez and Windle: Textbook of histology, New York, 1953, McGraw-Hill Book Co.)

29

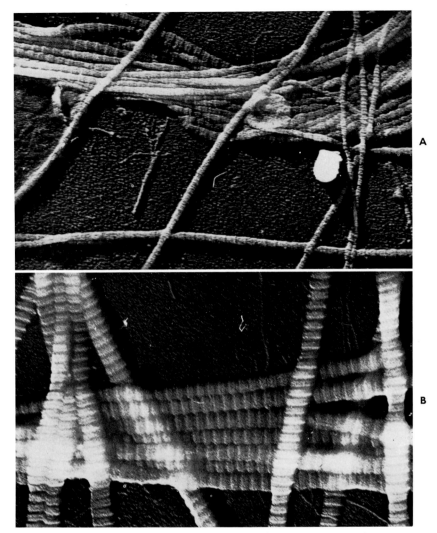

Fig. 3-2. Electron micrograph of connective tissue of skin: **A,** reticular fibers (2 days); **B,** collagenous fibers (90 days). Reticular fibers are smaller in diameter than are collagenous fibers but apparently have the same periodicity. (×45,000.) (Courtesy Dr. J. Gross, Boston, Mass.)

interval of 640 Å in the mature fibrils (Figs. 3-2 and 3-3). Information derived from electron microscope and x-ray diffraction studies have shown that the unit molecule of collagen is made up of long polypeptide chains and is known as tropocollagen. It measures approximately 2,600 to 3,000 Å in length and about 15 Å in width. These molecules arranged side by side in a staggered fashion make up collagen exhibiting an average periodicity of 640 Å.

Reticular fibers. Reticular fibers are similar to collagenous fibers in that they exhibit the same 640 Å periodicity present in collagenous fibers. They are finer in caliber, do not stain appreciably with eosin, but have an affinity for silver. Accordingly they are not readily distinguished in sections prepared in the ordinary way. On boiling they yield reticulin, which differs slightly from gelatin obtained from collagenous fibers. Reticular fibers also resist peptic

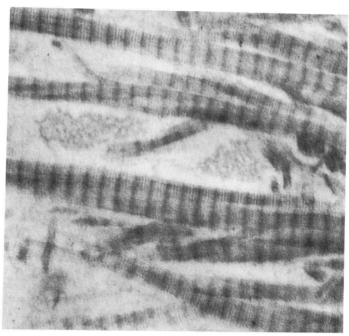

Fig. 3-3. Electron micrograph of several collagen fibrils from rat dentin showing the dark, 640-Å bands and also the interperiodic bands between them. (×75,000.)

digestion longer than do the collagenous fibers.

Elastic fibers. Elastic fibers occur singly or in the form of sheets. In ordinary preparations they are hardly distinguishable from the collagenous fibers. If the sections are stained with resorcin, however, the elastic fibers will be sharply differentiated, since this dye colors them deeply but leaves the collagenous fibers pale. In such slides the elastic fibers appear as stout, branching structures, heavier than the individual collagenous fibrils or reticular fibers. On boiling they yield elastin and they show a greater resistance to acids than do the collagenous fibrils. As their name implies, their most important physical characteristic is their elasticity, but this is not apparent in histologic preparations.

GROUND SUBSTANCE

The ground substance of connective tissue is a homogeneous semifluid material that coexists with the tissue fluid and forms the fluid environment of the cells and fibers. The tissue fluid–ground substance complex is generally discernible only in especially well-preserved tissues. In the latter condition, the ground substance stains metachromatically with toluidine blue. It has been shown by chemical analysis to contain several polysaccharides, including hyaluronic acid. The enzyme hyaluronidase hydrolyzes hyaluronic acid, which, in turn, causes a reduction in viscosity and a consequent increase in the permeability of the tissues.

The process by which intercellular structures are formed was for a long time controversial. Electron microscopy has now shown in a fairly conclusive manner that the fibers are elaborated by modified portions of the endoplasmic reticulum and the Golgi apparatus, which are prominent cell constituents of the connective tissue–forming cells, such as fibroblasts and chondrocytes.

The elements composing the tissues of this group have in varying degree the function of binding together the parts of the body and furnishing it with a supporting framework. Less obvious are other functions performed by the connective tissues. The fluid intercellular substance of connective tissue plays a part in the nutrition of the body. Connective tissue of the loose variety contains many cells belonging to the defense system of the body (leukocytes, macrophages, and so on) and is active in limiting the process of local infections and in the healing of tissues and organs. For the present we shall consider the connective tissues in relation to their connective and supporting qualities. From that point of view one may arrange them in order of their degree of differentiation and their solidity, although it must be emphasized that any classification is difficult and cannot be adhered to rigidly, since the different varieties have transitional forms.

MUCOUS CONNECTIVE TISSUE

Mucous connective tissue, usually found in the embryo and not to be confused with mucus-secreting epithelium, retains much of the appearance of mesenchyme, the primitive tissue from which it is derived. The cells are spindle shaped or branching. The intercellular fluid of mesenchyme is replaced by a mucoid jellylike mass from which the tissue derives its name. Fibers of the white or collagenous variety are present, lying in proximity to the cells (border fibrils or fibroglia). In microscopic preparations the jelly stains faintly, the fibers more deeply. In the adult body, mucous connective tissue is present in the vitreous humor of the eye. It is usually studied in sections of the umbilical cord (Wharton's jelly) and is of interest chiefly because it illustrates a relation between fibers and cells that is less evident in the more highly differentiated tissues.

RETICULAR TISSUE

In ordinary preparations reticular tissue also has an appearance somewhat similar to that of mesenchyme. The cells composing it are sometimes called primitive reticular cells. They are branching cells, the process of which are generally in contact with each other. The intercellular substance consists of a viscous fluid and fine reticular fibers. The latter take the same color as the cell processes when the preparation is stained with eosin, and this makes it difficult to distinguish them. By careful examination, however, among the slightly granular cytoplasmic processes one may see other fine hyaline strands, which are intercellular fibers. With special stains (silver nitrate) the fibers may be more clearly demonstrated. They then appear as short fine fibers, for the most part closely associated with the cells.

Reticular tissue such as has just been described is illustrated in Figs. 3-4 and 3-5. It forms the basis of the lymphoid organs, such as the lymph nodes, where it is combined with lymphocytes and other blood cells. The latter are present in such numbers as to obscure the reticular network in parts of the preparation, and care must be taken to avoid such regions in finding a place to study the fundamental tissue.

A more attenuated form of reticular tissue is found immediately subjacent to the epithelium of many organs (for example, the digestive tract). Here the cells are more widely separated, and the appearance presented is like that of fine areolar tissue. Stains specified for the reticular fibers must be used in such cases to distinguish between the two kinds of tissue.

FIBROUS TISSUE

All fibrous tissues (areolar, irregular, regular dense fibrous, and elastic) are composed of cells, intercellular fluid, and fibers. In the looser tissues there are relatively few fibers irregularly arranged, a large amount of intercellular fluid, and numerous cells. In denser tissues there is an increase in the number of fibers and a corresponding decrease in intercellular fluid as well as cells.

Areolar tissue

In an earlier discussion it was indicated that reticular tissues appear as a typically loose fibrous type. In this discussion we shall consider areolar tissue (Fig. 3-8), in which collagenous fibers predominate but in which elastic fibers are also present. This type of tissue is found in mesenteries, in omenta of the alimentary canal, in the subcutaneous tissues (under the skin), and immediately below the mucosal epithelium of

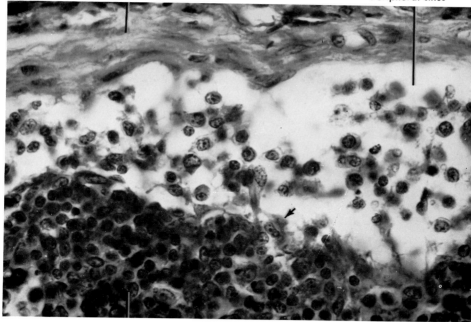

Fig. 3-4. Section of lymph node showing peripheral sinus. Arrow indicates reticulocyte. (×640.)

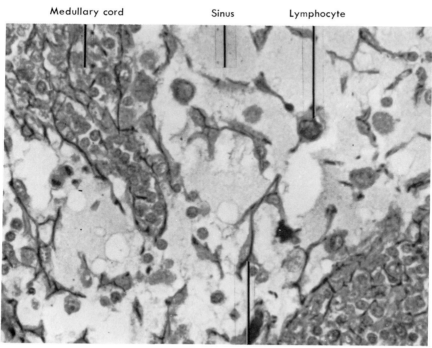

Fig. 3-5. Section of lymph node showing distribution of reticulocytes and reticular fibers in sinus. (Bielschowsky method: ×640.)

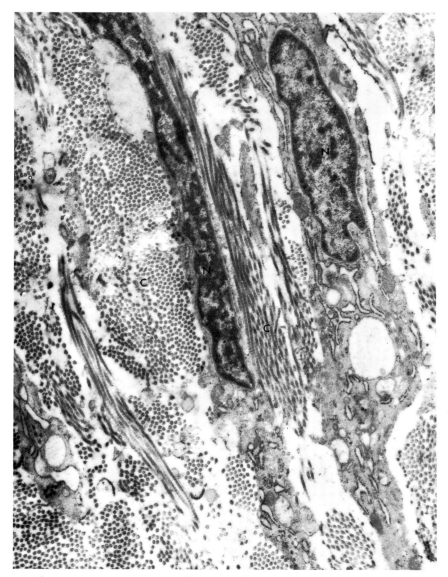

Fig. 3-6. Electron micrograph showing dense irregular connective tissue from human perifdental membrane. *N,* Nucleus of fibroblast; *C,* collagen fibrillae. (×15,000.)

the alimentary canal. The predominating collagenous fiber bundles branch and are of variable thickness. They also intertwine to form a network. In sections they are cut in all possible planes, and since they twist and interlace, bundles can be traced for only short distances. Elastic fibers are usually nearer the surface of the tissue and, when stretched, form a network of straight fibers that give rise to Y-shaped branches, often curling at the free ends. In hematoxylin and eosin–stained sections, elastic fibers are not generally distinguishable from the white fibers. Sectioned materials stained with elastic tissue stain show elastic fibers as scattered short single pieces cut obliquely. The fibrous elements, produced and maintained by cells, called fibroblasts, form the main morphologic component of connective tissue proper utilized in binding organs together to resist stress, strains, and displacements (Fig. 3-6). The intercellular fluid fills in the spaces between fibers and cells and provides transport for nutrients and metabolic wastes. This fluid does not ordinarily stain and is usually conveyed to and through areolar tissue by small blood vessels and drained by the blood and lymphatic capillaries. Since tissue spreads of mesenteries are the usual source of areolar tissue for study, a description of cells follows. The reader is cautioned to distinguish between cells that are properly a part of fibrous connective tissues everywhere and epithelial types that happen to be located around or passing through areolar tissue.

Fibroblasts. Fibroblasts are present in all types of fibrillar tissue, from the finest areolae to the tendons and elastic membranes. In loose areolar tissue, when seen in surface view, they appear as rather large branching cells with pale oval nuclei. The cytoplasm is so lightly stained as to be often barely perceptible, so that one may distinguish the nucleus alone. Often the cells lie in such a position that they are seen from the side. In that case they are fusiform and somewhat easier to see. In fully formed areolar tissue there are no fibrils connected with the fibroblasts. The cells sometimes lie very close to the fibers, especially in the denser kinds of tissue, but careful examination makes it evident that cells and fibers are actually separate. The fibroblasts are the most common cells of areolar tissue and usually the only kind to be found in the dense fibrillar tissues (Figs. 3-7 to 3-9).

The fibroblasts that form the fibers are present in all forms of fibrous tissue (Fig. 3-7). There are, in addition, cells that have no part in carrying out the connective function of the tissue. They are fairly constant elements in the tissue, and their morphologic characteristics will be described in this chapter, since they are to be distinguished from the fibroblasts, but their significance, like that of the cells of reticular tissue, will be discussed in a later section.

Mesothelial cells. The nuclei of mesothelial cells occur in mesenteries and are frequently confused with the nuclei of fibroblasts. Mesothelial nuclei are much larger, somewhat lighter staining, and appear as elongated ovals, never fusiform in tissue spreads (Fig. 3-10). In addition, the mesothelial cytoplasm does not usually stain. These cells are not a regular feature of areolar tissue but belong to the epithelium that forms the boundary of mesenteric and serous membranes.

Macrophages. Macrophages are one of the so-called wandering cells of fibrous tissues. The active phagocytic cells are frequently detected after the ingestion of insoluble stain particles or carbon particles. Whereas the cytoplasm may extend for some distance, these cells are smaller than fibroblasts. They have darker staining and smaller nuclei, frequently indented on one side. The cytoplasm is irregular in outline, containing numerous vacuoles and granules that require special staining techniques for adequate demonstration. They occur less frequently than fibroblasts. These cells are active in inflammatory conditions and are part of the reticuloendothelial system. They are also called clasmatocytes, histiocytes, pyrrol or "dust" cells, and resting wandering cells (Fig. 3-10). The so-called inactive, or resting, macrophages are oval shaped with an irregular outline. The nuclei of the latter are as previously described, but they do not appear to ingest particles unless mobilized and activated.

Plasma cells. Plasma cells (Figs. 3-11 and 3-12) are comparatively rare in most connective tissue. They may be found in considerable numbers in the tunica propria of the digestive tract and in the loose connective tissue surrounding the secretive portions of the lactating mammary gland. They are smaller than macrophages and differ from them and from fibroblasts in having a definitely rounded or oval shape without cytoplasmic processes. The cytoplasm is basophilic and nongranular. The nucleus is small and eccentrically placed. The chromatin of the nucleus is gathered in large

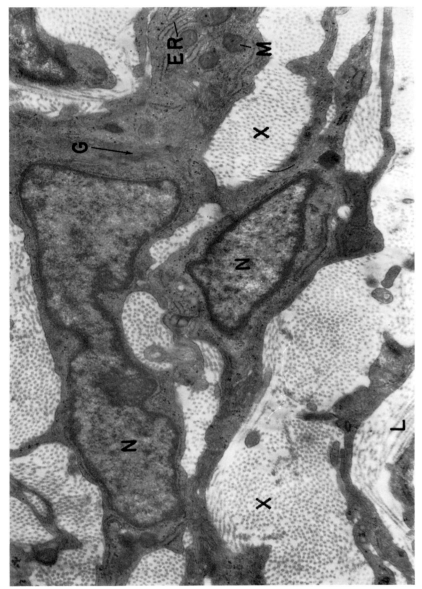

Fig. 3-7. Electron photomicrograph of collagenous connective tissue in mouse. *ER,* Rough endoplasmic reticulum; *L,* longitudinal section of collagen fibrillae; *M,* mitochondria; *N,* nucleus of fibroblast; *G,* Golgi complex; *X,* transverse section of collagen fibrillae. ($\frac{2}{3}$×27,000.) (Courtesy Dr. F. Gonzales, Chicago, Ill.)

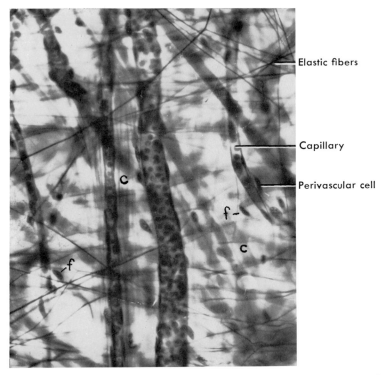

Elastic fibers

Capillary

Perivascular cell

Fig. 3-8. Stretch preparation of omentum showing areolar connective tissue. *f,* Fibroblast; *c,* collagen fibers.

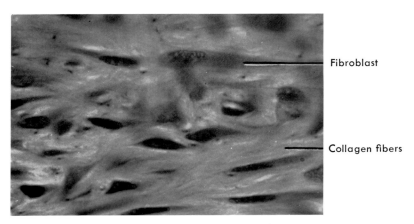

Fibroblast

Collagen fibers

Fig. 3-9. Dense connective tissue.

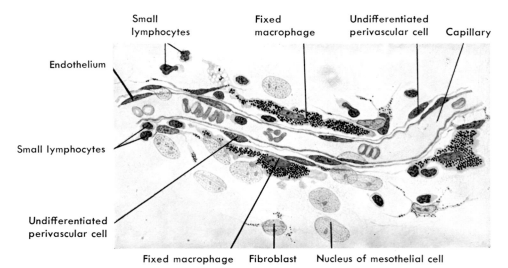

Endothelium

Small
lymphocytes

Fixed
macrophage

Undifferentiated
perivascular cell   Capillary

Small lymphocytes

Undifferentiated
perivascular cell

Fixed macrophage   Fibroblast   Nucleus of mesothelial cell

Fig. 3-10. Stretch preparation of omentum of rabbit vitally stained with lithium carmine. (Hematoxylin stain; ×500.) (From Maximow and Bloom: A textbook of histology, Philadelphia, 1952, W. B. Saunders Co.)

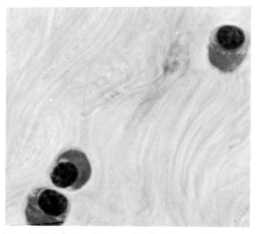

Fig. 3-11. Photomicrograph of plasma cells in connective tissue of mammary gland. Note eccentrically placed nucleus. (×1,600.)

granules along the nuclear membrane (so-called cartwheel nucleus). The cytoplasm near the nucleus stains less intensely and appears as a perinuclear halo (Plate 2). The plasma cells produce antibodies and are part of the tissue-based defense system.

Mast cells. Mast cells exhibit basophilic and metachromatic cytoplasmic granules composed partly of polysaccharide. They are large round cells with pale nuclei frequently obscured by the abundant granules (Figs. 3-13 and 3-14). In hematoxylin and eosin preparations they are sometimes referred to as tissue basophils. They are frequently found in the vicinity of blood vessels and should not be confused with flattened cells known as undifferentiated perivascular cells. Mast cells contain heparin, an anticoagulant polysaccharide, and histamine. These cells may influence blood flow through capillary beds and are probably damaged during anaphylaxis. The properties of mast cells mimic those of the basophilic leukocytes (see Chapter 6). Species that have large mast cell populations tend to have very few basophils. It is presently thought that these two cell types, the mast cell and the blood basophil, supplement each other. During an infection, infiltration of a tissue by basophils may represent a quick response to foreign proteins (an antigenic stimulus), while in more long-lasting processes (chronic inflammation, parasite infestation, neoplasia) in which interaction between the host and foreign antigens is prolonged, basophils

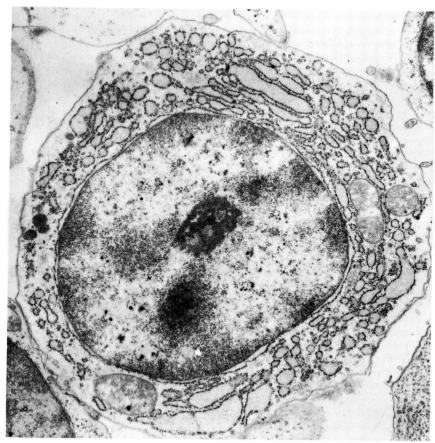

Fig. 3-12. Electron micrograph of a plasma cell from a cat. In addition to the large nucleus, the characteristic feature of the cytoplasm is the extensive system of cisternae studded with ribosomes on which antibody synthesis occurs. (×17,000.)

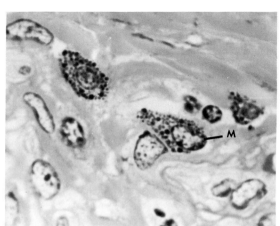

Fig. 3-13. Photomicrograph of mast cells from gingival connective tissue, *M*, containing metachromatic granules. (×1,200.)

may gradually give way to new mast cells arising in the tissues.

Blood cells. Fully formed leukocytes and red blood cells are often found in areolar tissue. Of these, tissue eosinophils are of frequent occurrence in some animals but not in others and may be associated with allergic reactions. Lymphocytes occur frequently in regions of inflammation. To be certain of the various kinds of cells observed one must use special stains. Many authors do not consider these cells part of the connective tissue but rather an invasion from blood and lymphatic capillaries.

Fat cells. Occasional fat cells are seen in areolar and other kinds of connective tissue. Details of fat cells are presented later in this discussion.

Dense fibrous tissue

Irregular. In irregular dense fibrous tissue the number of collagenous fibers is increased tremendously, whereas there is a definite decrease in intercellular fluid and number of cells. The thick collagenous bundles are arranged in an intertwining network (Fig. 3-15). In routine hematoxylin and eosin–stained sections the whole mass stains a bright yellowish pink or red;

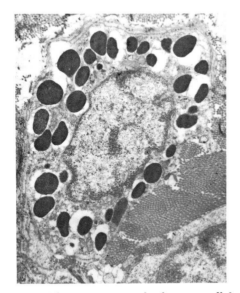

Fig. 3-14. Electron micrograph of a mast cell from the small intestine of a mouse. Note the numerous large electron dense granules. (×10,000.)

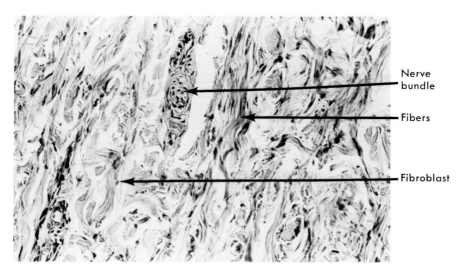

Nerve bundle

Fibers

Fibroblast

Fig. 3-15. Dense fibrous tissue, irregularly arranged, from dermal layer of the skin. Note nerve bundle.

Collagen fibers

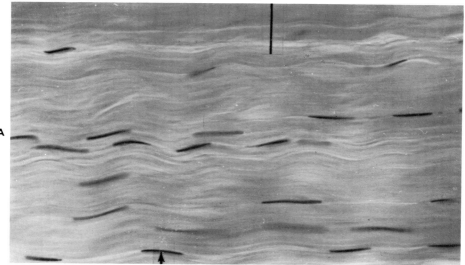

A

Fibroblast nucleus

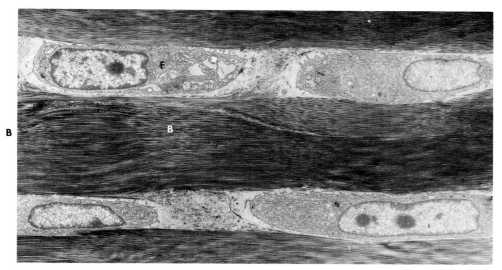

F

B

B

Fig. 3-16. Longitudinal section of tendon. *B,* Collagen fibers; *F,* fibroblast. (×640.)

widely scattered fusiform fibroblast nuclei are also a feature of this tissue. This tissue occurs in the form of sheets. Examples of the latter variety occur in the perichondrium, periosteum, dermis, and capsules of many organs. In certain encapsulated organs, pillars of dense irregular connective tissue known as trabeculae penetrate and subdivide the structure. The trabeculae usually bear blood vessels, nerves, and sometimes the ducts of glands. The trabeculae are composed almost entirely of collagenous fibers but, in some instances, may include elastic and reticular fibers and even smooth muscle.

Regular. Regular dense fibrous tissue occurs in cords or bands and is typified by tendons, ligaments, and aponeuroses. In the tendon the fibers are densely arranged in thick, parallel, unbranching bundles. These bundles are so closely crowded that the cells between them are flattened to a platelike form (Fig. 3-16). The cells lie in rows parallel to the fibers. In profile the nuclei are very long and thin, whereas in surface view the individual nuclei are elongated ovals. In cross section the cells are so compressed that they appear as winglike projections between adjacent bundles. Tendons are composed almost entirely of collagenous fibers.

Elastic tissue

Elastic fibers are of rather general occurrence in connective tissue, but they are not considered elastic tissues. In certain situations the elastic fibers predominate, whereas the collagenous fibers are sparse. In the walls of arteries, elastic fibers have developed and fused to such an extent that they form an incomplete (fenestrated) membrane, enclosing cells and a few collagenous fibers. As such, this arrangement might be termed dense irregular elastic tissue. A form of dense regular elastic tissue is found in the neck ligament of the ox (ligamentum nuchae) and in the smaller ligaments found between the vertebrae (ligamentum flavis). In this type, thick, long, branching elastic fibers lie in nearly parallel arrangement in association with very few cells and an extremely small number of fine collagenous fibers. In such a dense arrangement the fibers, especially in older animals, appear yellow in color, hence the now obsolete term *yellow fibers.*

ADIPOSE TISSUE

Adipose tissue is commonly included in the groups of connective and supporting tissues, although it differs from the other members of the group in several respects. The cells composing it do not form intercellular fibers or matrix but are specialized for the storing of fat. They thus form a reserve of foodstuffs as well as supporting pads of tissue. The cells are mesenchymal in origin, like those of connective tissue. They lose their protoplasmic processes early in the course of their transformation and become round, with abundant cytoplasm and central nuclei. The fat is de-

posited in the cytoplasm in minute droplets that gradually increase and unite in one large drop, which pushes the nucleus to one side of the cell. As still more fat accumulates, the nucleus becomes flattened and the cytoplasm is reduced to a mere film enclosing the fat globule. In tissues that have been treated with ordinary fixatives followed by alcohol, the fat is dissolved out, leaving the cytoplasm of the cells in the form of large irregular rings, each having a dark flat nucleus at one side. In preparations made with osmic acid the fat resists the action of the alcohol and appears as a deeply stained mass occupying the center of each cell. There is no intercellular substance elaborated by adipose tissue cells. They lie embedded in reticular or areolar tissue, the fibers among them being the product of reticular cells or fibroblasts. Adipose tissue is illustrated in Fig. 3-17.

Fat is made up of glycerol esters and fatty acids. They are synthesized from carbohydrates and may be stored or called upon as a reserve source of food in time of bodily need. Adipose tissue serves as a padding for organs, mechanically protecting them from shock, as a reserve food supply, and lastly as an agent in thermoregulation by aiding in the conservation of body heat, particularly in the newborn.

SEROUS MEMBRANES

Serous membranes, the pleura, peritoneum, and pericardium, consist of a thin layer of loosely arranged connective tissues covered by a layer of relatively flat mesothelial cells. The membrane is made up of loosely arranged collagenous fibers, scattered elastic fibers, fibroblasts, macrophages, mast cells, adipose cells, and a varying number of other cells. The amount of fluid exudate and the variety and number of cells suspended in it increase greatly in adverse physiologic or pathologic conditions.

RETICULOENDOTHELIAL SYSTEM

The reticuloendothelial system, sometimes referred to as the system of macrophages, has as its most significant function

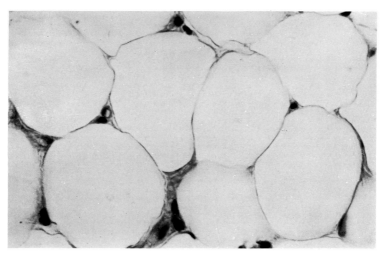

Fig. 3-17. Adipose tissue showing fibroblast nuclei between fat cells. (Hematoxylin and eosin stain.)

the ingestion and removal of particulate matter. These cells are found in the loose connective tissue, in lymphatic and myeloid tissues, in sinusoids of the liver, spleen, adrenal gland, and hypophysis, and also as "dust" cells in the lung and some perivascular cells.

The cells that occur in the sites mentioned here differ morphologically but react in a similar fashion when subjected to certain adverse conditions. When, for example, a weak solution of a dye such as trypan blue is injected into an animal, subsequent examination will show an appreciable accumulation of this dye in all the cells in the system to a degree not observed in any other cells. Whereas this experimental confirmation shows the simi-

larity in function of this group of cells, it has been shown that macrophages in specific tissues or organs phagocytize materials of a rather selective nature. The macrophages in the spleen and liver phagocytize degenerating red blood cells, retaining the iron for reutilization. In the lungs, dust and other particles of this nature are removed by the cells. Particulate matter of several kinds is removed by macrophages in the lymph nodes. The kinds of matter ingested by the macrophages may be relatively inert or noxious in character. The function of macrophages is accordingly concerned with the defense mechanism of the body. The cells of this system arise from primitive reticular cells, preexisting macrophages, lymphocytes, and monocytes.

4
Cartilage

In the connective tissues described in Chapter 3 the elements present consist of cells and fibers embedded in a viscid ground substance and tissue fluid. The noncellular elements are collectively known as the matrix. In the supporting tissues such as cartilage and bone, the character of the matrix varies. In cartilage the ground substance is semirigid and contains a protein-carbohydrate complex known as chondromucoid. On partial hydrolysis the latter yields chondroitin sulfuric acid. Chondromucoid is PAS positive and basophilic and stains metachromatically with toluidine blue. In older individuals, mineralization of cartilage, for example, in the larynx, may occur and is usually accompanied by degenerative changes of the cells. Cations, for example, calcium and strontium, are bound strongly to chondroitin sulfuric acid, and the cartilage in these regions stains orthochromatically with toluidine blue and appears intensely basophilic with hematoxylin and eosin.

Cartilage forms the skeleton of the embryo and is exemplified in the adult by the tracheal rings. Throughout the matrix collagenous fibers interlace much as they do in the fluid matrix of areolar tissue. The cells lie in minute spaces in the matrix called the lacunae (Fig. 4-1). These vary in shape according to their position in the plate of cartilage. They are thin and oval shaped near the edges of a cartilage plate and larger and rounder near the center of a plate. The cells, originally stellate like other mesenchyme cells, have lost their protoplasmic processes and have assumed the shape of the lacunae in which they lie. Unlike other connective tissue, cartilage contains no blood vessels, so that nourishment must reach the cells by seepage through the matrix.

Cartilage develops from mesenchyme, as do the other supporting tissues. Mesenchyme cells first elaborate the fibers and later lay down the solid matrix upon them. Each cell forms a circumferential layer of matrix, thus enclosing itself in a lacuna. As growth and development proceed, the amount of matrix between cells increases, pushing them farther apart, so that ultimately the condition is reached in which the cells lie in lacunae scattered through a relatively large amount of intercellular substance. For a time, at least, after the embryonic period, growth may be effected interstitially by the division of cartilage cells and the laying down of matrix around each daughter cell. Later, however, the increasing solidity of the matrix renders this type of growth more difficult, and increase in the size of the cartilage plate is caused by the addition of new layers at the periphery by the cells of the perichondrium (appositional growth). In adult cartilage one may, as we have said, find two or four lacunae close together separated by very thin walls of matrix. These and the lacunae that contain two cells indicate that interstitial growth is proceeding with difficulty.

FIBROCARTILAGE

Cartilage occurs in three forms, fibrous, hyaline, and elastic; these are distinguished

44

Collagen fibers   Chondrocytes

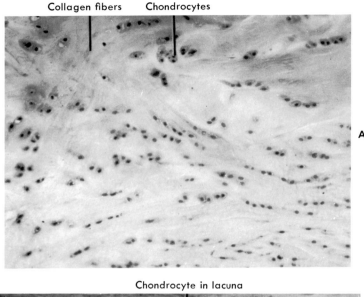

A

Chondrocyte in lacuna

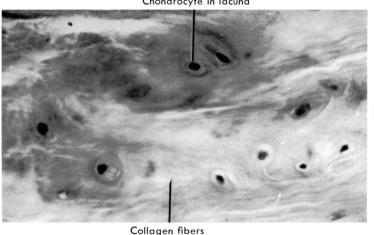

B

Collagen fibers

Fig. 4-1. Fibrocartilage from symphysis of rabbit. (**A,** ×160; **B,** ×640.)

by the character of their fibers and the relative proportions of fibers and matrix. Of the three types, fibrocartilage most nearly resembles connective tissue (Fig. 4-1). In the intervertebral disks, it blends on one side with connective tissue and on the other with hyaline cartilage, and, as we shall see, it is intermediate between the two kinds of tissue in qualities as well as in position. It consists of a network of coarse white fibers, which take the usual red color when stained with eosin. These

fibers are embedded in a solid matrix, which fills the interstices between them. The extent of the matrix varies somewhat in different specimens. In some cases it replaces the fluid matrix only partially and appears merely as fine purplish lines between the red fibers and as thin capsules surrounding the cells. In others its amount is greater and it forms darker lines among the fibers and definite branching islands containing lacunae. In the former condition it is not easily distinguished from dense connective tissue, but one characteristic feature is always to be seen: the round or oval lacunae that contain the cells. In connective tissue the cells are flattened by the pressure of the surrounding fibers; in cartilage, they are protected by the capsules of matrix in which they lie.

HYALINE CARTILAGE

The collagenous fibers of hyaline cartilage are not gathered in bundles but are dispersed throughout the tissue in a fine, close network completely filled in by the substance of the matrix. The union is so close as to form a mass that, though pliable, is very firm. The fibers and matrix have, moreover, the same staining capacity and refractive index, so that in ordinary preparations they are not morphologically distinguishable. Hyaline cartilage is so called because the matrix appears clear (glasslike), and special techniques are required to demonstrate that the intercellular substance consists of fibers and matrix.

Hyaline cartilage occurs in the form of definite plates, in each of which the cells and matrix exhibit a definite plan of organization. If one studies a cartilage plate from the trachea, for instance, certain regions may be distinguished, and the plan will be found to be typical of all cartilage plates. At the periphery of the plate there is a fibrous layer, the perichondrium. This is, on the outside, similar to the surrounding areolar tissue with which it blends. It is well supplied with blood vessels. Toward the cartilage the perichondrium becomes denser; that is, the fibers become heavier and more closely crowded, and the interfibrillar spaces containing the cells become smaller. The outer layer of the perichondrium is called the fibrous layer; the inner, the chondrogenetic layer. At the inner border of the chondrogenetic layer a condition is reached in which individual fibers are no longer distinguishable, their identity being obscured by the solid matrix in which they are embedded. Both fibers and matrix are pink in this region in well-stained hematoxylin-eosin prepara-

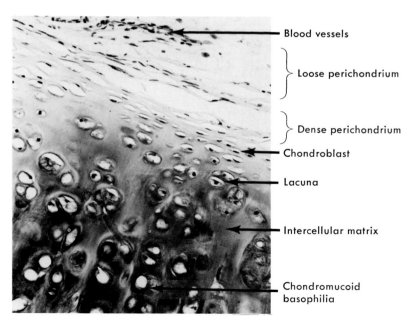

Blood vessels

Loose perichondrium

Dense perichondrium

Chondroblast

Lacuna

Intercellular matrix

Chondromucoid basophilia

Fig. 4-2. Hyaline cartilage from trachea.

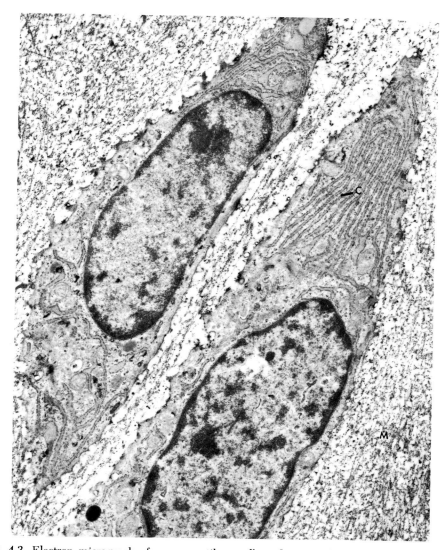

Fig. 4-3. Electron micrograph of young cartilage cells and surrounding cartilage matrix. The most characteristic features of these cells are the prominent arrays of cisternae, *C*, studded with ribosomes. The matrix, *M*, surrounding the cells shows delicate reticular fibers and dark granules, which are probably acid mucopolysaccharide. (×12,000.)

Connective tissue

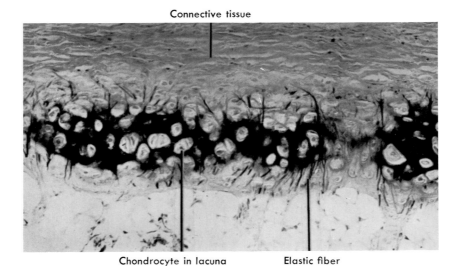

Chondrocyte in lacuna   Elastic fiber

Fig. 4-4. Elastic cartilage. (Verhoeff's method; ×160.)

tions. The cells are no longer free as in the fluid matrix of the perichondrium but are enclosed in spindle-shaped lacunae.

Toward the center of the plate, changes occur in cells and matrix. The latter becomes chemically basic and accordingly stains blue rather than pink (territorial matrix). The matrix between the cell groups known as interterritorial matrices becomes increasingly nonbasophilic with age because of loss of chondroitin sulfate and increase in albuminoid substances chemically related to keratin. The color is pale except immediately around the lacunae, where it is often very dark. The shape of the lacunae also changes toward the middle of the plate; they become round rather than flattened. Often they are found in pairs or groups of four with the sides toward each other flattened. The cells (*chondrocytes*) occupying these central lacunae are spherical and in the living tissue fill the entire space. They are separated from the matrix by a fine capsule, which rarely may be distinguished. In fixed preparations the cytoplasm is usually shrunken, and the only prominent feature is the nucleus. This is surrounded by an irregular cytoplasm. The shrinkage occurs because the fixatives penetrate slowly through the matrix and do

not reach its center until after postmortem changes have taken place there and because the cartilage cells contain large amounts of glycogen and fat that are lost in processing. When cartilage cells are well preserved, they are roughly spherical and have a prominent, centrally placed nucleus. The cytoplasm is granular and basophilic. Large mitochondria, varying amounts of glycogen, numerous vacuoles, and lipid droplets are present. At the electron microscope level, the surface of the cell is irregular and the rough endoplasmic reticulum occupies the greater part of the cytoplasm. The appearance of hyaline cartilage is illustrated in Figs. 4-2 and 4-3.

ELASTIC CARTILAGE

Elastic cartilage is similar to hyaline cartilage in the arrangement of perichondrium, matrix, cells, and lacunae. The difference is that elastic cartilage contains, besides the invisible collagenous fibers, a network of elastic fibers, which may be readily demonstrated by the use of the appropriate stain. This type of cartilage occurs in the epiglottis and is present also in the external ear (Fig. 4-4). The areas in which elastic cartilage will be found in the embryo exhibit connective tissue fibers and fibroblasts. The fibers are wavy and do not react characteristically for either collagen or elastin. These peculiar fibers apparently transform into elastic fibers and then chondrocytes develop. A perichondrium located on the periphery of the growing cartilage subsequently initiates appositional growth during the ensuing embryonic period.

FUNCTIONS OF CARTILAGE

The function of cartilage varies and serves the organism in many ways. Hyaline cartilage forms a large part of the temporary skeleton of the embryo. This variety of cartilage makes up the articulating surface of movable joints: in this capacity it exhibits properties of unusual strength for support and also allows the bones to move freely. In the respiratory system the cartilage prevents the collapse of passageways. Hyaline cartilage participates in and contributes to the growth and calcification of long bones. Nutritional and vitamin deficiencies and hormonal imbalance modify the normal participation of cartilage in bone development and result in the production of abnormalities of the skeletal system.

5

Bone

The connective and supporting tissues hitherto described are found as components of various organs. Bone, on the other hand, forms a complete system of supporting structures, the skeleton. Like the other members of the group, it consists of cells and matrix. In this tissue the matrix becomes mineralized. The proportion of organic matter is greatly reduced so that, when it is destroyed by drying, the matrix appears but little altered from the living condition.

DEVELOPMENT

The subject of the development and adult structure of bone is complicated by the fact that there are two types of ossification and two kinds of arrangement of the tissue in its fully formed state. It is advisable to consider the interrelations of these before describing any of them in detail. Differences in development arise because in the embryo some of the bones are laid down in undifferentiated mesenchyme, whereas in other parts of the body a temporary supporting system of cartilages precedes bone formation. The first type of ossification (intramembranous) is comparatively simple. In the second type (cartilage replacement), stages of cartilage erosion and of bone formation are intimately associated and form a more confusing picture. The essential process by which a bony matrix is formed is, however, the same in both cases. The difference between intramembranous and cartilage replacement bone lies entirely in the tissue that precedes each in the place where it de-

velops. The immediate result is also the same in both cases: the formation of a mass of irregular trabeculae of bone penetrated by blood vessels and connective tissue. Such bone is called spongy or cancellous bone.

In whatever manner it has been formed, the newly developed spongy bone undergoes secondary changes. These consist of (1) erosion and (2) rebuilding. Differences in the manner and extent of rebuilding in different parts of the bone result in the development of two types of adult structure. In some regions the bone is eroded and rebuilt in its original form (spongy). In others rebuilding follows a new pattern and is more extensive so that the tissue has the arrangement called compact bone. Compact and spongy bone are alike in their essential elements but differ in the arrangement and relative amounts of matrix, blood vessels, and marrow spaces.

In the following outline the development of bone has been divided, for convenience, into four steps: spicule formation, confluence of spicules, erosion, and rebuilding.

A. Formation of spicules of matrix
　1. Intramembranous — spicules laid down directly in mesenchyme
　2. Cartilage replacement
　　a. Bone formed around the outside of the cartilage (perichondrial)
　　b. Erosion of the center of the cartilage
　　c. Bone laid down on fragments of disintegrating cartilage (endochondrial)

B. Confluence of spicules to form spongy bone
C. Secondary erosion
D. Rebuilding
   1. In the form of new spongy bone
   2. In the form of compact bone

The division is arbitrary, and it should be remembered that different parts of the same bone may be in different stages of development at any one time and that the steps merge gradually into each other. Although all the processes involved are most active during fetal and early postnatal life, they continue slowly until old age is reached and any one of them may be accelerated by metabolic or traumatic

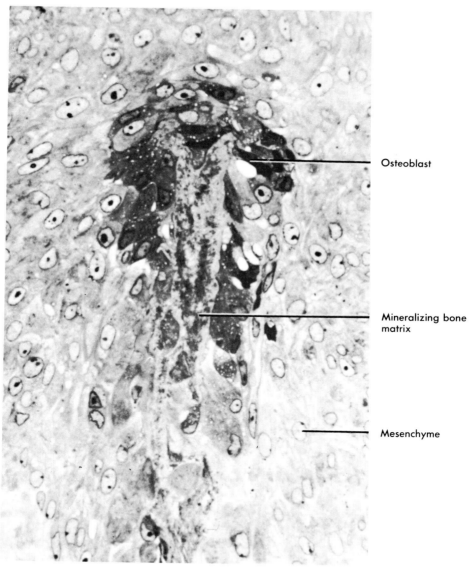

Osteoblast

Mineralizing bone matrix

Mesenchyme

Fig. 5-1. Developing bone spicule. (×800.) (From Bevelander: Outline of histology, ed. 7, St. Louis, 1971, The C. V. Mosby Co.)

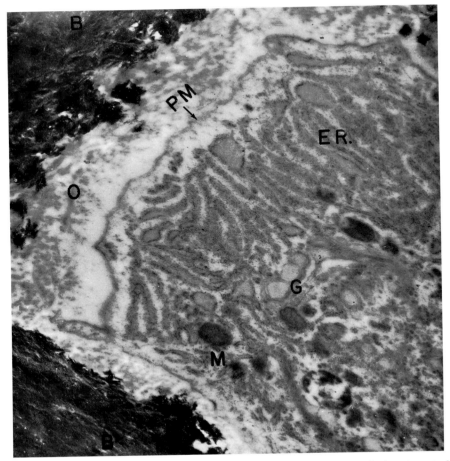

Fig. 5-2. Electron photomicrograph of an osteoblast in rat. *B*, Bone; *ER*, endoplasmic reticulum; *G*, Golgi complex; *M*, mitochondria; *O*, osteoid; *PM*, plasma membrane. (×30,000.) (Courtesy Dr. F. Gonzales, Chicago, Ill.)

changes. In the following account of the development of bone we shall trace the histogenesis of intramembranous bone and cartilage replacement bone, respectively, through the stages leading to the formation of adult bone.

Intramembranous bone

The regions in which the process of intramembranous bone formation occurs are determined by the proximity of blood vessels. In an area where bone will develop, mesenchymal cells differentiate to form fibroblasts. The cells are connected with one another by their processes and are sur-

rounded by delicate bundles of reticular fibers. The cells and fibers are loosely arranged in a semiviscid ground substance.

The initiation of bone formation consists of the production of an increased amount of ground substance between the cells, often trapping some of the cells within it. At the same time, the cells increase in size, assume a polyhedral form, and maintain, meanwhile, the numerous processes by which they are connected with adjacent cells. At this stage they are known as osteoblasts (Figs. 5-1 and 5-2), and the bone in the nonmineralized state is sometimes referred to as osteoid.

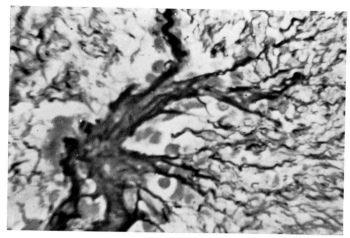

Fig. 5-3. Developing spicule of membrane bone showing origin and incorporation of fibers before mineralization occurs. (Reticulum stain.)

Osteoblasts, as their name implies, are associated with bone formation and are invariably found on the margin of growing bones (Fig. 5-4). During the period of growth they are arranged in an epithelioid layer of cuboidal or low columnar cells joined together by slender processes. The nucleus, usually located in the basal region, exhibits a prominent nucleolus. By appropriate staining methods a diplosome and well-developed Golgi apparatus can be observed adjacent to the nucleus. Mitochondria are numerous and usually elongated. The cytoplasm of the active cell is intensely basophilic and also contains PAS-staining granules, as well as considerable amounts of alkaline phosphatase. At the electron microscope level (Fig. 5-2) the osteoblast exhibits an extensive, rough endoplasmic reticulum; numerous free ribosomes; well-developed Golgi membranes and vesicles, lysosomes, and other inclusions. The general appearance of the cell is similar to other cells known to be engaged in protein synthesis.

When certain conditions are attained in the elaboration of this complex of cells and matrix, the tissue undergoes calcification; that is, the mineral is deposited in the matrix in the form of hydroxyapatite (Ca_3 $[PO_4]_2)_3$–$Ca(OH)_2$. In addition, bone mineral may contain other cations such as

sodium, magnesium, carbonate, and citrate. The mineral or inorganic part of a bone may vary from 35% dry weight in young bones to 65% in adult bones.

The organic or interstitial component of bone contains numerous reticular fibers (Fig. 5-3), which are surrounded by an amorphous ground substance. In the embryonic state this substance is PAS positive and metachromatic, the latter property being correlated with the presence of a sulfated polysaccharide.

Following the initial stages of bone formation just described, subsequent changes occur: osteoblasts arrange themselves on the surface of the developing bone in a continuous layer. Reticular fibers are added to the matrix from the surrounding mesenchyme to give rise to the so-called osteogenic fibers upon which calcification subsequently takes place. As mineralization occurs, these fibers become collagenous. The bone increases in thickness by adding successive layers of matrix resulting from osteoblastic activity. During this process, some of the osteoblasts with their processes become entrapped in the matrix and, when calcification occurs, they occupy a space in the matrix known as a lacuna. These are the true bone cells, or *osteocytes* (Figs. 5-4 and 5-5).

An osteoblast, after it is surrounded by

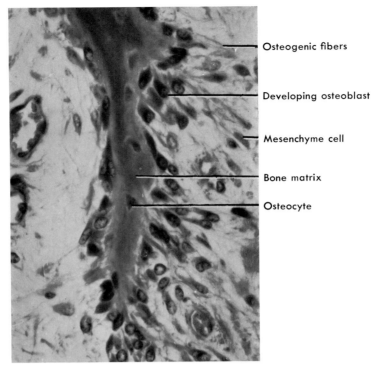

Osteogenic fibers

Developing osteoblast

Mesenchyme cell

Bone matrix

Osteocyte

Fig. 5-4. Developing intramembranous bone. Note that peripheral osteoid is lighter than central portion.

bone matrix, remains in the tissue as a bone cell. The spicule thus formed contains all the essential elements of the bone: fibers, a calcified matrix, and cells situated in lacunae. It differs from cartilage in two respects: the chemical composition of the matrix and the shape of the lacunae. In cartilage the lacunae are round or oval and are entirely separate from each other. The fibers of a new spicule are arranged in a woven pattern (woven bone) while the fibers of adult bone are usually arranged in layers (lamellar bone).

Osteocytes, or bone cells, occur in lacunae within the calcified matrix. The main portion of the cell is flattened, conforming to the shape of the lacuna that it occupies. Numerous slender processes extend from the cell body into canaliculi of the surrounding matrix. Although the extent of these processes is controversial, it is generally believed that they do not make contact with the processes of adjacent cells.

Since the osteocytes were originally osteoblasts, it is not surprising that the cytoplasm resembles osteoblasts. The osteocyte differs, however, in that it is a less active cell and, accordingly, the organelles are not as prominent as those occurring in the osteoblast (Fig. 5-5). The osteocyte is not concerned with bone formation but rather with metabolic activities necessary for the maintenance and modification of the bone matrix.

As each spicule grows by the addition of new layers, or lamellae, of bone substance, it encroaches on the surrounding mesenchyme, and soon adjacent spicules come in contact and fuse with each other. Thus by union of originally separate masses, a latticework of bony trabeculae is formed. It is characterized by the irregular shape and arrangement of its parts and of the enclosed spaces. The latter contain embryonic bone marrow, which has developed from the mesenchyme in this region.

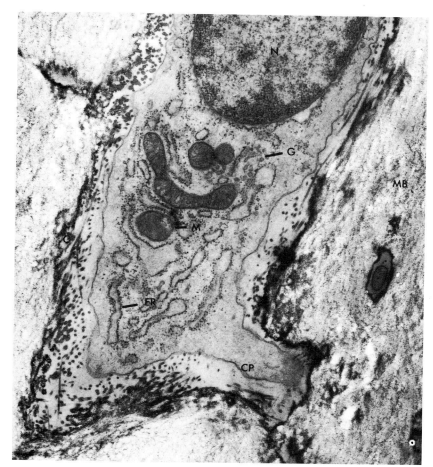

Fig. 5-5. Electron micrograph of portion of an osteocyte from calvarium of rat. *C,* Collagen; *CP,* cell process; *ER,* endoplasmic reticulum; *G,* Golgi vesicles; *M,* mitochondrion; *MB,* bone matrix; *N,* nucleus. (×23,000.)

Cartilage replacement bone

Bone in the condition just described (spongy bone) is ready for the processes of erosion and rebuilding, which may transform a part of it into compact bone. Before discussing these changes, however, we must consider the way in which spongy bone develops in situations where cartilage precedes it as a temporary supporting structure. In many parts of the embryo a kind of model of the skeleton is laid down in cartilage. This must be replaced by bone in a gradual manner so that the part will not be left unsupported at any time. The process is well illustrated in the femur, which exemplifies a long bone.

Before actual replacement of the cartilage is begun, a cylinder of intramembraneous bone is formed around its outside. This is the so-called perichondrial bone, laid down in a collarlike band around the shaft of the cartilage, the ends of which are left free for growth (Fig. 5-6). In longitudinal sections of a developing bone of this type, the perichondrial bone appears as a fairly dense strip of bone on each side of the cartilage. As soon as the perichondrial bone is well established,

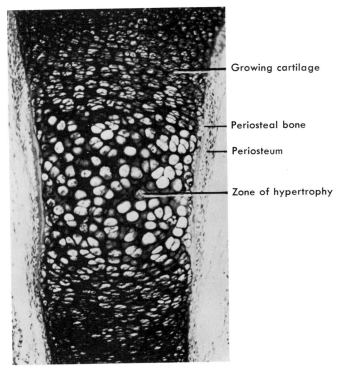

Growing cartilage

Periosteal bone

Periosteum

Zone of hypertrophy

Fig. 5-6. Central part of shaft of developing long bone.

changes occur in the part of the cartilage that is covered by it. A mass of mesenchymal tissue called the periosteal bud invades the cartilage, breaking down the matrix as it grows (Fig. 5-8). The periosteal bud contains blood vessels, osteoblasts, and osteoclasts. By its action on the cartilage matrix it forms a cavity in the central portion of the model, which is the primitive marrow cavity. Jagged spicules of cartilage matrix are left projecting into the cavity, and it is along these that the osteoblasts line up and begin the formation of bone, which, because it lies within the outlines of the cartilage model, is called endochondrial bone (Figs. 5-7 to 5-9). The essential process of endochondrial bone formation is like that occurring in intramembranous bone. Fibers are formed and matrix is deposited upon them, giving rise to separate spicules, which later become confluent, resulting in a mass of bony trabeculae. The difference between the spic-

ules of the two kinds of bone is that in endochondrial ossification each spicule is laid down around a fragment of calcified cartilage matrix that may be seen at its center for some time after bone formation has begun, whereas in intramembraneous bone spicules no such substrate is present. The timing of these events varies with the different bones.

If one examines a section of a cartilage that is being replaced by bone, he will see zones that represent different stages of development (Figs. 5-7 and 5-9). At each end the cartilage is normal. Toward the middle, near the beginning of the region surrounded by perichondrial bone, is a zone of rapid growth, which is adding to the length of the model. This zone is characterized by the arrangement of the lacunae in rows lying in the long axis of the model. The lacunae in each row are flattened and separated from each other by thin plates of matrix, while the matrix be-

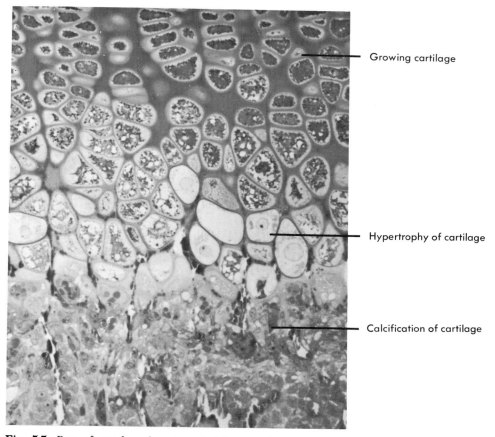

Growing cartilage

Hypertrophy of cartilage

Calcification of cartilage

Fig. 5-7. Part of epiphyseal region of 4-day rat femur showing cellular differences during growth. (Plastic section; ×250.)

tween adjacent rows forms solid columns or bands. Still farther toward the center, the lacunae are enlarged, and, at the border of the marrow cavity, they are confluent and the matrix is reduced to jagged trabeculae. This is the place at which the erosive action of the invading marrow cells is apparent. The cartilage cells are said by some writers to be destroyed along with the matrix. Other workers claim that they are transformed into osteoblasts. Calcium salts are laid down in the remains of the cartilage matrix in this part of the model, with the result that it stains more deeply with hematoxylin than does the normal matrix in other parts of the section. It is upon the bits of calcified cartilage, as previously mentioned, that the bone is laid

down. In properly stained sections, one may see spicules of dark purple, partially calcified cartilage matrix coated with one or more layers of red bone. The whole is surrounded by osteoblasts (Fig. 5-9). This latter region, the primary spongiosa, has undergone mineralization and is known as the zone of provisional or preliminary calcification. It affords a certain amount of rigidity to the junction between hyaline cartilage and spongy bone.

The foregoing discussion describes the formation of the shaft or diaphysis of a long bone in which there is, at first, only one center of ossification. Later, however, new and independent centers develop in the ends of the cartilage model without the preliminary formation of perichondrial

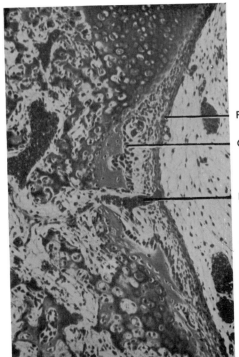

Periosteum

Osteoblasts

Periosteal bud

Fig. 5-8. Section through center of shaft of developing long bone showing periosteal bud and associated structures.

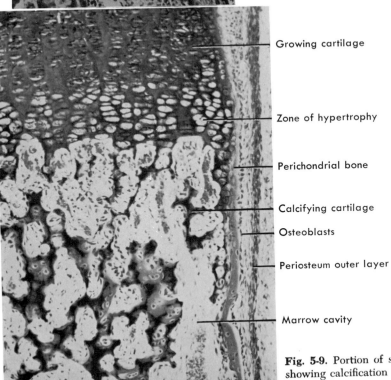

Growing cartilage

Zone of hypertrophy

Perichondrial bone

Calcifying cartilage

Osteoblasts

Periosteum outer layer

Marrow cavity

Fig. 5-9. Portion of shaft of developing long bone showing calcification of cartilage.

bone. These new centers, in the epiphyses, spread radially. The growth zone of cartilage on which the increase in length of the bone as a whole depends thus comes to lie between two centers of ossification, which encroach on it from opposite directions. The growth zone persists, however, during the early years of life, and so long as it remains, the stature of the individual increases. Ultimately, at about the twentieth year of life, ossification outruns cartilage growth and the epiphyses and diaphysis unit. After this has occurred, growth in length of bone ceases, but additions in thickness may be made by osteoblasts in the surrounding periosteum. The importance of this layer, as well as its structure, will be discussed in connection with the histology of the adult bone.

The process of erosion of bone actually begins soon after the first trabeculae of spongy bone have been laid down and continues actively as long as the bones are growing. It starts at the point where bone

formation began: at the borders of the primary marrow cavity. Thus as mineralization of the diaphysis of a long bone moves toward the ends of the cartilage model, it is followed by a secondary breaking down and resorption of part of the newly formed tissue. The result is an enlargement of the marrow cavity, which prevents the bone from becoming too heavy and solid. During the internal reconstruction of the bone, the tips of the trabeculae of the spongiosa are constantly being resorbed. This is necessary for the overall growth of the bone. This process tends to maintain a spongiosa of a constant length, increasing the length of the bone meanwhile. The portion of the spongiosa that undergoes resorption is known as the *secondary spongiosa*.

Osteoclast

Large multinucleated cells, the osteoclasts, are associated with bone resorption and often are located in concavities of the bone surface (Howship's lacunae) (Fig.

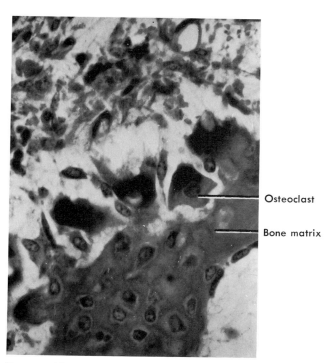

Osteoclast

Bone matrix

Fig. 5-10. Erosion of bone showing osteoclasts in depressions (Howship's lacunae).

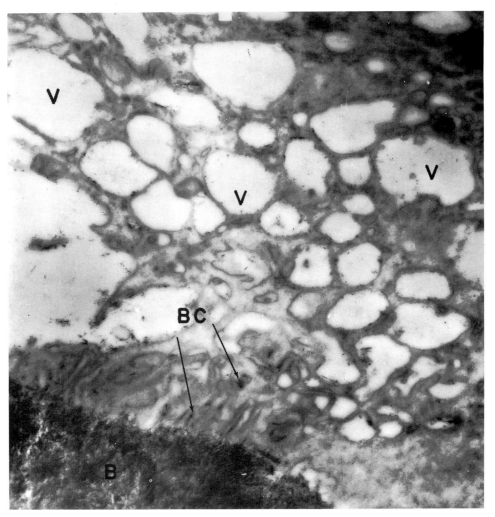

Fig. 5-11. Electron photomicrograph of an osteoclast showing crystals. *B,* Bone; *BC,* bone crystals; *V,* vacuole. (×20,000.) (Courtesy Dr. F. Gonzales, Chicago, Ill.)

5-10). The cytoplasm is only slightly baso-philic and exhibits a vacuolated appear-ance. The nuclei are similar in appearance to those of the osteoblasts. At the electron microscope level, it has been shown that the surface of the cell adjacent to the bone appears to be characterized by numerous infoldings of the cell membrane, giving rise to clefts (Fig. 5-11). Evidence sug-gests that bone salt crystals are loosened from the bone matrix by enzymatic activity and taken up by the folds in the surface,

then by vesicles in the cytoplasm where they undergo demineralization. The mech-anism whereby the collagen fibers and matrix are degraded is, according to sug-gestive evidence, accomplished by proteo-lytic enzymes elaborated by the osteoclasts.

Erosion is not confined to the central portion of the bones where, as we have said, its effect is a progressive enlargement of the marrow cavity. It occurs throughout the mass of all bony tissue, but in all places except the marrow cavities it is followed

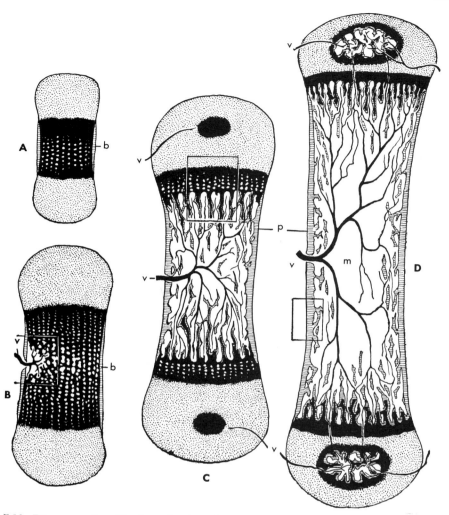

Fig. 5-12. Diagrams of ossification of a long bone. **A,** Early cartilaginous stage; **B,** stage of eruption of periosteal bone collar by an osteogenic bud of vessels; **C,** older stage with a primary marrow cavity and early centers of calcification in epiphyseal cartilages; **D,** condition shortly after birth with epiphyseal centers of ossification. Calcified cartilage in all diagrams is black. *b,* Periosteal bone collar; *m,* marrow cavity; *p,* periosteal bone; *v,* blood vessels entering centers of ossification. (From Nonidez and Windle: Textbook of histology, New York, 1953, McGraw-Hill Book Co.)

by rebuilding. In the ends of the long bones and in the central portions of other bones the rebuilding keeps pace with erosion and follows the pattern of the original formation of the tissue, resulting in a renewal of spongy bone. In the peripheral parts of all bones, however, rebuilding is more rapid than erosion, and a compact layer of bone is established.

Formation of haversian systems. Compact bone is more regular in its arrangement than spongy bone. Its development may be described as follows. The marrow spaces, containing reticular tissue and blood-forming cells, are penetrated throughout by a rich vascular network. The vessels at the periphery of the bone follow a more or less regular pathway parallel to

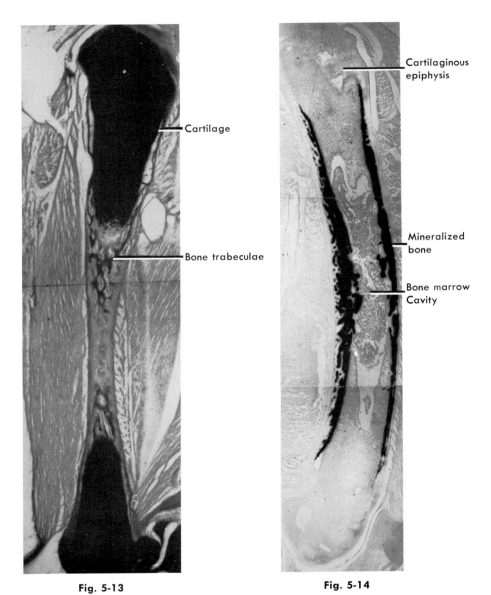

Cartilage

Bone trabeculae

Cartilaginous
epiphysis

Mineralized
bone

Bone marrow
Cavity

Fig. 5-13   **Fig. 5-14**

Fig. 5-13. Radioautograph of femur of 14-day-old chick injected on thirteenth day with ^{35}S. Note uptake in cartilage matrix and to lesser degree in bone matrix. Black areas are metachromatic. Compare with Fig. 5-14.

Fig. 5-14. Radioautograph of longitudinal section of femur of 14-day-old chick injected with ^{45}Ca on thirteenth day. Black areas show regions of ^{45}Ca uptake. Practically no endochondral ossification is present in the chick bone at this time.

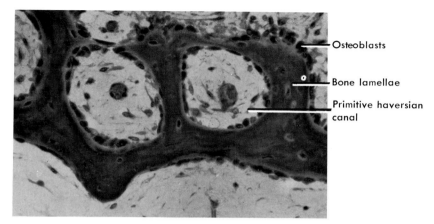

Osteoblasts

Bone lamellae

Primitive haversian canal

Fig. 5-15. Remodeling of bone to form haversian systems.

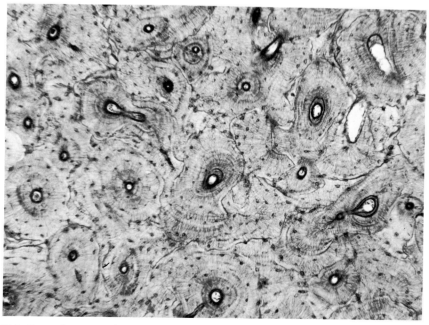

Fig. 5-16. Ground section of compact bone showing arrangement of haversian systems. (×100.)

the surface. In long bones, they run mainly in the long axis of the bone. In places where compact bone is to be formed, erosion follows a definite plan, rounding out the marrow spaces so that they form cylindrical cavities around the blood vessels (Fig. 5-15). After the marrow spaces have been thus reshaped, they are lined by successive concentric layers (lamellae) of new bone. The process continues until the space is almost filled with lamellae and it eventually persists as a central canal containing blood vessels, nerves, and connective tissue. Such a grouping of layers of bone, with its central canal, is called a haversian system.

The remodeling of bone does not end when the primary haversian systems are laid down but continues into adult life. The primary systems are partially destroyed to provide space for new ones in response to changes in mechanical requirements. The final result is a mass of bone composed of secondary and tertiary haversian systems embedded in the remains of earlier systems. The lamellae that form the background for the haversian systems, holding them together in a solid mass, are called interstitial lamellae. The surface of the bone is formed by circumferential lamellae that have been laid down by the osteoblasts of the periosteal tissue. This region contains no haversian systems. Endosteal lamellae of the same character line the shaft where it borders the marrow cavity.

ADULT BONE

Since the development of bone has been so fully discussed, little remains to be said about its adult structure. Gross examination of adult bone that has been sawed in half will show that it is composed of both spongy and compact tissue. In the long bones the spongy arrangement is confined to the epiphyses and inner part of the shaft, and there is a central marrow cavity entirely devoid of bone matrix. In flat bones the spongy tissue forms trabeculae crossing from one side to the other, so that there is no large marrow cavity but several small irregular marrow spaces. Either form of bone has an outer layer, or cortex, of

compact tissue that is, in turn, covered by a tough fibrous coating called the periosteum.

Microscopically, sections of decalcified spongy bone present a picture much like that of developing intramembraneous bone except for the greater extent of the trabeculae. Osteoblasts and osteoclasts are less common but may be found in portions of the tissue that are undergoing changes in arrangement. The matrix stains red with eosin and is lamellated; the cells are dark in color and disposed, one in each lacuna, between adjacent lamellae. With special techniques, one may demonstrate the canaliculi and the fibers on which the matrix was deposited, but these are not ordinarily visible in hematoxylin-eosin preparations.

Ground sections of bone do not show the cellular elements of the tissue, since these are destroyed in the making of the preparation. Such sections are useful in studying the architecture of compact bone. In transverse ground sections the following features are to be noted (Figs. 5-17 to 5-19). The haversian canals appear as empty circular spaces, each of which is surrounded by six to fifteen concentric lamellae of matrix. The lacunae and the canaliculi radiating from them are readily visible. Between haversian systems is the packing of interstitial lamellae, and a piece taken from the periphery of the bone will contain periosteal lamellae. Canals running diagonally or at right angles to those of the haversian systems are the canals of Volkmann. They provide for transverse connections and anastomosis between the blood vessels and are distinguished from haversian canals by their direction through the tissue and by the fact that they are not surrounded by concentric lamellae. The vascular pattern of bone is best seen in longitudinal sections in which, however, the concentric arrangement of lamellae is not to be observed. The appearance of decalcified bone is shown in Fig. 5-20.

It will be seen from the description of bone that, despite its physical rigidity, it is a tissue that retains considerable ability to respond to environmental changes. The most obvious of these are traumatic

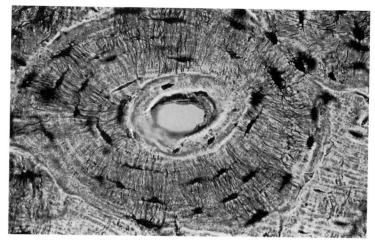

Fig. 5-17. Ground section showing haversian system (osteone) with concentrically arranged lamellae and centrally located haversian canal.

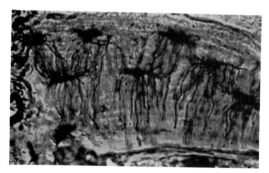

Fig. 5-18. Higher magnification of portion of Fig. 5-17 to show detail of lacunae and canaliculi in bone matrix.

changes such as fractures, which are repaired by the osteoblasts in the periosteum and at the border of the marrow cavity. Some disturbances of the ductless glands provide a stimulus to the osteoblasts of the periosteum that results in the laying down of additional cortical layers of bone (acromegaly). Also the skeleton serves as a storehouse for calcium, and the rates of erosion and rebuilding respond to variations of the mineral metabolism of the body. It is essential to life that a certain amount of calcium be present in the body fluids. When this amount is not supplied by the diet, it may be withdrawn from the bones, or, con-versely, excess calcium may be stored in them.

The skeletal system is under the influence of several hormones. Parathyroid hormone and vitamin D are responsible for the maintenance of normal levels of calcium in the blood. The activity of the parathyroid gland appears to depend upon calcium levels in the circulation. When blood calcium is low, secretion of the gland is stimulated. In hyperparathyroidism, bone is resorbed to an unusual degree and is replaced by fibrous tissue; this condition is known as *osteitis fibrosa* or von Recklinghausen's disease. *Calcitonin* is a hormone that is derived from the thyroid gland. It has an action antagonistic to that of parathyroid hormone in that it lowers blood calcium and inhibits bone resorption. In addition to the two hormones mentioned, it has been shown that the growth hormone elaborated by the hypophysis is necessary for normal bone growth and that the gonadal hormones play a role in the rate of skeletal maturation.

It is obvious that normal bone growth and maturation are dependent on several nutritional factors. This is especially true of the adequate supply and availability of minerals such as calcium and phosphorus, which are the main inorganic components

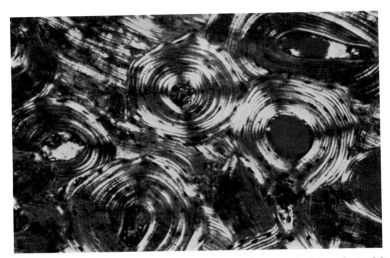

Fig. 5-19. Cross section of compact bone; ground section photographed in polarized light. This photograph indicates the high degree of orientation of the fibers and crystals of bone.

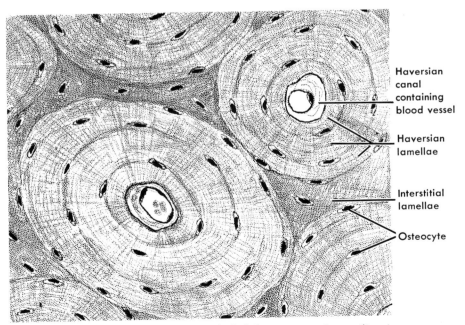

Haversian
canal
containing
blood vessel

Haversian
lamellae

Interstitial
lamellae

Osteocyte

Fig. 5-20. Compact bone decalcified showing organic constituents.

of bone. It has been shown that a dietary insufficiency of either calcium or phosphorus leads to a rarefaction and brittleness of bones. In situations where dietary calcium and phosphorus are adequate but vitamin D is deficient, interference with mineral absorption occurs and mineralization of the growing epiphysis is inhibited, giving rise to a condition known as *rickets.* When subjected to stress, bones in this state become deformed.

Adult rickets (*osteomalacia*) is a condition in which bone exhibits considerable amounts of osteoid tissue. The situation is caused by a long-term deficiency of dietary minerals and vitamin D. Deficiency in vitamin A results in an inhibition of the rate of growth of the skeleton by interfering with the ratio of osteoblasts and osteoclasts responsible for growth and resorption respectively. Retardation of growth and of healing of fractures is correlated with a deficiency of vitamin C resulting from insufficient production of the elements needed to form the bone matrix.

Periosteum

The periosteum is a connective tissue layer covering the bone except at the articular surfaces. It is divisible into two layers. The outer of these is a network of densely packed collagenous fibers with blood vessels. The inner layer provides the penetration fibers (of Sharpey), which are inserted into the bone and attach the periosteum to it. In the inner layer of the periosteum, one may also find fine elastic fibers loosely arranged. Osteoblasts occur here also whenever appositional growth of the bone is taking place. The endosteum is a thin layer of connective tissue lining the marrow cavity and the smaller cavities within the bone. In addition to the more obvious function that the periosteum performs, such as anchorage for tendons and ligaments, it is also concerned with repair and regeneration of bone.

BLOOD SUPPLY AND NERVES

The blood supply of bone comes by two routes. Near the middle of the shaft there is a medullary or nutrient canal that pierces the bone and leads to the marrow cavity. The nutrient artery passes through this canal, giving off branches to the haversian canals on the way. In the marrow cavity, it divides into an ascending and a descending branch, both of which supply the marrow.

The other sources of blood for the bone tissue are by way of the numerous arteries of the periosteum. These enter the substance of the bone through Volkmann's canals, which, in turn, lead to haversian canals.

Veins leave the bone through the nutrient canal, and it is here also that the medullated and nonmedullated nerves enter. The latter accompany the blood vessels into the haversian canals.

MARROW

Although marrow is not actually a part of bone as a tissue, it is included in sections of decalcified bone and should be mentioned here. It is of two kinds, named red and yellow marrow, respectively, according to their color in the fresh state. Both kinds have a framework of reticular tissue. Red marrow is the chief site of the formation of certain types of blood cells including the red corpuscles and contains a great number of blood vessels. The details of its structure will be considered in the following chapters. In yellow marrow the blood-forming elements have been replaced by adipose tissue and the amount of reticular tissue is reduced. Red marrow is present in the cavities of all bones during fetal life and early childhood. It is gradually replaced by yellow marrow and is found in the adult chiefly in the epiphyses of long bones and in the ribs, vertebrae, cranial bones, and sternum.

BONE REPAIR

After bone fracture, the following events occur in connection with the repair of the injured bone. First, there is a hemorrhage caused by the rupture of blood vessels, which is soon followed by the formation of a clot. Subsequently, fibroblasts and capillaries migrate into the area formed by the clot, which results in the formation of gran-

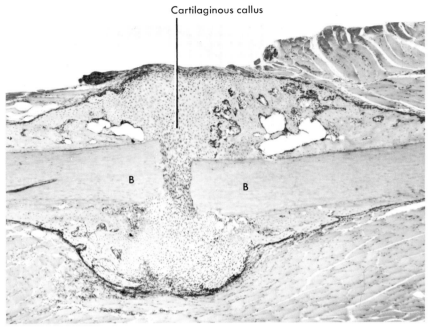

Cartilaginous callus

Fig. 5-21. Partial repair of bone fracture (rabbit rib). The space between the fractured ends of the bone, *B,* is filled in with fibrous tissue. On the periphery a cartilaginous callus, later replaced by bone, has developed. (×40.)

ulation tissue. The granulation tissue then becomes infiltrated with dense fibrous tissue, giving rise to a fibrous union *(procallus)*. The fibrous tissue soon is transformed to cartilage, which constitutes a temporary union or *callus* (Fig. 5-21). The cartilaginous callus is gradually replaced by bone because of the potential activity of the cells in the periosteum. Finally, excess bone present in the callus is partially or completely resorbed. The repair of bone as described here is dependent on an adequate blood supply, on the activity of the bone-forming cells in the periosteum, and also on adequate vitamin and mineral supplies.

JOINTS

The bones are joined together to form the skeleton by a series of articulations, the structure of each varying with the degree of movability of the joint. Articulations that are nearly or quite immovable are called synarthroses. In the skull, for instance, the bones are held together by ligaments composed of short fibers, of which some are elastic and others are continuations of the fibers of Sharpey. The vertebrae are less closely joined, allowing a limited amount of movement, and the spaces between them are occupied by intervertebral disks of fibrocartilage.

The movable joints or diarthroses are characterized by a space between the bones, which is the articular cleft. Each bone bordering on this space has at its end a cap of articular cartilage, which is the remainder of the embryonic cartilage model of the bone. This cartilage is of the hyaline type but has no perichondrial fibrous layer (Fig. 5-22).

The capsule that encloses the articular cartilages and the space between them has two layers. The outer part is the stratum fibrosum, composed of dense fibrous tissue continuous with the outer layer of the periosteum of the bones. The stratum fibrosum is blended with the tendons and ligaments

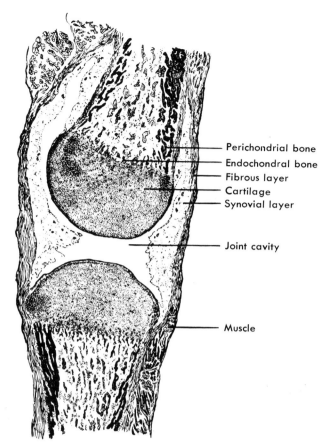

Perichondrial bone
Endochondral bone
Fibrous layer
Cartilage
Synovial layer

Joint cavity

Muscle

Fig. 5-22. Joint from finger of a newborn child. The process of cartilage replacement is still going on, and one may distinguish between endochondral and perichondral bone.

of the muscles attached at this point. The inner, or synovial, layer is of looser and more vascular connective tissue. Where it borders on the articular cavity, it is lined with a layer of dense connective tissue. This consists of fibers and fibroblasts arranged around the border of the cavity. The synovial layer sometimes forms pro-jections into the joint cavity, which may contain fibrocartilage. The synovial fluid, or synovia, is believed to be secreted, at least in part, by cells of the synovial membrane. It is a yellow viscid fluid containing mucoproteins and cellular debris. It serves to lubricate and thus facilitate the smooth movement of the articulating surfaces.

6

Blood and blood formation

Mesenchyme, an embryonic connective tissue derived from the mesoderm, contains characteristic cells that are stellate in shape and connected one to the other by their cellular processes. These cells undergo many changes, which result in the elaboration of blood, lymph, blood vessels, connective tissue proper, cartilage, and bone. In blood and lymph the intercellular substance is fluid; in the connective tissues, fibers occur; in cartilage the intercellular substance is semirigid and contains fibers; whereas in bone the fibers present are impregnated with mineral salts.

The various connective tissues in the adult tend to blend together in some respects. For example, the fibers of the connective tissue proper become incorporated into cartilage and bone; similarly, certain chemical substances such as acid polysaccharides are found in the intercellular areas of connective tissue as well as in cartilage and bone. In the case of blood cells the constant exchange between them and the cells of the connective tissue makes sharp distinctions between these tissues difficult.

Blood and lymph are the fluid tissues of the body. Their function is to distribute oxygen, nutritive substances, and the products of the endocrine glands to all parts of the body and to remove waste substances and toxins. Both consist of a fluid matrix, called the plasma, and cells of various types.

The cells or corpuscles of blood are of two types: red and white. Together they are about equal in bulk to the plasma. Red cells are more numerous than white; there

are 4 to 5 million of them in a cubic millimeter of normal blood compared to only 8,000 or 10,000 white cells.

BLOOD
Red blood corpuscles (erythrocytes)

When a drop of freshly drawn blood is examined under the microscope, red corpuscles are seen as biconcave disks having a diameter of approximately 8 μ. In the fresh state they appear greenish in color rather than red. The depression in the center of each corpuscle makes a light spot that might at first sight be mistaken for a nucleus. Adult red cells are, however, nonnucleated in mammalian blood. Often they stick together in rows, or rouleaux. As a drop of blood dries at its edges the red cells lose fluid and change their shapes. Some are cup shaped, others are very irregular in outline. In sections of organs and tissues stained with hematoxylin and eosin, the red blood cells have a bright orange or red color. The disk shape is the most common in such preparations; but, especially in small vessels, the cells are sometimes cup shaped, sometimes compressed into angular forms. The usual method of preparing blood for microscopic study is to spread a drop on a slide so that it forms a thin smear and then to stain it with a special stain. Wright's stain is commonly used. The red corpuscles when so treated lose volume without changing shape. Those at the center of the smear, when there have been no changes caused by rapid drying, have the form of biconcave disks, which average about 7.5 μ in diameter. The cells

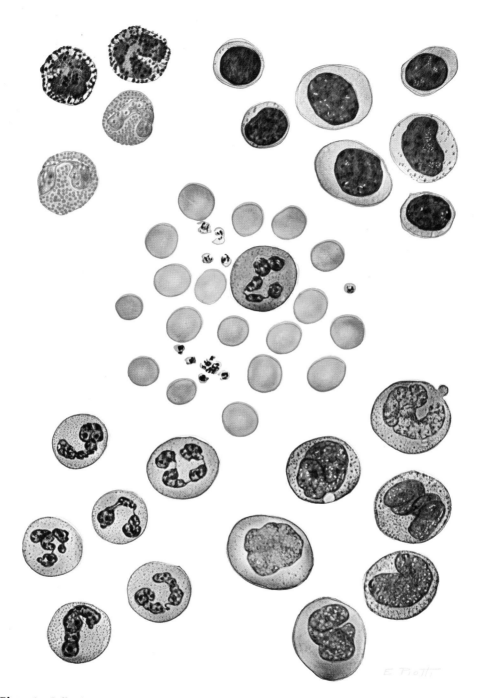

Plate 1. Cells from smear preparation of normal human blood. Center: Adult red blood corpuscles, blood platelets, and a polymorphonuclear neutrophil. Left above: Two polymorphonuclear basophils and two polymorphonuclear eosinophils. Right above: Three large and four small lymphocytes, some with granules in protoplasm. Left below: Polymorphonuclear neutrophils. Two of these cells, the uppermost and the lowermost of the group, are young, with merely crooked nuclei, sometimes known as band, stab, or nonfilamentous forms; mature cells have multilobed nuclei. Right below: Six monocytes, some containing more protoplasmic granules than others. In the younger cells nuclei tend to be rounded and in the adult cells they are horseshoe shaped, indented, or lobed. (Wright's stain.) (From Bremer and Weatherford: A text-book of histology, New York, 1948, The Blakiston Co.)

are nongranular and colored pale brown or pink by the stain.

About 1% of the erythrocytes examined in a smear, although having lost their nuclei, have a diffuse bluish stain and are somewhat larger than the red-staining cells. When stained with cresyl blue, a network of reticulum appears in the cytoplasm; they are accordingly known as *reticulocytes*. They are immature erythrocytes.

Because the red blood cells are nonnucleated, it is sometimes said that they should not be called cells. The name erythroplastid may be used, but erythrocyte is the more common term. The cytoplasm of the red corpuscles contains a substance called hemoglobin, which combines with oxygen and is transformed to oxyhemoglobin. In the body tissues, where the oxygen tension is less than in the lungs, the oxyhemoglobin is reduced and the oxygen is utilized in metabolic processes of the cells. Hemoglobin is also important in the transport of carbon dioxide from the tissues to the lungs.

Hemoglobin imparts a reddish tint to cells containing it if the latter are stained with Wright's stain. This fact is important in recognition of early stages of development of red blood cells. (See discussion on bone marrow later in the chapter.)

White blood corpuscles (leukocytes)

The leukocytes as a group respond differently from the red cells to the treatment involved in making a smear. Erythrocytes lose a slight amount of volume and are therefore smaller in the smear than in the fresh state. Leukocytes, on the contrary, are flattened by the treatment and acquire a greater diameter.

The colorless leukocytes are true cells and contain a nucleus and cell organelles. They exhibit a limited degree of ameboid movement and, for convenience, may be divided into two main groups: the granular variety and the nongranular or lymphoid types. In sections stained with hematoxylin and eosin the leukocytes stand out among the erythrocytes because of their darkly stained nuclei. It is sometimes possible to identify lymphocytes, granulocytes, and monocytes in such preparations, but for critical examination of white cells one must use preparations made with special stains.

GRANULAR (POLYMORPHONUCLEAR) LEUKOCYTES

An outstanding feature of the granulocytes is the presence of granules in the cytoplasm. Each variety of granulocyte has a different kind of granule readily identified at both the optic and the electron microscope levels. A second characteristic feature of these cells is the nucleus, which is multilobed. Although several criteria may be used to distinguish and classify the granulocytes, the one most commonly used is based on the morphologic characteristics of the nucleus and the size, shape, and tinctorial properties of the granules. The granulocytes make up from 60% to 70% of the white cells. In a blood smear treated with Wright's stain the types of cells illustrated in Plate 1 may be distinguished.

Neutrophilic (heterophilic) leukocytes. The nucleus of neutrophilic leukocytes consists of from three to five irregular oval lobes connected by thin chromatin strands. In dry smear preparations an appendage appears on one of the lobes in approximately 3% of the cells. This chromatin appendage, known as a "drumstick" (not to be confused with irregularities on the margin of the nuclei), represents the chromatin material in which the female (XX) chromosomes are located. The cytoplasm (except for a clear homogeneous peripheral zone) is slightly acidophilic and contains numerous fine granules, which appear purple or lavender. These cells measure about 8 μ in the fresh state and attain a size of 12 μ in a dry smear preparation. At the electron microscope level the granules appear diverse in size and shape (Fig. 6-1).

Acidophilic (eosinophilic) leukocytes. The acidophilic leukocytes, which are approximately spherical, measure 9 μ in diameter in the fresh condition and in dry smears may attain a diameter of nearly 12 μ. They make up from 2% to 5% of the total leukocytes in the peripheral blood. In contrast with the nuclei of the neutrophils, the nuclei of the acidophils usually consist

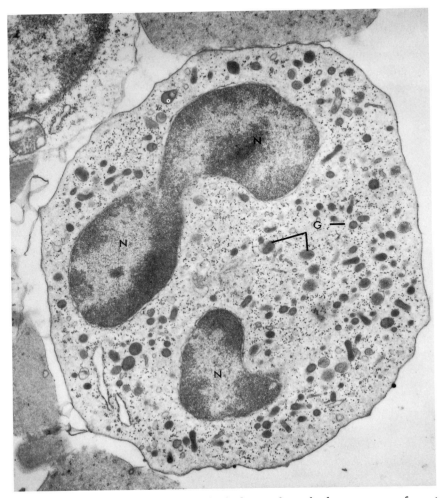

Fig. 6-1. Electron micrograph of neutrophilic leukocyte from the bone marrow of a cat. The granules are bounded by a membrane and vary in density. They contain hydrolytic enzymes. Ribosomes are scattered throughout the cytoplasm. G, Specific granules; N, lobes of nucleus. (×19,000.)

of two oval lobes connected by chromatin strands. Except for a centrally located area occupied by the cytocentrum, the cytoplasm contains numerous coarse granules, which in man are spherical. When stained with acid dyes, the granules vary in appearance from pink to bright red. When observed with the electron microscope, the granules exhibit dense crystalline bodies that vary in appearance in different species (Figs. 6-2 and 6-3).

Basophilic leukocytes. The basophils are

least numerous of the leukocytes and comprise less than 0.5% of the total count. They are approximately the same size as the neutrophils. The nucleus often appears S-shaped, is constricted in two or more regions, and stains less intensely than the other varieties. The granules are extremely coarse and with Wright's stain appear a dull blue. They also give the impression of being partially extruded from the cell surface and often partially obscure the nucleus. Viewed with the electron microscope,

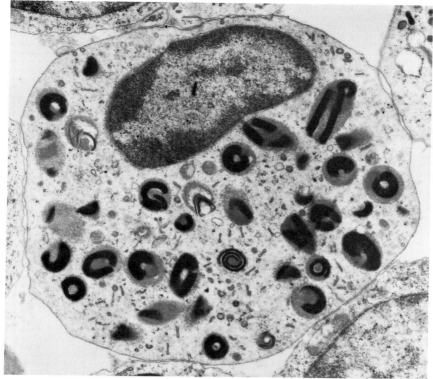

Fig. 6-2. Electron micrograph of eosinophilic leukocyte from bone marrow of cat. Note that the granules are dense and contain dark organic crystals of varying shapes and sizes. (×17,000.)

the granules appear membrane bound; the material enclosed by the membrane varies in appearance in diverse species. Scattered mitochondria and Golgi vesicles are usually present (Fig. 6-4).

NONGRANULAR LEUKOCYTES

Lymphocytes. In the human the lymphocytes make up from 20% to 25% of the total number of white cells of the blood. They are spherical and measure from 6 to 8 μ in diameter, although some of them may be slightly larger. The most characteristic morphologic feature of these cells is the presence of a large, dense nucleus with a distinct indentation on one side, which is not, however, observed in dry smear preparations. Prominent nucleoli may be observed in well-prepared sections at both the optic and the electron microscope levels. The cytoplasm appears as a thin rim surrounding the nucleus. It is homogeneous and basophilic, which is referable to numerous ribosomes observed at the electron microscope level. Occasionally, purple *azurophilic* granules may be observed in the cytoplasm but these are inconstant features that represent early stages in granule development.

The larger lymphocytes are relatively few in number, and their increase in size results from the presence of a greater amount of cytoplasm. The cytoplasm usually contains a few scattered mitochondria and granules.

Monocytes. The monocytes resemble the lymphocytes, especially in forms that appear to be transitional. A typical monocyte measures from 9 to 12 μ in diameter. In dry smear preparations, however, they may appear to be 20 μ or larger. The mature monocyte exhibits considerably more cyto-

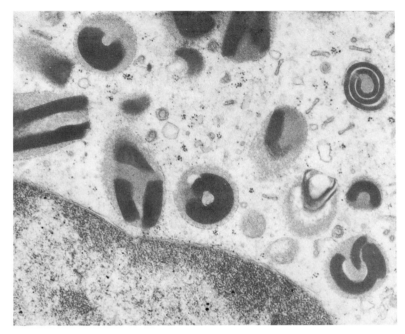

Fig. 6-3. Electron micrograph of part of eosinophilic leukocyte from bone marrow of a cat showing detail of organic crystals in membrane-bound granules. (×33,000.)

plasm than does the lymphocyte and often, though not invariably, has an eccentrically placed nucleus that is oval or kidney shaped. It stains less intensely than the lymphocytes. Organelles such as mitochondria and a Golgi apparatus are usually observed. The monocytes comprise from 3% to 8% of the leukocytes of the circulating blood.

FUNCTIONS OF LEUKOCYTES

The leukocytes in the bloodstream appear to be inactive, and their function is not well understood. Outside the bloodstream, they exhibit ameboid movement. Leukocytes constantly migrate from the vessels to the tissues. This is particularly noticeable at the site of local injury or infection, where the granulocytes migrate in response to chemotactic stimulation. Later, monocytes also accumulate in these areas. Among the granulocytes only the neutrophils exhibit phagocytosis. Many types of bacteria are ingested by this process. During this process the specific granules of

the cell break down and disappear, meanwhile liberating hydrolytic enzymes, which are responsible for the destruction of bacteria. Various other enzymes are present in leukocytes, but their function is not known at present.

Platelets

In addition to the cells just described, blood contains groups of very minute cytoplasmic fragments that are called platelets, or thrombocytes, and are not generally included under the head of corpuscles. The individual platelet, about 2 μ in diameter, is composed of a cytoplasm, which stains blue with Wright's stain. It has a dark granular center, the chromomere, and a light peripheral area, the hyalomere.

Thrombocytes, or platelets, are believed to liberate the enzyme *thromboplastin* involved in the clotting of blood (Fig. 6-5). Thromboplastin transforms prothrombin to thrombin, which, in turn, transforms fibrinogen to fibrin. Thromboplastin also has been identified in blood plasma. Platelets

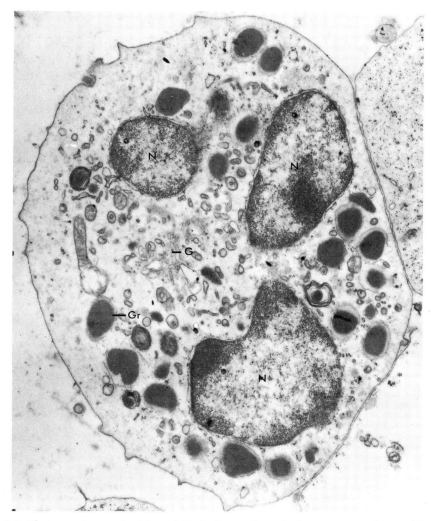

Fig. 6-4. Electron micrograph of basophilic leukocyte from the bone marrow of a cat. This cell contains three nuclear lobes, *N*, but does not show connecting strands of chromatin. Also shown are the Golgi apparatus, *G*, and the large dense membrane-enclosed granules, *Gr*. (×17,000.)

are formed by the budding off of cellular fragments from megakaryocytes in bone marrow.

Plasma

The fluid part of blood containing dissolved electrolytes and plasma proteins is called *plasma*. One liter of plasma contains 940 ml. of water; the rest of the volume is occupied by 60 gm. of protein. Plasma makes up about 55% of the blood volume and cells make up the remainder. The relative amounts of blood cells and plasma (the hematocrit) vary under different physiologic conditions. In addition to electrolytes and proteins, plasma contains a number of dissolved substances such as nutrients, gases, hormones, and clotting factors. One of the constituents of plasma, *fibrinogen,* is converted upon standing to a

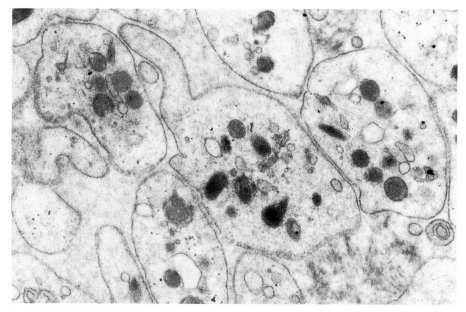

Fig. 6-5. Electron micrograph showing several blood platelets (thrombocytes). (×29,000.)

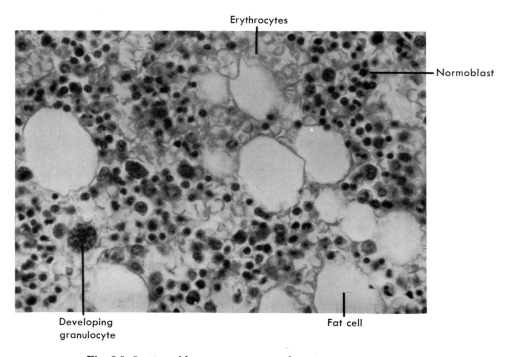

Fig. 6-6. Section of bone marrow in monkey. (Eosin-azure; ×640.)

fibrous clot in which erythrocytes and platelets become enmeshed. Clots help to control blood loss during hemorrhage. The clear, straw-colored fluid from which cells and clotting factors have been removed is called *serum*. Plasma transports the nutritive substances derived from food, the waste products of various tissues, and secretions of the endocrine glands.

LYMPH

Lymph is of less interest to the student of histology than blood. It consists of a fluid plasma that is somewhat different chemically from blood plasma. In it are floating leukocytes, principally lymphocytes and large mononuclear leukocytes. In sections of lymph vessels one sees only a fine granular coagulum with occasional nucleated corpuscles.

BLOOD FORMATION

In the adult body, blood cells are normally formed in two organs that are alike in having a framework of reticular tissue but different in the kinds of corpuscles that they produce. Bone marrow is the normal source of the red blood cells and the granulocytes, and probably also the monocytes, and lymph nodules of the lymphocytes.

Bone marrow

It will be remembered that, in the formation of a bone, a space is left at the center by the resorption, first, of the cartilage and, later, of endosteal bone. This space is invaded by mesenchyme, which develops into an organ having no part in the supportive function of the bone itself. This is the red bone marrow, which in the adult is the source of the majority of the blood corpuscles. The primitive mesenchyme of the embryo develops in this location into three main types of cells: (1) framework of reticular tissue, (2) adipose tissue, and (3) hematopoietic or blood-forming cells (Fig. 6-6). In early life all three kinds of cells are present in the marrow of any bone (Fig. 6-7). Later the hematopoietic cells disappear from the marrow of some of the bones, leaving only reticular tissue and fat cells, which make up the yellow marrow. In other bones the marrow continues to form blood cells throughout life, and their presence makes the tissue red.

Marrow may be studied in smear preparations or in sections. For critical examination, a blood stain must be used. In such a preparation, one may recognize the cells shown in Plate 2.

Reticular tissue cells. In sections, reticular tissue cells are somewhat obscured by the hematopoietic cells, but they may be distinguished in smears or thin sections.

Adipose tissue cells. Adipose tissue cells are generally scattered in red marrow and appear under the low power of the microscope as holes in the marrow because of the loss of lipid during fixation. About half of normal bone marrow is occupied by fat cells (Fig. 6-6).

Hematocytoblasts (stem cells). Hematocytoblasts are from 10 to 12 μ in diameter and have a basophilic, usually nongranular, cytoplasm. The form of the cell is pear shaped or polygonal, without cytoplasmic processes. The nucleus is large and is situated at the widest part of the cell. As the name implies, these are regarded as the cells from which the blood cells are derived.

Promyelocytes, myelocytes, metamyelocytes. There are three intermediate stages between the hematocytoblast and the granular leukocyte. They are characterized in general by the development of cytoplasmic granules, which are neutrophilic, eosinophilic, or basophilic, according to the kind of leukocyte destined to develop from each. It is possible, with sufficient care, to recognize three main types or stages of this group. The youngest (promyelocyte) is a spherical cell with a basophilic cytoplasm much like that of the hematocytoblast except that it contains a few granules. The nucleus of the promyelocyte is large and pale. The second stage (myelocyte–marrow cell) is the most common of the group and is the most easily distinguished. The myelocytes divide rapidly, giving rise to successive generations of cells in which one may trace a gradual increase in the number of specific cytoplasmic granules

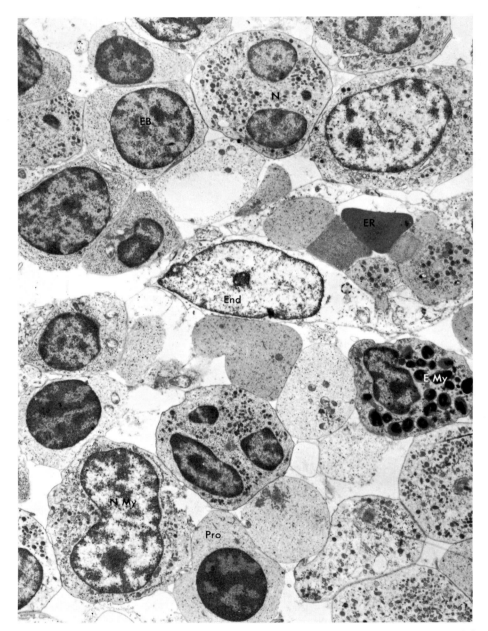

Fig. 6-7. Electron micrograph of bone marrow from cat. *EB*, Erythroblast; *EMy*, eosinophilic myelocyte; *End*, endothelial cell of capillary; *ER*, erythrocyte; *N*, neutrophil; *NMy*, neutrophilic myelocyte; *Pro*, proerythrocyte. (×5,500.)

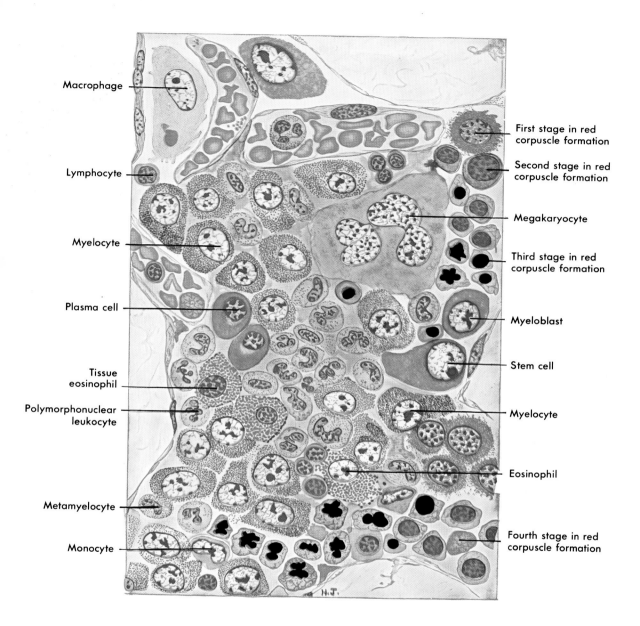

Macrophage

Lymphocyte

Myelocyte

Plasma cell

Tissue
eosinophil

Polymorphonuclear
leukocyte

Metamyelocyte

Monocyte

First stage in red
corpuscle formation

Second stage in red
corpuscle formation

Megakaryocyte

Third stage in red
corpuscle formation

Myeloblast

Stem cell

Myelocyte

Eosinophil

Fourth stage in red
corpuscle formation

Plate 2. Normal vertebral bone marrow, male adult. In one field, representative cells have been brought together in the proper proportion and relation one to another in order to illustrate typical normal picture. (Zenker fixation, decalcified and stained with phloxine-methylene blue.) (From Bremer and Weatherford: A text-book of histology, New York, 1948, The Blakiston Co.)

and an accompanying loss of affinity for basic stains. Also, as divisions occur, there are slight loss of size and increase of density of the nucleus. The products of the last divisions of the myelocytes are the metamyelocytes. These cells develop without further division into polymorphonuclear leukocytes. Metamyelocytes are, in fact, early stages of granulocytes that are not sufficiently mature to enter the circulation under normal conditions.

Proerythroblasts, erythroblasts, normoblasts. The proerythroblast is the earliest recognizable stage in the development of the red blood cell. It differs from the promyelocyte in the following ways. It is slightly smaller and has a more chromatic nucleus; hemoglobin is beginning to develop in its cytoplasm; at this stage the cytoplasm is basic, like that of the hematocytoblast and the promyelocyte, but the presence of hemoglobin gives it a slightly purplish or grayish tinge. In the next stage, the erythroblast, a series of changes develops gradually as the cells divide. These changes are of two kinds: an increase in the amount of hemoglobin in the cytoplasm and a decrease in the size of the cell and its nucleus. The former change is expressed morphologically as a shift in color from the grayish blue of the proerythroblast toward the pink that is characteristic of the erythrocyte. When the pink color is fully developed, the cells are called normoblasts. A normoblast is only slightly larger than an erythrocyte but differs from it in having a nucleus. Normoblasts undergo several divisions, during which their nuclei become progressively smaller and darker. Ultimately the nucleus of the normoblast is reduced to a compact, deeply staining mass, and, when this is extruded from its surface, the cell is a fully developed red blood corpuscle.

Giant cells or megakaryocytes. Megakaryocytes are the largest cells of bone marrow and the most readily recognized. They have a rather dense reddish cytoplasm and a polymorphic nucleus. In size and color they resemble the osteoclasts, which will be found at the margin of the marrow. Osteoclasts, however, have many separate nuclei (polykaryocytes), whereas the parts of the nucleus of a giant cell are connected by strands of nuclear material. It is from the cytoplasm of the giant cell that the blood platelets are formed. In addition to the cells just described, all types of blood corpuscles are to be found in bone marrow.

Development of blood cells in embryo. While the most important permanent source of blood cells is the red bone marrow, there are several other sites of blood formation that occur during embryonic development.

The first area in which this occurs is in the yolk sac of the embryo. Other sites of origin are the mesenchyme, thymus, liver, spleen, and the lymph nodes.

Germinal centers of lymph nodes

Lymphoid tissue contains centers of lymphocyte production. These consist of areas that stain more lightly than the surrounding tissue because they are composed of large, pale cells with vesicular nuclei. These are hematocytoblasts, which differ from the hematocytoblasts of bone marrow in that they are destined to produce only one type of corpuscle, the lymphocyte. Some authors prefer to give to them the name *lymphoblast* on this account. Surrounding such a center of pale cells is a ring of densely packed lymphocytes, which, with their deeply stained nuclei and scanty cytoplasm, form a marked contrast of color in the germinal center.

7

Muscle

The fibers of muscle differ from those of connective tissue in structure and in function. In the connective tissues the fibers are intercellular and noncontractile and serve the purpose of binding or padding. In muscular tissue the cells are called fibers and are composed of elongated cells in which the property of contractility is highly developed. The function of muscle is to move parts of the body by its contraction. Only a small amount of intercellular substance is present in muscle, except as it is intermingled with connective tissue cells and fibers.

The morphologic characteristics common to all types of muscle are as follows: the cells are elongated with well-defined nuclei; the cytoplasm (sarcoplasm) stains red with eosin and contains fibrils (myofibrils) made up of contractile proteins that run parallel to the long axis of the cell; and the fibers (cells) are surrounded by a limiting membrane, the sarcolemma. Three types of muscle are morphologically distinguishable: smooth muscle, skeletal muscle, and cardiac muscle. Of these, the first and last are under the control of the autonomic nervous system and are called involuntary muscle. Skeletal muscle is innervated directly by the central nervous system and can, for the most part, be controlled by impulses from the higher centers of the brain. It is accordingly called voluntary muscle.

In examining the three basic muscle types, one should keep in mind certain basic structural differences. The muscle types will differ among themselves in the mode of attachment of the individual muscle cells to each other and to the connective tissue framework that provides support for the muscle mass. They will also differ in the surrounding connective tissue framework and also in the extent and arrangement of the vascular bed, lymphatic drainage, and nerve supply. Diversity will also be noted in the number and location of nuclei per cell, the visible details of the contractile apparatus (myofibrils), and the distinctness of the membranes and intercellular matrix at the light microscope level.

SMOOTH MUSCLE

Smooth muscle is derived from mesenchyme, the cells of which are not originally different in their appearance from those that give rise to the connective and supporting tissues. The muscle-forming cell, however, soon assumes a peculiar shape. It elongates into a spindle, elaborating at the same time a small amount of intercellular substance. At an early stage in the development of the connective tissue cell, fibers are visible along its border, to which the name *fibroglia* is given. In a similar way the developing smooth muscle cell is seen to have fibers along its border, here called myoglia. As the cells increase in size and become closely applied to each other, intercellular fibers become very difficult to demonstrate and will not be seen in ordinary sections.

Smooth muscle cells are spindle shaped and vary in length from 0.02 to 0.5 mm. They have a diameter at their thickest portion of about 4 to 7 μ. The cells may be best seen in preparations made by shaking

80

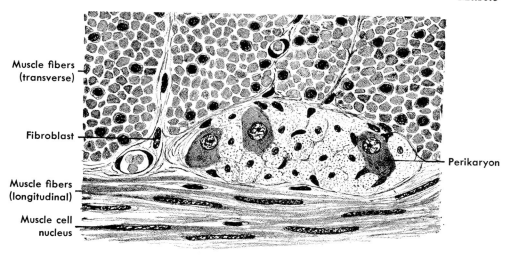

Muscle fibers (transverse)

Fibroblast

Muscle fibers (longitudinal)

Muscle cell nucleus

Perikaryon

Fig. 7-1. Smooth muscle from wall of intestine of monkey showing longitudinal and transverse sections of fibers. Compare nuclei of muscle cells with those of fibroblasts of connective tissue among muscle fibers. Also illustrated are perikaryon, fibers, and supporting cells of Auerbach's nerve plexus.

Cell (fiber) with centrally located nucleus

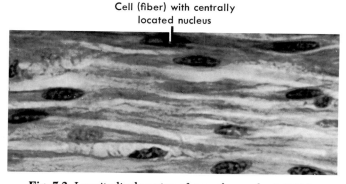

Fig. 7-2. Longitudinal section of smooth muscle. (×640.)

a bit of muscle in a weak acid solution. This dissolves the intercellular substance and makes it possible to study the form of the isolated fiber. The myofibrils in the cells of smooth muscle are fine and not easily seen. The nucleus of the cell is elongated and centrally located at the thickest portion of the spindle. It lies in a small area of granular cytoplasm, and the myofibrils diverge to pass around this area. The sarcolemma is so thin that it is imperceptible in ordinary preparations. Branch-

ing fibers are very rare; they have been found in a few parts of the body but are to be regarded as exceptional.

Many of the features just described are imperceptible in longitudinal sections of smooth muscle (Figs. 7-1 and 7-2). The fibers normally occur in sheets, closely packed together, and an entire cell can seldom be seen. In thick sections it is often difficult to make out the boundaries of the adjacent fibers, since several of them are included overlapping in the depth of a sec-

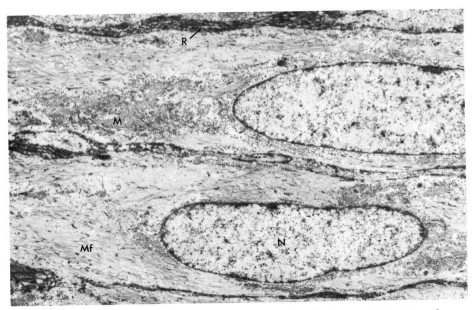

Fig. 7-3. Electron micrograph of parts of two smooth muscle cells from small intestine of mouse. *M*, Mitochondrion; *Mf*, myofibrillae; *N*, nucleus; *R*, reticular fibers. (×6,500.)

tion. One may see only the long nuclei and the cytoplasm, faintly marked by the myofibrils. Longitudinal sections are best studied at the edge of a band or sheet where the muscle shades off into the surrounding connective tissue, and individual cells may be distinguished.

In transverse section the smooth muscle cells appear as disks of cytoplasm having various diameters. The largest of the disks are cut through the middle of the fibers and include the nucleus of the cell. The smaller sections pass through the ends of the fibers and therefore have no nuclei in them. The characteristics peculiar to smooth muscle in cross section are the small size and round shape of the individual fiber, the homogeneous appearance of the cytoplasm, and the fact that the nuclei are centrally located in the cells (Fig. 7-1). Smooth muscle occurs in bands or sheets surrounding glandular organs and forming a part of the wall of tubular organs. Such sheets are not surrounded by definite coverings but mingle with the areolar or reticular tissue around them. Isolated fibers of

smooth muscle also may be found in the tunica propria of the digestive tract.

The smooth muscle fiber (Fig. 7-3) is enveloped by a plasma membrane studded with vesicles believed to be concerned with pinocytotic activity. External to the membrane is a homogeneous coat or layer similar to the basal lamina commonly observed in epithelial cells. External to the basal lamina, scattered reticular fibers occur. In certain regions of the cell surface, specializations occur that suggest by their appearance and relation to adjacent cells that they may be specialized desmosomes.

The myofilaments are delicate structures usually oriented in the direction of the long axis of the cell. Mitochondria occur in the region of the nuclear poles, beneath the cell membrane, and also between the myofibrils. The endoplasmic reticulum and Golgi apparatus, also located at the nuclear poles, are poorly developed and not closely related to the contractile apparatus spatially as are the intracellular membranes of striated muscle.

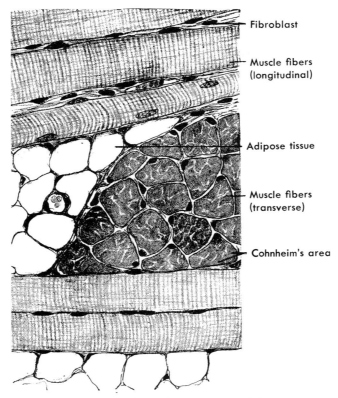

Fibroblast

Muscle fibers (longitudinal)

Adipose tissue

Muscle fibers (transverse)

Cohnheim's area

Fig. 7-4. Striated muscle from tongue of dog.

SKELETAL MUSCLE

Skeletal muscle, or striated voluntary muscle, presents a different appearance from the type just described. It develops from solid masses of mesoderm cells known as myoblasts. Some authors contend that striated fibers develop by an elongation of the myoblast, which undergoes rapid mitotic nuclear division and, in turn, results in an elongated multinucleated cell. Other authors state that the elongated muscle cell or fiber is the result of the fusion of the growing myoblasts, giving rise to a syncytial arrangement. The latter view is apparently correct. Another view is that both of these methods of development occur. The striated muscle fiber is longer and thicker than the smooth muscle fiber, maintains a uniform diameter throughout its length, and ends bluntly. Early in de-

velopment the nuclei migrate from the center to the periphery of the cell, where they are to be found in adult muscle of this type.

The sarcolemma, which is barely perceptible in smooth muscle, can be observed with the light microscope. It is now apparent from electron microscope studies that the film investing the muscle fiber and visible with the optic microscope is not a single structure but consists internally of the plasmalemma of the muscle fiber and a coating of mucopolysaccharide and delicate reticular fibers. Sarcolemma is currently considered the plasmalemma of the muscle fiber.

The most striking morphologic characteristic of striated muscle is the appearance of transverse markings that extend across the cell body of the muscle cell. These striations are caused by the fact that the cell contains numerous thick bundles of contractile protein called *myofibrils*. These myofibrils are in turn made up of slender threadlike units of the proteins actin and myosin and are called *myofilaments.* (Fig. 7-7). The alternate arrangement of thick and thin filaments exists in register across the cell, giving rise to the striped appearance visible at the light microscope level. Each myofibril is composed of a succession of bands with different refractive indices.

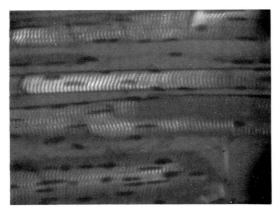

Fig. 7-5. Longitudinal section of striated muscle photographed through crossed Nicol prisms. *Light bands,* isotropic, and *dark bands,* anisotropic parts of muscle fiber. (×160.)

One set of these, the A bands, appear dark and are doubly refractile or anisotropic. The A bands alternate with light or I bands, which are isotropic (Fig. 7-6). When the fibers are viewed with polarized light, the A bands appear light and the I bands appear dark (Fig. 7-5). In specially stained preparations, a dark transverse line bisecting the I band has been observed and is called the Z band. When myofibrils are gently treated with acid, the bundles of contractile protein break apart at the Z bands. Local application of neural transmitter in the vicinity of the Z band results in a brief contraction between two Z bands. Because of this, the distance between two Z bands has been called the structural and functional unit of the muscle contractile protein and is known as the *sarcomere.* The sarcomere includes one A band and parts of the two I bands extending from the adjacent Z lines.

At the electron microscope level the bands can be observed more clearly than at the optic levels (Figs. 7-6 and 7-7). The I band, as previously noted, is bisected by the dark Z band. Between the Z band and each margin of the I band a less distinct line occurs, marking the limits of the N band. The A band is bisected by a dark M band. On both sides of the M band is a

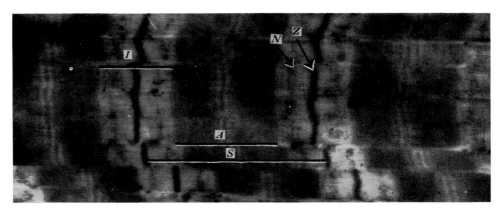

Fig. 7-6. Electron photomicrograph of striated muscle. Longitudinal section of rest length of rabbit psoas. *I,* I band; *A,* A band bisected by a light area, the H band that is, in turn, divided by a thin dark disk, the M band; *N* and *Z,* disks, respectively; *S,* sarcomere. Note that myofibrils are further divided into myofilaments. (×45,000.) (Courtesy Dr. Spiro, New York, N. Y.)

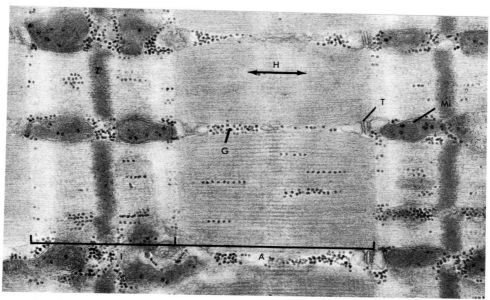

Fig. 7-7. Electron micrograph of striated muscle. Longitudinal section of Capuchin diaphragm. Note thick myofilaments in A band, thin myofilaments in lateral part of I band. *G*, Glycogen; *H*, H band; *A*, A band; *I*, I band; *Mi*, mitochondrion; *T*, triad; *Z*, Z band. (×32,000.)

somewhat lighter and broader area marking the H band.

The myofibrils, the smallest contractile elements visible with the light microscope, are shown by the electron microscope to be divided into smaller units, the *myofilaments*. These are of two kinds and differ in their size and chemical composition. The thicker filaments, containing *myosin*, are approximately 100 Å in diameter and 1.5 μ long. These filaments are the chief constituent of the A band. The thinner filaments contain *actin*, measure 50 Å in diameter, extend approximately 1 μ in either direction from the Z line, give rise to the I band, and continue for some distance into the A band. The length of the actin filaments observed in the A band is dependent upon the degree of contraction exhibited by the fiber. The arrangement and variation in the size of the filaments are responsible for the banding appearance observed in these structures. The I band contains thin filaments and appears light.

The central region of the A band contains only thick fibrils and is somewhat darker in appearance than is the I band.

The portions of the A band adjacent to the I band contain both thick and thin fibers, which are densely packed and appear denser or darker than other parts of the fibril.

With the electron microscope, one may observe that the sarcoplasm or cytoplasm fills the spaces between the myofibrils and is most abundant in the region of the nucleus. Located within the sarcoplasm are mitochondria, which are large, abundant, and most numerous at the poles of the nucleus. They also occur between the myofibrils, where they are usually arranged with their long axis parallel to the long axis of the myofibrils (Fig. 7-6). In addition, a small Golgi network is located at the pole of the nucleus, and lipid droplets and particles of glycogen occur between the myofibrils.

The sarcoplasmic reticulum, which corresponds to the endoplasmic reticulum of other cells, is visible only with the electron microscope. It is a continuous system of fine, membrane-bound, interconnecting tubules forming a meshwork around each myofibril (Fig. 7-8). The system exhibits

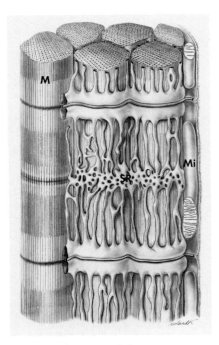

Fig. 7-8. Three dimensional drawing of a group of myofibrils *(M)* from skeletal muscle surrounded by a net sarcoplasmic reticulum *(SR)*. *Mi*, Mitochondrion. Each myofibril is made up of many myofilaments. (From Bloom and Fawcett: A textbook of histology, ed. 9, Philadelphia, 1968, W. B. Saunders Co.)

a constantly repeating pattern. It is longitudinally arranged in reference to the A and I bands and exhibits three transversely arranged channels located near the A-I junction in mammalian muscle (Fig. 7-7). This complex is known as a *triad.* The triad is believed to facilitate the transmission of excitatory impulses to the muscle fibers.

The appearance of ordinary sections of skeletal muscle is represented in Figs. 7-4, 7-9, and 7-10. The important points are as follows. In longitudinal section the myofibrils are marked by alternating light and dark transverse bands. There are many nuclei in one fiber, lying at its periphery immediately beneath the sarcolemma. Occasionally one sees a nucleus that seems to be in the center of a fiber. Careful focusing of the microscope will show, however, that in such a case one is looking down on the surface of a tangential section and that the nucleus is on the outside of the cell (Fig. 7-10). In transverse sections it is apparent that the fibers are larger than those of smooth muscle, having diameters that range from 17 to 87 μ. Their shape is round or polygonal, and the peripheral position of the nucleus is noticeable. It is also possible to see the cut ends of the myofibrils, which give the cytoplasm a finely stippled appearance. In transverse section, one may

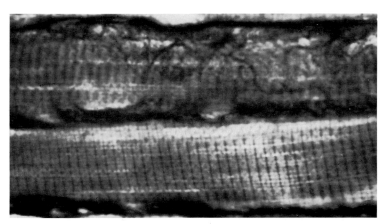

Fig. 7-9. Longitudinal section of striated muscle; upper fiber shows arrangement of reticular connective tissue. (Silver stain.)

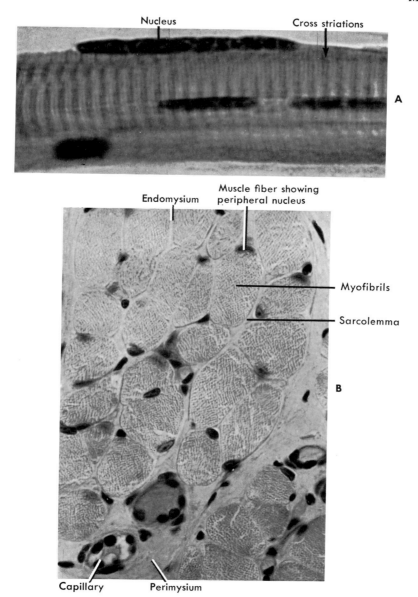

Fig. 7-10. Human striated muscle. A, Longitudinal section; B, transverse section. (A, ×2,000; B, ×640.)

see that the myofibrils are gathered in groups rather than being evenly distributed throughout the cytoplasm. Large fibrils are sometimes called a muscle column of Kölliker. In a cross section of a muscle fiber, one may sometimes see such a group of fibrils separated from adjacent groups by clear sarcoplasm. Such cross sections of muscle columns are called Cohnheim's areas. It is now believed that these areas are fixation artifacts.

Skeletal muscle, as the name implies, is attached to the bones, the attachment being made through the tendons. At the point where the muscle joins the tendon, the nuclei are especially numerous, indicating that this is the region of the most rapid growth. The myofibrils may be traced to the sarcolemma, which covers the end of the fiber, and tendon fibers may be seen in close contact with the outside of the membrane. It is thought by some writers that the tendon fibers actually pierce the sarcolemma and are continuous with the myofibrils. However, such a continuity cannot be observed in sections.

The fibers that compose a muscle are gathered together in fascicles or bundles. Fine connective tissue surrounds the individual fibers; this is called the endomysium. The covering of a fascicle is the perimysium, and the sheath surrounding a group of such bundles is the epimysium.

Muscle of exactly the same morphologic appearance as the skeletal muscle is found in various places where it is not attached to the bones. In such situations it has no surrounding connective tissue sheath but merges with the connective tissue about it. Such muscle is not truly skeletal, since it does not move parts of the skeleton. In the tongue, for instance, it is more accurately described by the name voluntary muscle. In other regions, muscle of this type is not,

strictly speaking, either skeletal or voluntary. The wall of the esophagus contains, in its upper portion, striated muscle that is neither under the control of the voluntary centers of the nervous system nor attached to bone. It is morphologically indistinguishable from skeletal muscle, however, and is therefore called by the same name.

CARDIAC MUSCLE

The third type of muscle is that of the heart. The functional peculiarity of cardiac muscle is its ability to contract rhythmically and continuously. The contraction is entirely independent of the will. Morphologically, cardiac muscle may readily be distinguished from smooth and skeletal muscle, although it shares some of the characteristics of each.

The fibers branch freely and anastomose (Fig. 7-11). This arrangement is evident under the low power of the microscope. The nuclei of cardiac muscle are centrally located like those of smooth muscle. The myofibrils are transversely striated in somewhat the same way as those of skeletal muscle, but the striations are not so marked. The sarcolemma and the external coating material are also less noticeable than that

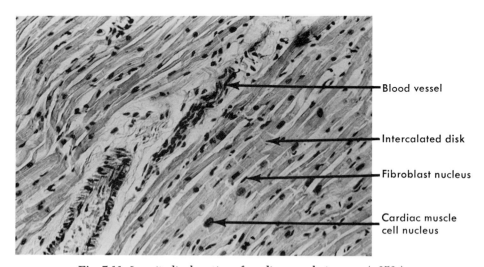

Blood vessel

Intercalated disk

Fibroblast nucleus

Cardiac muscle cell nucleus

Fig. 7-11. Longitudinal section of cardiac muscle in man. (×250.)

Branching fiber   Nucleus   Intercalated disc

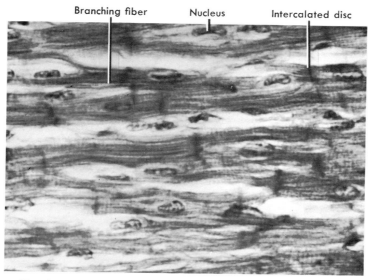

Fig. 7-12. Longitudinal section of cardiac muscle of dog. (×160.)

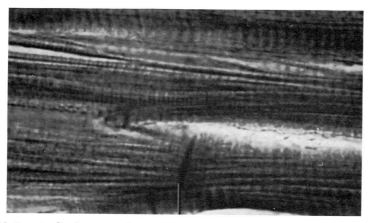

Fig. 7-13. Longitudinal section of intercalated disk cardiac muscle fibers of dog. (×640.)

of skeletal muscle. In longitudinal sections the fibers are recognizable because of their branching. They are distinguished from sections of striated muscle by the central position of their nuclei. In some preparations of cardiac muscle, one may see transverse markings on the fibers, which are different from the striations of the myofibrils. These are the intercalary disks. They are peculiar to cardiac muscle and often appear as steplike formations in the fibers.

Electron microscope studies have shown that the intercalated disks are composed of membranes marking the cell boundaries at the junction of the fibers. This observation demonstrates that the cells, or fibers, of cardiac muscle are not of the syncytial type as was formerly believed (Figs. 7-11 to 7-15). They are often mentioned as a diagnostic feature of cardiac muscle, but, since a special technique is required to demonstrate them, the student should not

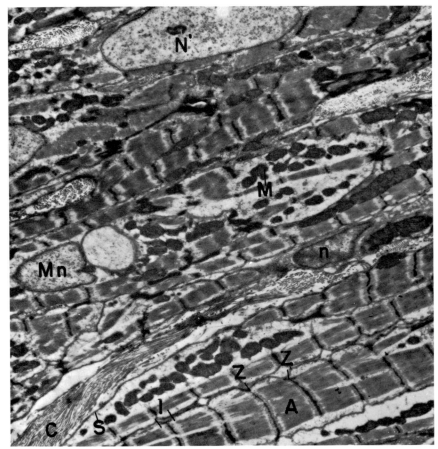

Fig. 7-14. Electron photomicrograph of cardiac muscle of snake. *A*, A disk; *C*, collagen fibrillae; *I*, I disk; *M*, mitochondrion; *Mn*, muscle cell nucleus; *N'*, nucleolus; *n*, nucleus of fibroblast; *S*, sarcolemma; *Z*, Z disk. (×6,000.) (Courtesy Dr. F. Gonzales, Chicago, Ill.)

rely on their presence in distinguishing cardiac from other kinds of muscle. The presence of transverse markings on the myofibrils, together with central nuclei and branching fibers, is a sufficient means of identification.

In transverse as in longitudinal section, the position of the nuclei differentiates cardiac from skeletal muscle (Fig. 7-11). In distinguishing cardiac muscle from cross sections of smooth muscle, one must observe the extent and character of the cytoplasm. The fibers of cardiac muscle are thicker than those of smooth muscle, having diameters of from 9 to 20 μ. It is possible to see in cross sections the cut ends of

the myofibrils, which give the cytoplasm a stippled appearance, except in the region immediately around the nucleus, which is occupied by membranes and lipid.

The most important diagnostic features of the three types of muscle are given in Table 2.

MUSCLE-TENDON JUNCTION

At the termination of a muscle, many of the fibers are attached to a tendon. The nature of the muscle-tendon attachment was not clarified until recently. With ordinary staining methods the impression obtained was that the muscle fiber and the tendon fibers were continuous and blended with

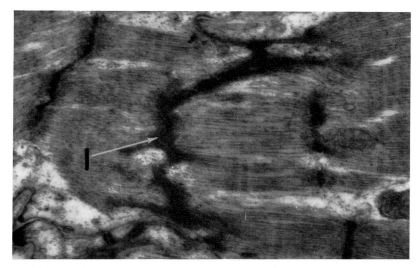

Fig. 7-15. Electron photomicrograph of cardiac muscle (snake) showing junction of fibers at intercalary disk *(I).* (Courtesy Dr. F. Gonzales, Chicago, Ill.)

Table 2. Most important diagnostic features of muscles

Type	Nucleus	Myofibrils	Sarcolemma and external coating	Shape and size
Smooth				
Longitudinal section	Central	Faint; no striation	Very thin	Spindle
Cross section	Central	Invisible	Very thin	Circular, 7 μ
Skeletal				
Longitudinal section	Peripheral	Well-marked striations	Definite sheath	Uniform thickness
Cross section	Peripheral	Visible as dots in groups	Definite sheath	Rounded polygons, 17 to 87 μ
Cardiac				
Longitudinal section	Central	Lightly striated	Thin sheath	Branching
Cross section	Central	Visible as dots	Thin sheath	Round, 9 to 20 μ

one another. Recent studies have shown that this concept is not correct. It has been shown that fine argyrophilic fibers thicken near the end, run parallel to the axis of the muscle fiber, and then converge over its termination to form a strand that is continuous with the fiber bundles of the tendon. It has also been shown in electron microscope studies that the connective tissue fibrils are inserted into indentations of the sarcolemma of the muscle fibers.

CIRCULATION AND INNERVATION OF MUSCLE

All muscle has a plentiful supply of blood vessels and nerves. In striated muscle the network of capillaries is so extensive that each fiber lies in contact with at least one blood vessel. The innervation consists of myelinated fibers from the central nervous system, and each muscle fiber is in connection with a nerve fiber. In smooth muscle, which is composed of smaller fibers, the individual cell is not so well supplied. Capillaries ramify through the tissue but not to the extent of reaching every cell. Similarly the nerve supply does not reach every smooth muscle fiber.

The capillaries of cardiac muscle are supplied through the coronary artery. Its nerve supply is derived from the sympathetic and parasympathetic systems.

8

Nervous tissue

The nervous system is divided into two parts: (1) the central nervous system (CNS), composed of the brain and spinal cord, and (2) the peripheral nervous system (PNS), consisting of all other nervous tissue, that is, ganglia and nerves. This system is composed of functional units known as *neurons* (nerve cells), which are arranged in chain formation extending throughout the body. Neurons are highly differentiated in that they are hyperirritable but have lost the ability to move and to reproduce and usually have limited powers to repair damage. It is this combination of irritability and arrangement that permits the nervous system to receive impulses, integrate them, and transmit them in such a way that coordinated activity occurs.

Neurons consist of a cell body or *perikaryon;* one or more branching afferent processes known as *dendrites,* which transmit impulses toward the perikaryon; and one efferent process known as the *axon,* which conducts impulses away from the perikaryon. The dendrites and axons are collectively called processes or *nerve fibers.* Branches occurring along the length of nerve fibers are called *collaterals,* those at the ends are called *terminal arborizations.* A *synapse* is a region in which the terminal arborizations of the axon of one neuron come in proximity to the dendrites or perikarya of succeeding neurons. Synapses are not regions of protoplasmic continuity, since minute but definite gaps between adjoining plasma membranes are demonstrable. (See Fig. 8-17.)

PERIKARYON

The perikaryon is a cytoplasmic thickening that includes a nucleus (karyon). The nucleus is usually a large, lightly staining, vesicular structure with a single prominent nucleolus and several fine chromatin granules (Fig. 8-1, *A*). The cytoplasm contains a conspicuous number of angular pieces of basophilic, metachromatic, RNA-containing, *chromophil substance,* usually referred to as Nissl or tigroid bodies. With toluidine blue the Nissl substance stains a purplish color and gives the cytoplasm a mottled appearance (Fig. 8-1, *B*). Chromophil substance extends into the dendrites but is absent in a well-defined funnel-shaped area adjacent to the axon known as the *axon hillock,* as well as in the axon itself. The amount of chromophil substance in the perikaryon varies considerably. By the use of special stains (for example, silver), minute *neurofibrils* (Fig. 8-1, *C*) may be demonstrated as a fine network embedded in the clear cytoplasm or *neuroplasm.* The neurofibrils are found in perikarya, as well as in both dendrites and axons. The fibrils are most readily visible in the axon hillock. With special techniques the Golgi apparatus and mitochondria may be demonstrated.

FINE STRUCTURE OF MOTOR NEURON

At the electron microscope level, the structure of the neuron may be observed in greater detail than at the optic level. The nucleus is relatively large and has, as

92

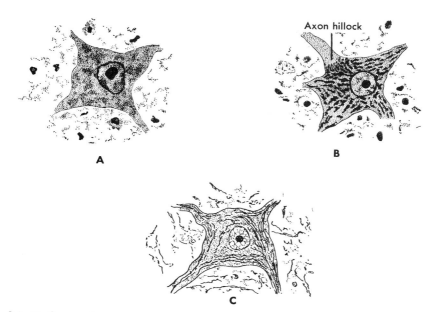

Fig. 8-1. Perikarya of motor neurons in the spinal cord stained in three different ways. **A,** Hematoxylin and eosin; **B,** toluidine blue, to show Nissl substance; **C,** silver nitrate, showing neurofibrils.

a rule, a single nucleolus and sparsely distributed chromatin material. The Golgi apparatus is usually prominent and may be present in the form of cisternae, vesicles, or both. The chromophil substance, or Nissl bodies, are prominent features of the cytoplasm and are widely distributed throughout the cell (Fig. 8-2) except at the periphery of the cell body. They are composed of short parallel cisternae of the endoplasmic reticular system and densely packed ribonucleoprotein granules. Neurofilaments appear as a fine meshwork extending throughout the cell. Aggregations of neurofilaments make up the neurofibrils. The mitochondria are usually rod shaped and are scattered among the several organelles present. In addition to the organelles mentioned, there may be granules and vacuoles of a transitory nature. The function of these inclusions is not clear at present.

Perikarya are sometimes classified according to the number of processes they bear. The so-called *unipolar* perikarya found in the dorsal root ganglion of the spinal cord bear a single process, which soon branches into an axon and dendrite (Fig. 8-3). *Bipolar* perikarya bear one axon and one dendrite as in the retina of the eye. (See Fig. 21-9.) *Multipolar* perikarya bear several dendrites and one axon, as in the ventral horn of the gray matter of the spinal cord (Fig. 8-1). Perikarya occur exclusively in *ganglia* of the PNS (Figs. 8-4 to 8-6) and in the gray matter of the CNS (Fig. 8-7).

NERVE FIBERS

Histologically, nerve fibers are of four types: (1) fibers without observable sheaths, (2) fibers with a prominent fatty myelin sheath only, (3) fibers with a cellular sheath enclosing a minute quantity of myelin, and (4) fibers with a cellular sheath enclosing a thick layer of myelin.

Both axons and dendrites may or may not bear these sheaths, and one cannot differentiate between these processes in routine histologic preparations of nerves (PNS). By the use of Nissl body stains—for example, toluidine blue—one can fre-

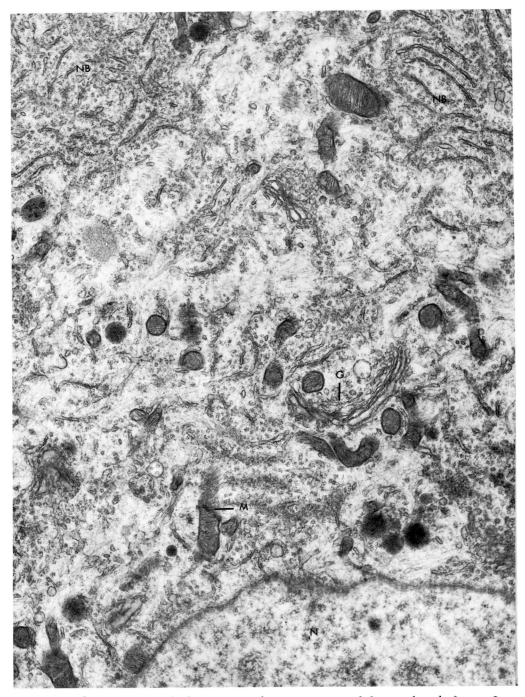

Fig. 8-2. Electron micrograph showing part of a motor neuron of the spinal cord of a rat. In addition to the characteristic organelles in this cell such as the nucleus, *N;* the Golgi apparatus, *G;* and mitochondrion, *M,* several Nissl bodies, *NB,* are also shown. These last structures are composed of parallel cisternae of endoplasmic reticulum and numerous ribonucleoprotein particules, some in contact with the membranes of the reticulum, others dispersed in the cytoplasmic matrix. (×17,300.) (Courtesy Dr. R. Yates, New Orleans, La.)

quently distinguish between axons and dendrites in the gray matter of the CNS. Because of this difficulty in histologic identification, it is customary to describe all "fibers" as one would an axon.

The axonic protoplasm itself is called the *axis cylinder* and consists of argyrophilic *neurofibrils* embedded in neuroplasm or *axoplasm*. The axoplasm shrinks considerably in routine preparations so that it frequently appears as a thin acidophil structure with hematoxylin and eosin stains. The term *axon* is frequently used interchangeably with axis cylinder. In the gray matter of the spinal cord, where visible sheaths are absent, the axis cylinder is usually referred to as a *naked axon*. The axis cylinder also appears exposed, that is, without a visible covering, near the sites of or within effectors (for example, muscles and glands). In gray matter, freely branching dendrites may sometimes be distinguishable from the single axon. Naked fibers frequently give rise to collateral branches along their length and form the freely branching terminal arborizations.

In the white matter of the spinal cord the axis cylinder is surrounded by a *myelin sheath*, a phospholipid-containing component that appears black when treated with osmic acid (osmiophilia). The periodic acid–Schiff test reveals that simple sugars are a component of myelin. When the mye-

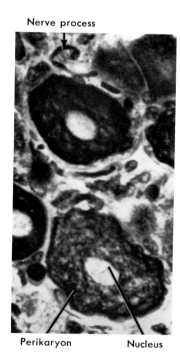

Fig. 8-3. Sensory neurons from dorsal root ganglion of cat. (Cajal method; ×640.)

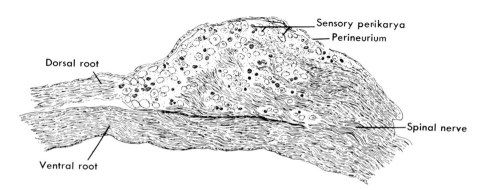

Fig. 8-4. Longitudinal section of spinal ganglion.

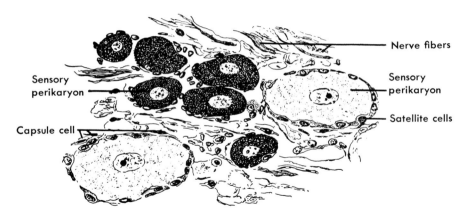

Fig. 8-5. Sensory cells of spinal ganglion.

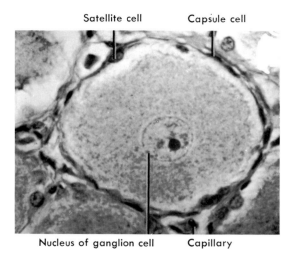

Fig. 8-6. Sensory neuron from spinal ganglion of monkey. (×640.)

lin is removed by fat solvents, such as absolute alcohol or xylene, certain stains indicate that myelin is penetrated by a protein-containing network of *neurokeratin*. In longitudinal sections of these nerve fibers, one may observe interruptions in the myelin sheath. They are known as the *nodes of Ranvier* (Figs. 8-8 and 8-14). In fresh tissue preparations myelin sheaths appear as white glistening coverings. The presence of this substance gives the characteristic color to the white matter of the CNS.

In the autonomic division of the peripheral nervous system the so-called gray fibers contain only a small amount of myelin surrounding the axis cylinder. These are still referred to as "nonmyelinated" fibers. They are found in the vagus nerve, sciatic nerve, and the nerve plexi in the digestive tract and peritoneal cavity. These fibers are enclosed in a cellular covering known as *Schwann's sheath,* and the cells are called *Schwann's cells* (Figs. 8-9 and 8-10). In gray fibers the Schwann cells are flat and overlap each other so that the sheath appears discontinuous. In longitudinal sections the nuclei of these cells may be seen in irregular rows following the wavy contours of the axis cylinders. In hematoxylin and eosin preparations these nuclei may be confused with those of the surrounding connective tissue cells. The attenuated cytoplasm of Schwann cells is visible only in special preparations and is also known as the *neurilemma.* In cross sections through certain nerves, several axis cylinders may lie in a small amount of myelin enclosed within one and the same Schwann cell (Fig. 8-9). The latter are nevertheless considered nonmyelinated fibers.

The fourth type of fiber consists of a single axis cylinder surrounded by a thick myelin sheath, as well as a smooth, definitely delineated neurilemma (Schwann's sheath) (Fig. 8-14). This type of white fiber is found in the peripheral nervous

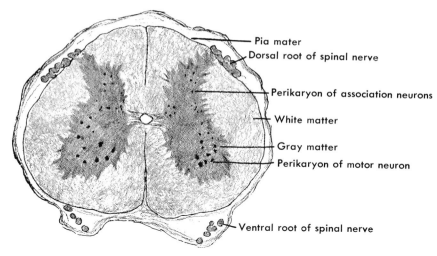

Fig. 8-7. Spinal cord of cat. (Low magnification.)

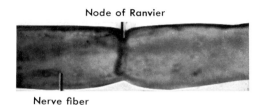

Fig. 8-8. Nerve fiber, teased preparation. (Silver stain; ×160.)

system. As in all heavily myelinated fibers, there are periodic interruptions in the myelin where the neurilemma dips to touch the axis cylinder at the *nodes of Ranvier*. These nodes are observed only in longitudinal sections or in teased preparations. In routine preparations the nodes appear as slender transverse striations. In silver preparations a black precipitate forms on the node and on the axis cylinder for a short distance on each side of it, so that the fibers are marked at intervals by small black crosses. In osmium preparations the blackened myelin region is seen to be interrupted at the site of the node. When visible, the Schwann's cell nucleus may appear to lie in an indentation of the myelin. In fixed preparations of peripheral

nerves the myelin of each segment is interrupted by oblique incisions, the Schmidt-Lanterman clefts.

FINE STRUCTURE OF MYELIN SHEATH

Electron microscopy has shown that the myelin sheath consists of a system of concentric lamellar membranes approximately 30 Å thick, varying in number from a few to fifty or more. The membrane is derived from the Schwann cell membrane, which wraps around the nerve fiber in concentric layers. It consists of lipids and alternating layers of neurokeratin (Fig. 8-11).

In the CNS, the oligodendrocytes form myelin by wrapping their plasma membrane around the nerve fiber in a manner similar to that described for the peripheral nervous system.

In fibers bearing both myelin and neurilemma, collaterals arise only at nodes, whereas branches of the axis cylinder may arise anywhere along a naked axon. It should be emphasized that with rare exception the descriptive terminology set forth previously in reference to axons is equally applicable in describing dendrites.

In passing it should be noted that some fibers are but a few millimeters long,

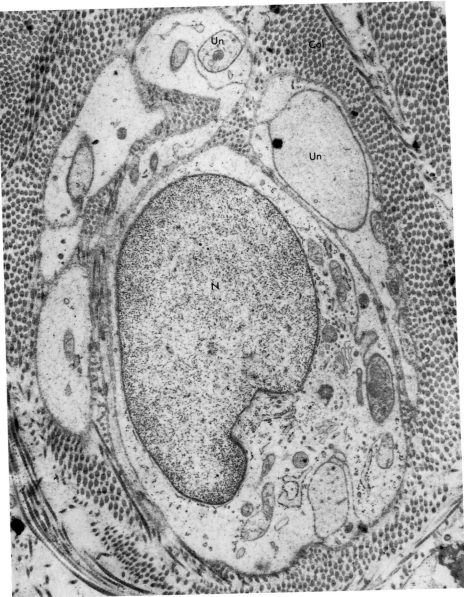

Fig. 8-9. Electron micrograph of a Schwann cell and associated nonmyelinated axons. *N,* Nucleus of Schwann cell; *UN,* nonmyelinated axon; *Col,* collagen. (×18,000.)

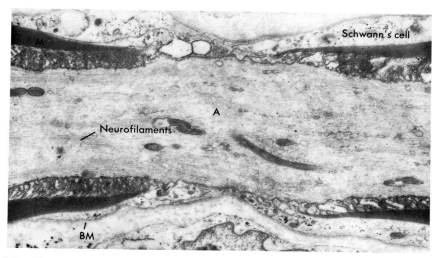

Fig. 8-10. Electron micrograph of longitudinal section of a human myelinated nerve fiber in region of a node of Ranvier. *A,* Axis cylinder; *BM,* basement membrane of Schwann cell; *M,* myelin. Note that myelin is lacking in region of node. (×17,000.)

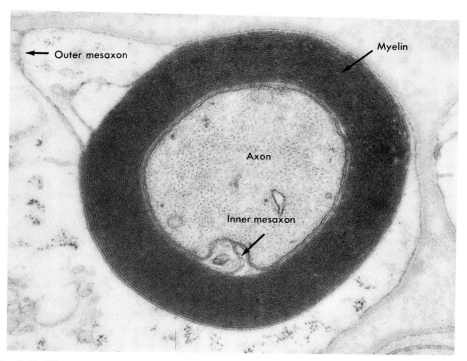

Fig. 8-11. Electron micrograph of transverse section of a myelinated nerve from the gingiva of a monkey. (×38,000.)

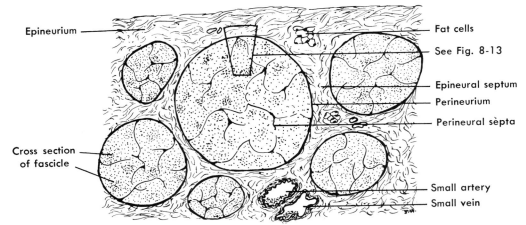

Epineurium — Fat cells — See Fig. 8-13 — Epineural septum — Perineurium — Perineural septa — Cross section of fascicle — Small artery — Small vein

Fig. 8-12. Portion of transverse section of nerve trunk.

while others are greater than 1 meter in length. The sum of protoplasm in the fibers of a neuron is many times greater than the amount of protoplasm in the perikaryon. White, or myelinated, fibers conduct impulses at a higher rate than do gray, or slightly myelinated, fibers. This would account for the fact that somatic reflexes (involving myelinated fibers and striated or skeletal muscles) are more rapid than visceral reflexes (involving slightly myelinated fibers and smooth muscle fibers). Fibers possessing a neurilemma can slowly regenerate if damaged, but the fibers of the CNS, lacking a neurilemma, do not regenerate.

NERVES

Nerves, or nerve trunks, are groups or bundles of fibers (axons, dendrites, and their collaterals) bound together by connective tissues and invested with blood capillaries. Nerves per se do not include perikarya. A single discrete bundle of nerve fibers and connective tissue is called a *fascicle* (Fig. 8-12). Some of the larger nerve trunks are composed of numerous fascicles, with an attendant increase in the amount of connective tissue and capillaries. The terminology used to designate the topography of the connective tissue associated with the nervous system is similar to that established for connective tissues found in skeletal muscles.

In nerve trunks comprised of several fascicles the entire structure is enclosed by a loosely arranged covering of collagenous and elastic fibers known as the *epineurium* (Figs. 8-12 and 8-13). In the large nerve trunks the epineurium is frequently prominent and contains many blood vessels. It also may give rise to extensions, known as epineural septa, occupying spaces between adjacent groups of fascicles. As the nerve trunk divides, the epineurium is reduced until it can no longer be distinguished from fine areolar tissue (Figs. 8-13 and 8-14).

A single fascicle is held together by a concentrically arranged layer of dense collagenous fibers called the *perineurium*. The perineurium varies from a thick prominent structure in large nerves to a very thin one in small nerves. Branches, or trabeculae, of the perineurium (perineural septa of some authors) penetrate the fascicle and give rise to the *endoneurium,* which in turn separates the individual nerve fibers. The endoneurium is composed of fine connective tissue sheaths that completely enclose and are intimately associated with the neurilemma of individual fibers. These sheaths are known as the *sheaths of Henle* or *endoneural sheaths* (Fig. 8-14).

Small nerve trunks occurring in connec-

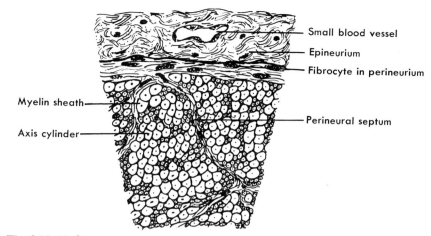

Small blood vessel

Epineurium

Fibrocyte in perineurium

Myelin sheath

Axis cylinder

Perineural septum

Fig. 8-13. Medium-power view of nerve fibers and surrounding connective tissue.

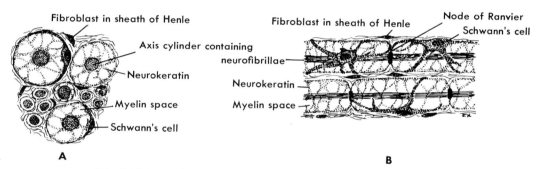

Fibroblast in sheath of Henle

Axis cylinder containing neurofibrillae

Neurokeratin

Myelin space

Schwann's cell

Fibroblast in sheath of Henle

Node of Ranvier

Schwann's cell

Axis cylinder containing neurofibrillae

Neurokeratin

Myelin space

A

B

Fig. 8-14. Nerve fiber. **A,** Transverse section; **B,** longitudinal section.

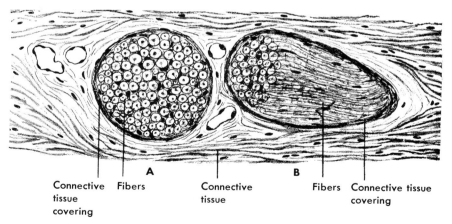

Connective tissue covering

Fibers

Connective tissue

Fibers

Connective tissue covering

A

B

Fig. 8-15. Myelinated nerve fibers forming small trunks in areolar tissue. **A,** Cut transversely; **B,** cut tangentially.

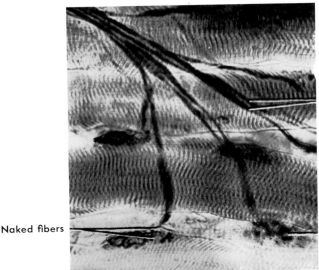

Fig. 8-16. Motor end plate. (Whole mount silver preparation.)

tive tissue are distinguishable from the fibers of connective tissue by the following features (Figs. 3-15 and 8-15). In longitudinal section, nerves appear as groups of fine fibers arranged regularly and parallel. The myelin sheaths may be completely dissolved, and, if this is true, each axis cylinder is then separated from its neighbor by a space bounded by the neurilemma sheath. The axis cylinder and neurokeratin are less eosinophilic (or more basophilic) than the surrounding connective tissue fibers. Sections through nerves containing a majority of nonmyelinated fibers are somewhat more difficult to distinguish and may even be confused with smooth muscle fibers by the novice. In nonmyelinated fibers the neurolemma sheaths are irregular and nearly in contact with the somewhat basophilic axis cylinders.

NERVE FIBER ENDINGS
Motor endings

The motor endings are the terminal parts of the *efferent neurons,* which are in contact with either muscles or glands. Striated muscles may exhibit two types of motor endings. (1) The motor end plate, shown in Fig. 8-16, consists of a terminal ramification of a naked fiber that ends on a mass of granular modified sarcoplasm. These structures appear in whole mounts as elevated areas, which measure from 40 to 60 μ in diameter. They are demonstrated with difficulty in sectioned material. (2) In some cases the motor terminations consist of a simpler bulblike arrangement of small loops that end on the surface of the sarcolemma.

The efferent fibers that supply cardiac muscle, smooth muscle, and glands are part of the autonomic nervous system. These fibers are usually nonmyelinated and often terminate in nodular thickenings. In muscle these terminations end near the nucleus of the muscle fiber; in glands the fibers reach to the base or sides of the gland cell where they end freely in an expanded terminal loop.

Sensory endings

Aside from those located in specialized organs, such as the eye and ear, the sensory endings, terminations of afferent fibers, consist of the following types: free endings, encapsulated endings, and muscle spindles.

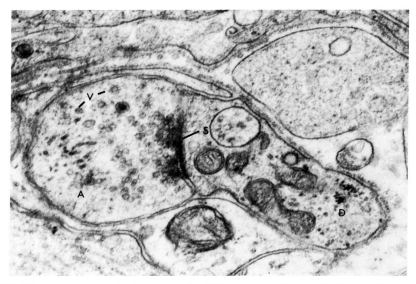

Fig. 8-17. Electron micrograph of an axon-dendritic synapse of sympathetic ganglion of guinea pig. *A,* Axon showing presynaptic vesicles, *V; D,* dendrite; *S,* synaptic cleft. (×32,000.) (Courtesy Mrs. N. Sulkin, Winston-Salem, N. C.)

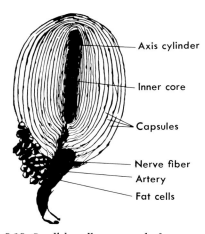

Fig. 8-18. Small lamellar corpuscle from mesentery of cat. The nuclei of the capsule cells appear as thickenings. The myelin of the nerve fiber may be traced to the inner core. (×50.) (From Bremer and Weatherford: A text-book of histology, Philadelphia, 1948, The Blakiston Co.)

Axis cylinder

Inner core

Capsules

Nerve fiber
Artery
Fat cells

Free endings. Free endings are the simplest type from the structural standpoint. They consist of terminal branches of delicate fibers that often show slight enlargements. These endings have been observed is stratified epithelia, tendon, and other connective tissue.

Encapsulated endings. Encapsulated endings are characterized by the presence of a central naked fiber or several branches embedded in tissue fluid, which is enclosed within a connective tissue capsule. From their structure and location, one may infer that these might function as pressure receptors. There are several varieties of encapsulated endings: (1) the tactile corpuscles of Meissner, (2) the genital corpuscles, (3) bulbous and cylindrical corpuscles of Krause, and (4) the lamellar corpuscles of Pacini (Fig. 8-18). The last named are so large as to be visible with the unaided eye.

Muscle spindles. Muscles have sensory fibers that terminate about slender bundles of muscle fibers, which are poorly developed. The terminal parts of the nerve fibers are arranged spirally around these muscle cells. This complex of nerve and

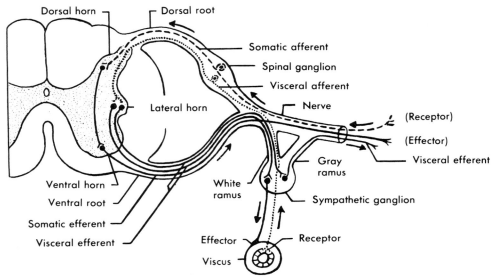

Fig. 8-19. Diagram showing relationship of somatic and visceral neurons to spinal cord, sympathetic ganglia, and viscera. (From Bevelander: Outline of histology, ed. 7, St. Louis, 1971, The C. V. Mosby Co.)

muscle is enclosed within a dense connective tissue sheath and is known as a muscle spindle. Structures analogous to muscle spindles also occur in tendons.

NEURON INTERRELATIONS

On the basis of function and anatomic relations neurons fall into three groups:

1. *Sensory* (first order or afferent) neurons, which are so situated and constructed as to respond to stimuli arising from within or outside the organism and to send impulses to association neurons.
2. *Association* (second order, intercalated, or internuncial) neurons, which serve as links between sensory neurons and neurons of the third group.
3. *Motor* (third order or efferent) neurons, which convey impulses to muscles or glands, stimulating them to action.

The sensory and motor neurons have long axons and are known as Golgi I type; the association neurons have short axons and are known as Golgi II type.

The most rapid responses to stimuli in higher organisms occur through the so-

called reflexes that involve neuron pathways called *reflex arcs*. These are divided into two major kinds, *somatic reflexes*, resulting in contraction of skeletal or striated muscle, and several varieties of *visceral reflexes*, usually resulting in contraction of smooth muscle fibers associated with the viscera.

In the most common type of reflex arc all three groups of neurons are involved in sequence, that is, sensory, association, and motor.

Reflex mechanism

The simplest manner in which the central and peripheral divisions of the system act to respond to environmental change is shown diagrammatically in Fig. 8-19. An impulse arises in a sensory end organ by stimulation of the latter. From there is it carried by the peripheral fiber of the sensory neuron to its perikaryon, which is located in the spinal ganglion. It then travels by way of the central process of this cell to the spinal cord. The impulse then passes through the dendrite and perikaryon of an intercalated (association) neuron, which is located in the dorsal horn of the gray matter of the spinal cord. The axon of the intercalated neuron is in synaptic relation with one of the dendrites of the third, or motor, neuron of the chain. This cell lies in the ventral horn of the gray matter. The impulse leaves by way of the axon of the motor neuron, passing through the ventral root of the spinal nerve and one of the peripheral nerves to an effector or organ that performs an action as a result of the impulse it receives.

The pathway just described illustrates a simple somatic reflex arc, or circuit. It serves to produce quick reaction to a change of external conditions without the intervention of conscious processes.

The part of the peripheral nervous system that serves to distribute impulses to the viscera is known as the autonomic system. This subdivision of the nervous system is made on a functional rather than a morphologic basis, but there is a difference between the number of neurons involved in the efferent pathways of the two divisions. Fibers of the cerebrospinal nerves pass directly from their central origins to the muscles they control. Those fibers of the autonomic system, on the other hand, have two neurons in the efferent arm. The perikaryon of the first is located within the central nervous system and gives rise to a preganglionic fiber. The second is located in a peripheral ganglion and gives rise to a postganglionic fiber that, in turn, reaches the effector. The fibers that constitute the craniosacral outflow are known as the parasympathetic system; those of the thoracolumbar region, the sympathetic system.

The course of a sympathetic reflex is illustrated in Fig. 8-19. An impulse arises in the epithelium of the gut, for instance, and travels by way of the peripheral process of a visceral afferent neuron through the ramus communicans to the spinal ganglion. The central process of this sensory cell conveys the impulse to the lateral horn of the spinal cord, where it synapses with the dendrites of a visceral motor neuron. The impulses leaves the spinal cord through the axon of the latter (preganglionic fiber),

which goes by way of the ventral root and the ramus communicans to synapse with a cell located in a sympathetic ganglion. The impulse is picked up by a neuron in this ganglion and carried by its axon to the effector of the viscus. In the case illustrated, this would be the smooth muscle of the gut. The axon of the ganglion cell is called the postganglionic fiber. Thus, in the autonomic system, there are two neurons involved in the pathway from the central nervous system to the viscera.

The two circuits just described are simple ones, requiring few neurons for the transmission of a stimulus from the receptor to the effector. The vast majority of responses to external stimuli, however, include much longer and more complicated chains of neurons. The study of such responses forms a separate branch of anatomy—neurology. We can mention in this text only a few facts concerning these processes.

A single sensory neuron may connect with several association (intercalated) neurons, some of which carry the impulse to the brain. A single association neuron usually receives impulses from several sensory and association neurons. The chains of neurons in the central nervous system are interconnected to form a network in which single neurons are brought under the influence of impulses arising from several different sources. In the spinal cord and brain, impulses are received from various parts of the body and are integrated so that the outflow of impulses along the efferent neuron is adjusted to the needs of the body as a whole.

It is evident from the foregoing description that perikarya are not evenly distributed throughout the nervous system but are collected into groups. The largest collection of these groups is in the gray matter of the brain and spinal cord, which contains the perikarya of motor and association neurons (Fig. 8-7). Sensory neurons have their perikarya in the spinal and cranial ganglia, while the visceral efferent neurons of the second order are gathered together in the autonomic ganglia. All these collections of nerve cells are connected among themselves by fibers, groups of which make up the nerve trunks. A nerve trunk consists of axons and dendrites of neurons, the perikarya of which are to be found in the ganglia, cord, or brain.

When the spatial relations of the nervous system and the various other parts of the body are considered, it is obvious that it would be impossible to study microscopically an entire neuron. For example, a motor neuron that sends impulses to a muscle of the foot has an axon that extends from the lumbar region of the spinal cord through the entire length of the leg. Other neurons, although not so extensive, have processes of such length that they cannot be dissected out and studied in their true relation to the cells. It is most convenient to divide the subject into two parts and study separately the nerve trunks and the collections of perikarya, but in so doing we must remember the true relation of these parts to each other.

NEUROGLIA (GLIA)

In addition to cells that are specialized for the transmission of stimuli, the nervous system contains many nontransmitting cells. We have previously described the connective tissue framework of nerve trunks, but the central nervous system does not have such an internal support. On the other hand, the meninges and an abundant arterial system (the latter containing relatively large amounts of elastic fibers and some collagenous fibers) form a tough external support for the CNS. Internally the support supplied by the presence of blood vessels is slight, and a type of interstitial cell known as an astroglial cell forms a pericapillary barrier that prevents the encroachment of blood vessel connective tissue on nerve cells. The astroglia form a part of the so-called internal support of the CNS collectively referred to as *neuroglia*. Another kind of neuroglia element, known as microglia, is believed by some authors to belong to the reticuloendothelial system and consists of inactive macrophages. The latter, however, do not seem to aid in support. Many investigators are of the opinion that the main internal support of the CNS is provided by the hydrostatic pressure of tissue fluid. This tissue fluid is believed to be eventually transformed to yield cerebro-

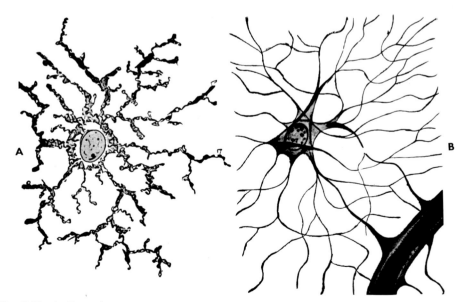

Fig. 8-20. A, Protoplasmic astrocyte. **B,** Fibrous astrocyte. (After Hortega; from Bremer and Weatherford: A text-book of histology, Philadelphia, 1948, The Blakiston Co.)

spinal fluid. Although glia may serve as mechanical support, they may also influence neuronal transmission and neural metabolism.

Astroglia

The most common type of neuroglia cell is the astroglia. These are branching cells, some of which (fibrous) have long, slender processes. Other astroglia cells (protoplasmic) are similar to the first except the processes are considerably thicker and perhaps more branched. Although different features have been described for the two types, the chief morphologic difference between them appears to be whether the processes are thick or thin, since they both contain neuroglia fibers within the processes. In either kind of astroglia the cells have specialized processes that are in close contact with the walls of the blood vessels of the nervous system. These "sucker feet" have been thought to enable the cell to derive nourishment from the blood; it is also stated, however, that their function is to provide a special limiting membrane around the vessels (Fig. 8-20).

Oligodendria

A second type of neuroglia cell is the oligodendria (or oligodendroglia). These cells have short beaded processes and no neuroglia fibrils. Their nuclei are smaller and darker than those of the astroglia cells. They are grouped around nerve cells and are aligned in rows along the fiber tracts in the brain and spinal cord.

Microglia

A third type is the microglia, the smallest of the neuroglia cells. They have deeply staining nuclei, are irregular in shape, and have no fibrils or "sucker feet." They are

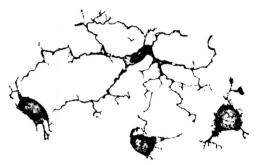

Fig. 8-21. Neuroglia cells from brain of rabbit. Microglia (above) and oligodendroglia. (Stained by Penfield's method.) (From Bremer and Weatherford: A text-book of histology, Philadelphia, 1948, The Blakiston Co.)

said to be phagocytic. Oligodendria and microglia are illustrated in Fig. 8-21.

Other types

The ependyma or layer that lines the central canal of the nervous system forms the fourth group of neuroglia cells. These are elongated cells that are arranged in a layerlike columnar epithelium. They contain fibrils and are sometimes ciliated.

The neurilemma and capsule cells are sometimes considered to be a fifth group of neuroglia cells.

It is of interest to note that these supporting cells, although similar in appearance and function to the simpler mesenchymal derivatives such as reticular tissue, are for the most part ectodermal in origin. This is certainly true of the ependyma and of the astroglia, which form the greater part of the tissue. The microglia are probably mesodermal in origin; the oligodendria are said to be ectodermal.

9

Circulatory system

Blood and lymph are the carriers of nutritive substances, hormones, and the products of metabolism. The circulatory or vascular system is the means by which blood and lymph are distributed throughout the body. The system includes the blood vessels, the heart, and the lymphatics.

BLOOD VESSELS

The blood vessels may be conveniently divided into three main groups for study: the capillaries and sinuses (or sinusoids), the arteries, and the veins.

Capillaries and sinuses

The capillaries have but one coat, which consists of simple squamous epithelium (endothelium) (Figs. 9-1 and 9-2). They are of fine caliber, some of them being so small that only one red blood cell at a time may pass through them. According to some authors, the tubule is clasped at intervals by Rouget's cells, or pericytes. These are branching cells that are said to be contractile and to cause the constriction of the capillaries. They are not ordinarily seen, however, and it is doubtful whether they should be considered to be a regular component of the capillary wall. Most of the capillaries are surrounded by connective tissue, and they form the connecting vessel between arteries and veins (Fig. 9-4). Their function is to provide a place for the exchange of oxygen and carbon dioxide; in them, the blood changes from arterial to venous (or vice versa in the lungs). Physiologically they are, therefore, an important part of the blood-vascular system.

Some capillaries do not connect arterioles and venules, and the substances passing through their walls are not oxygen and carbon dioxide. An example of this kind of vessel may be found in the glomerulus of the kidney. The vessel in the glomerulus is, structurally, a capillary; however, blood passing through it gives off nitrogenous wastes but not oxygen. Other vessels consisting only of endothelium are called sinusoids. Their walls are in close apposition with epithelial tissue, from which the blood

Nucleus of endothelial cell of capillary

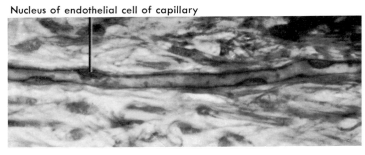

Fig. 9-1. Longitudinal section of capillary. (×640.)

108

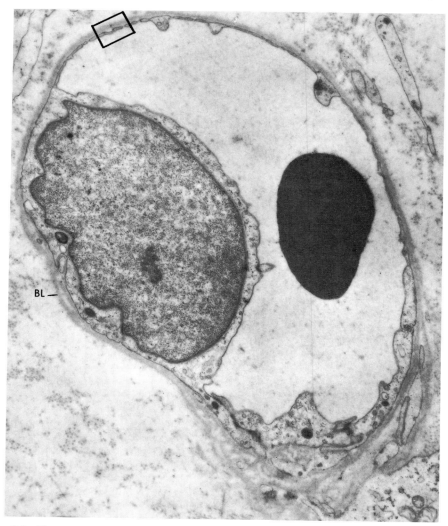

BL —

Fig. 9-2. Electron micrograph of a fenestrated capillary cut transversely. The wall of the capillary consists of an attenuated endothelial cell whose nucleus projects into the lumen. The cytoplasm of the endothelial cell contains many pinocytotic vesicles and is invested by a delicate basement membrane (lamina), *BL.* (×11,000.)

removes the secretion or to which it gives up substances for storage. They are relatively large in caliber, and the walls are irregular in shape. Some of them are lined with cells that exhibit the phagocytic properties of the reticuloendothelial system. The cells of the sinusoids are separated from the parenchyma of organs by a delicate network of reticular fibers.

The structure of the endothelial cells var-ies in capillaries that occur in different organs and tissues. In some, the cytoplasm is extremely attenuated and contains pores. They are known as fenestrated capillaries (Fig. 9-3). The number and size of the pores are accentuated in the endothelium of the glomerular capillaries. In others such as those found in muscle, glands, and other tissues, the endothelium forms a continuous layer around the lumen and thick-

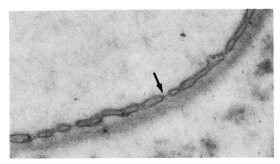

Fig. 9-3. Electron micrograph of part of the endothelial cell of capillary shown in area represented by box in Fig. 9-2. Arrow indicates pores. (×27,000.)

ens around the nucleus. In this continuous type, the adjacent endothelial cells are in very close contact, and the cell junctions often overlap or interdigitate.

The electron microscope has shown that both the luminal and the basal walls of the endothelial cells of the capillaries are studded with pinocytotic vesicles, which indicates that transport of materials may occur either into or out of the capillary lumen. This supposition, however, still needs additional confirmation.

Arteries

Blood is carried from the heart to the capillaries by arteries. The wall of an artery is generally characterized by the presence of a coat of smooth muscle spirally arranged and by considerable amounts of elastic tissue. Because of this, arteries retain their shape after death and appear circular in transverse section. In this system of vessels, there is a gradual change of structure as the caliber of the vessels diminishes. The changes in structure are neither abrupt nor can they be accurately correlated with the size of the vessels. It is convenient, however, to select for study and description the following groups of vessels: aorta, medium-sized arteries, small arteries, and arterioles.

Aorta. The intima of the aorta is lined with short polygonal endothelial cells. Below this lining there is a layer containing fine collagenous and elastic fibers and also a few scattered fibroblasts. The deeper portion of the intima also contains collagenous as well as longitudinally oriented muscle and elastic fibers. The internal elastic membrane consists of two or more lamellae that blend with similar membranes of the interna and media and is hence difficult to identify.

The second coat or media is by far the thickest layer, forming approximately four fifths of the thickness of the wall. It consists of a mixture of circularly arranged smooth muscle and elastic fibers. The latter predominate and mingle, on the one hand, with the elastic fibers of the intima and, on the other, with those of the outermost layer or adventitia. The smooth muscle fibers unite to form branching bands and, like the elastic fibers, appear spirally arranged. The muscle fibers are enclosed or surrounded by delicate reticular fibers.

The adventitia is a comparatively thin coat of connective tissue. Elastic fibers are concentrated at the outer border of the media, forming the external elastic membrane. Collagenous fibers merge with those of the connective tissue surrounding the vessel and are arranged in longitudinal spirals. In the adventitia and the outer portion of the media are small nutrient vessels (vasa vasorum) and nerves (nervi vasorum).

The aorta and a few other vessels like it are sometimes called the large arteries, or arteries of the elastic type. The common iliacs, axillaries, carotids, and pulmonaries belong in this group.

Medium-sized arteries. In the group of medium-sized arteries are included most of the vessels observed grossly in dissection to which names have been given. They are known as muscular or distributing arteries, in contrast to those like the aorta in which elastic tissue predominates. They are characterized by the presence of conspicuous media composed chiefly of smooth muscle. An artery of this group is shown in Fig. 9-4, and in it one may distinguish the following features: the intima consists of endothelium and a very small amount of subendothelial collagenous and elastic connective tissue (Fig. 9-5). The latter is

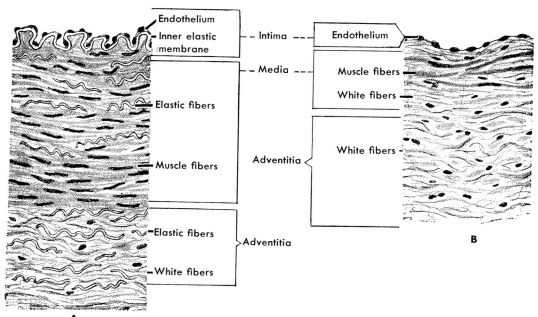

Fig. 9-4. Medium-sized artery, **A**, and vein, **B**, of dog.

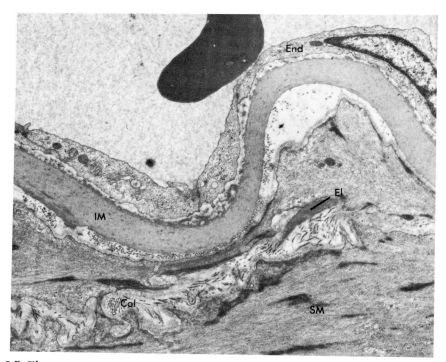

Fig. 9-5. Electron micrograph of part of wall of muscular artery of mouse. *Col,* Collagen fibers; *El,* elastic fiber; *End,* endothelium bordering lumen; *IM,* inner elastic membrane; *SM,* smooth muscle. (×10,000.)

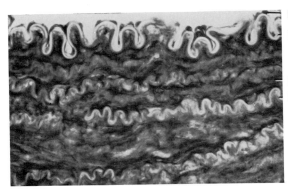

Endothelial nucleus

Inner elastic membrane

Fine collagenous fibers
Elastic fiber in media

Fig. 9-6. Medium-sized artery showing intima and media.

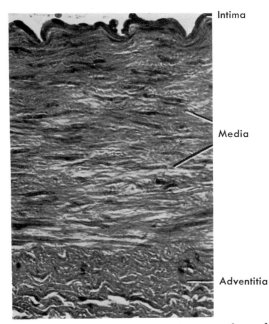

Intima

Media

Adventitia

Fig. 9-7. Medium-sized artery. (Hematoxylin and eosin stain.)

concentrated in the inner elastic membrane. In traverse section this looks like a continuous sheet of elastic tissue, but, in surface view, it exhibits open spaces (fenestrated membrane). Changes that occur at death cause the smooth muscle to contract, and this contraction throws the elastic membrane and its covering of endothelium into wavy folds (Fig. 9-6). This results in a scalloped appearance of the border of the lumen, as seen in traverse section of the vessel.

The media in vessels of this group, like that of the aorta, is the thickest of the three layers. It is composed mainly of smooth muscle circularly arranged. Interspersed among the muscle fibers are isolated strands of elastic tissue, distinguished by their wavy course and their highly refractive quality, as well as reticular and collagenous fibers and fibroblasts. The adventitia consists of an external elastic membrane and a layer of collagenous connective tissue containing small vessels and nerves. In some vessels of this group, strands of smooth muscle, longitudinally arranged, are observed in the adventitia.

The artery represented in Fig. 9-4 is fairly typical of the group. It must be emphasized, however, that a considerable variety of structure is included in the class of vessels that are called medium-sized arteries, or arteries of the muscular type. A vessel may have considerably more or considerably less elastic tissue than the one represented and still belong to the same group (Figs. 9-7 and 9-8).

Small arteries and arterioles. Small arteries and arterioles are the types of arterial vessels usually found in sections of organs (Figs. 9-9 to 9-13). They present intermediate forms between the vessels just described and the capillaries or sinusoids, which consist of a tube of endothelium alone. Elements are lost from the wall in the following order. First, the elastic fibers

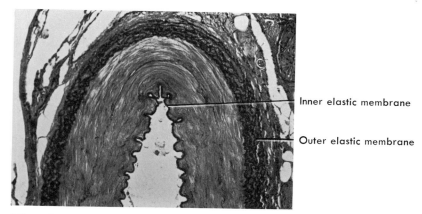

Inner elastic membrane

Outer elastic membrane

Fig. 9-8. Medium-sized artery showing distribution of elastic tissue. (Verhoeff's method.)

Capillary

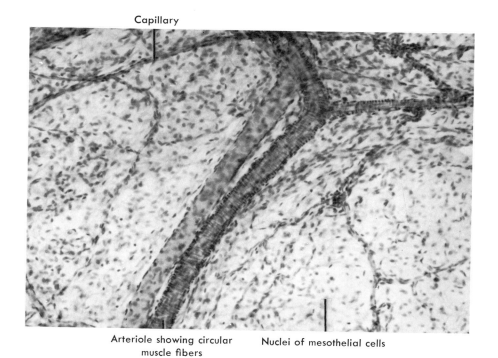

Arteriole showing circular muscle fibers   Nuclei of mesothelial cells

Fig. 9-9. Stretch preparation of mesentery, surface view. (×40.)

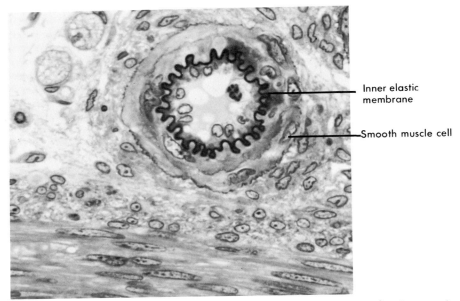

Inner elastic
membrane

Smooth muscle cell

Fig. 9-10. Transverse section of small artery from the wall of rat intestine showing prominent inner elastic membrane. (×800.)

scattered through the media disappear, leaving a middle coat composed entirely of smooth muscle. Then the external elastic membrane is lost, and the adventitia becomes a covering of collagenous fibers that are hardly distinguishable from the surrounding connective tissue. From this point on the vessel cannot be said to have the three typical coats: intima, media, and adventitia. In still smaller vessels the inner elastic membrane is first replaced by scattered elastic fibers and then disappears altogether. The muscle of the media also thins out to a few scattered fibers, and, finally, the blood passes into a tube consisting of endothelium alone. Precapillary arterioles and arterioles are vessels that have three distinct coats: the endothelium, a muscle coat from one to several cells thick, and an external connective tissue coat. The so-called small arteries are recognized by having a larger diameter and a definite internal elastic membrane in addition to those components present in the arterioles.

Veins

The veins, by which blood returns from the capillaries to the heart, have walls that are composed largely of collagenous connective tissue, with muscle and elastic fibers much less prominent than they are in the arterial wall. Because of the reduced amount of elastic tissue, veins do not retain their shape after death and appear in sections as irregularly rounded structures. In general, the wall of a vein is not so thick as that of the accompanying artery, but its lumen is larger (Fig. 9-14).

The organization of the tissues in three coats is frequently indistinct. Tracing the system back from the capillaries toward the heart one may observe small veins and venules, medium caliber veins, and large veins.

Small veins and venules. Small veins and venules occur in the connective tissue of organs (Fig. 9-12). The first addition to the endothelium that changes the vessel from a capillary to a venule is not muscle but collagenous fibers. These and the accompanying fibroblasts are oriented longitudinally with respect to the vessel. As the caliber of the venule increases, its wall includes first muscle and then, in still larger vessels, scattered elastic fibers. The elements are arranged as in arteries but in different proportions. The larger vessels of

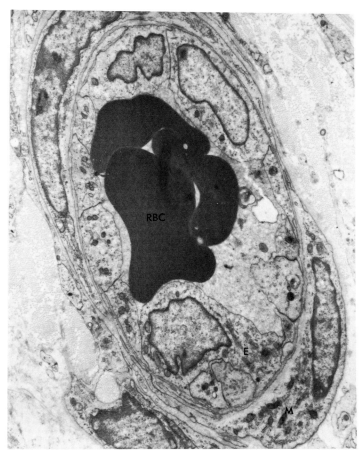

Fig. 9-11. Electron micrograph of transverse section of an arteriole. The vessel wall is made up of several endothelial cells, *E*, surrounded by a single layer of smooth muscle cells, *M*, and the lumen contains red blood cells, *RBC*. (×4,500.)

this group have three coats: the intima consists of endothelium, subendothelial collagenous fibers, and scattered elastic fibers. The latter do not form a complete membrane and are not present in sufficient number to cause the scalloping of the border of the lumen, which is characteristic of arteries. The media is a thin coat of muscle interspersed with collagenous fibers. The adventitia, which consists of collagenous tissue, is the thickest of the three coats.

Veins of medium caliber. Veins of medium caliber exhibit many of the characteristics just described. The adventitia of collagenous fibers is the thickest of the coats. The muscle of the media and the elastic tissue of the intima increase some-

what in amount, but there is no inner elastic membrane (Fig. 9-15). In some veins of this group longitudinal muscle fibers occur in the intima and in the adventitia. In the latter coat, there may be a complete layer of such muscle fibers placed next to the circular muscle fibers of the media. This is not, however, a common occurrence.

A typical vein of this group is illustrated in Fig. 9-4. As in the case of arteries, the group varies widely in structure.

Large veins. Large veins show an increase in the amount of longitudinal muscle in the adventitia and a slight increase in the amount of elastic tissue in the intima. The elastic tissue, however, is

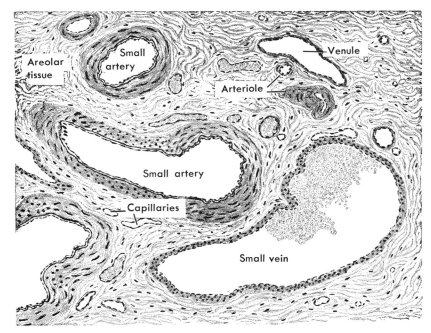

Fig. 9-12. Capillaries, arterioles, venules, small arteries, and small veins in submucosa of digestive tract.

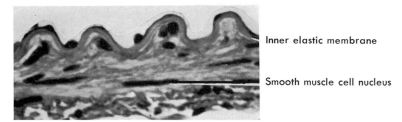

Fig. 9-13. Longitudinal section of small artery. (Hematoxylin and eosin stain.)

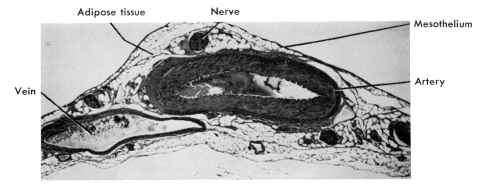

Fig. 9-14. Medium-sized artery, vein, and nerve. (Hematoxylin and eosin stain.)

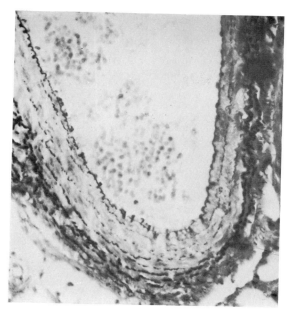

Fig. 9-15. Medium-sized vein showing distribution of elastic tissue.

not as prominent, even in the largest veins, as it is in quite small arteries. The circular muscle of the media is reduced in veins of this group and is lacking entirely in a few of them.

Some veins, particularly those of the extremities, also contain valves. They consist of a thin connective tissue membrane. The surfaces of the valves are covered by endothelium, which is reflected from the internal surface of the intima.

Comparison of veins and arteries

The difference between the smaller arterial and the venous vessels lies in the amount of muscle and connective tissue present in each. Muscle is the predominant tissue in arterioles; in the venules there is little muscle and the walls consist mainly of endothelium and connective tissue. The larger vessels of the two groups may be distinguished by the following: intima, media, adventitia, and size and shape of vessels.

Intima. In arteries the presence of a complete inner elastic membrane is a distinguishing feature. This membrane contracts after death, throwing the intima into small folds and allowing the endothelial nuclei to project into the lumen of the vessel. In the veins the endothelium remains smooth. The entire intima of some veins extends into the lumen at intervals in large folds or reduplications, which serve as valves to prevent the backflow of the blood.

Media. The media is the thickest coat of any artery and consists of muscle interspersed with elastic tissue. In veins the media is a thin coat of muscle; it usually contains all circular fibers, but occasionally has longitudinal fibers. It has more collagenous white fibers than the media of an artery and includes elastic tissue only in the largest vessels in the system.

Adventitia. In arteries the adventitia is less important than the media. It contains the outer elastic membrane, and there are seldom any muscle fibers in it. The adventitia of the vein is its thickest coat and often contains several longitudinal muscle fibers.

Size and shape of vessels. The lumen of the vein is larger than that of the accompanying artery, but its wall is thinner. Because of the relatively large amount of elastic tissue, arteries retain their round shape in sections more often than do the veins. The latter are likely to be collapsed in section.

HEART

The heart is a specialized portion of the vascular system and develops from an enlargement of two veins in the embryo. It has three coats—endocardium, myocardium, and epicardium.

Endocardium

The endocardium, which corresponds to the intima of the vessels, includes an endothelial lining and a relatively thick subendothelial layer, which is made up of connective tissue, smooth muscle, and elastic fibers. The valves of the heart are folds of the endocardium in which the fibroelastic elements are prominent. The annuli fibrosi are rings of dense connective tissue that surround the openings from one chamber to another.

Purkinje fibers

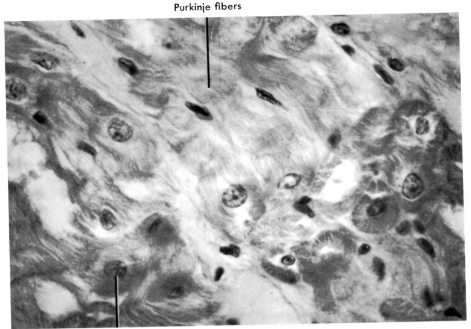

Nucleus of fiber

Fig. 9-16. Purkinje fibers of heart. (×640.)

Myocardium

The myocardium or muscular coat corresponds to the media of the vessels. It is made up of interlacing bundles of muscle. The tissue, however, is not like that of the media of the vessels. It is muscle of specialized type, cardiac, found nowhere else in the body. The nature of this muscle has been discussed in Chapter 7.

Epicardium

The epicardium is the visceral portion of the pericardial sac enclosing the heart. Its covering consists of a single layer of flattened mesothelial cells. Subjacent to the mesothelial cells is a fibrous layer containing scattered elastic fibers. The epicardium is attached to the myocardium by a layer of vascularized areolar connective tissue, the subepicardial layer.

Valves of the heart

The atrioventricular valves consist of a plate of connective tissue beginning at the collar of tough fibrous tissue surrounding the roots of the major vesels *(the annulus fibrosa)* and reinforced by strands of dense ligamentous tissue. The core of the valve consists mostly of dense cartilage-like (chondroid) tissue containing small spindle-shaped or rounded cells. Outside the core is a covering layer of endocardium that is thickened on the atrial side of each valve flap to resist the mechanical pressures that occur when the valves close. The connective tissue core is penetrated by the fibrous chordae tendinae that hold the valve flaps to the papillary muscles of the ventricles. Small slips of muscle penetrate into the bases of the valves. Normal valves do not contain capillary beds.

The semilunar valves are similar in structure except that they are thinner, have no chordae tendinae, and have a thicker chondral plate to provide more reinforcement in the absence of the chordae. Varying amounts of elastin are found, depending on the need for resilience in the valves.

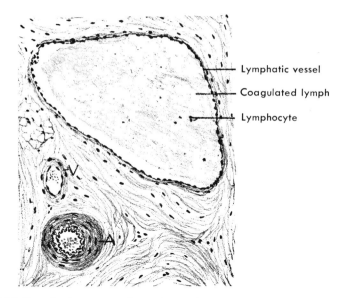

Lymphatic vessel

Coagulated lymph

Lymphocyte

Fig. 9-17. Lymphatic artery and vein from hilum of lymph node. *V,* Vein; *A,* artery.

Impulse conducting system

The heart contains modified cardiac fibers whose function is to coordinate the heartbeat by regulating the time of contraction of the atria and ventricles. The impulse that coordinates contraction normally begins at the *sinoatrial node,* which is located in the right atrium at the point of entry of the superior vena cava. From the sinoatrial node, the impulse spreads over the atrial muscle to the atrioventricular node, located in the posterior portion of the interventricular septum. From this point a bundle of modified cardiac muscle cells (the Purkinje fibers) bifurcates and a separate branch passes down through the subendocardial tissue of the right and left ventricles. The cells within the two nodal regions are spindle-shaped, highly branching cells separated from each other by bits of connective tissue. The bundles of Purkinje fibers *(bundles of His)* in the ventricular walls are indistinct in the human heart but can be distinguished from ordinary cardiac muscle by their foamy-appearing cytoplasm, reduced number of myofibrils, and increased cellular diameter. Comparison of cardiac muscle in Fig. 7-8 with that in Fig. 9-16 illustrates the marked reduction in the number of myofibrils occurring in the Purkinje fibers.

LYMPHATIC SYSTEM

The lymphatic system consists of lymph capillaries and vessels but is unlike the blood vascular system in that it does not form a complete circuit through which the fluid leaves and returns to a central propelling organ. Lymph capillaries begin blindly in the connective tissues from which they collect tissue fluid. The latter passes as lymph from the capillaries to larger vessels, which join together, forming ultimately the thoracic duct and the right lymphatic duct. The thoracic duct is the larger of the two, since it alone receives lymph drainage from the abdomen. It empties its contents into the bloodstream at the junction of the left internal jugular and left subclavian veins. In some cases there is a right lymphatic duct opening into the corresponding veins on the right side of the body, but the single duct on this side is often replaced by several smaller lymphatics.

Lymphatic vessels are thin walled and

less conspicuous than the blood vessels (Fig. 9-17). The structure of the larger lymphatics most nearly resembles that of the veins, but, rather than containing blood, they are filled with a granular coagulum containing a few lymphocytes. The large lymphatics are composed of three coats: (1) an intima of endothelium and subendothelial tissue, (2) a media of circular muscle with little elastic tissue, and (3) an adventitia of loose connective tissue with scattered bundles of longitudinal muscle. They have numerous valves and are distinguishable from veins chiefly through the absence of blood in them.

10
Lymphoid organs

In the group of lymphoid organs are included the lymph nodes, the spleen, the tonsils, and the thymus. Lymphoid tissue consists of reticular tissue infiltrated with lymphocytes. The reticular tissue is almost evenly distributed throughout the organs, but the lymphocytes are more concentrated in some regions than in others, such concentrations being known as nodules. These are to be found in the lymph node, the tonsil, and the spleen and are also widely distributed along the digestive tract, occurring singly or in groups.

Before considering the distribution and arrangement of lymphoid tissue in the organs just mentioned, it seems appropriate to emphasize that this tissue is widely distributed beneath moist epithelial membranes throughout the digestive and respiratory tracts and other parts of the body in a form not sharply outlined from the rest of the surrounding connective tissue. This is usually referred to as a *diffuse lymphoid tissue* in contrast to the denser form, such as the lymph nodules in which the lymphocytes are more closely aggregated.

LYMPH NODE

A lymph node or gland is a mass of lymphoid tissue enclosed in a capsule of connective tissue. Many such nodes are scattered along the course of the lymph vessels of the body, the most conspicuous groups lying in the cervical region, the axilla, and the groin. Each node is a small, bean-shaped organ (from 1 to 25 mm. in diameter) having an indented hilum (Fig. 10-1). The nodes are whitish in color in the fresh specimen. When stained with hematoxylin and eosin, a section of a node appears as a mass of purple tissue enclosed in a connective tissue capsule. The capsule sends trabeculae toward the center of the node from various points along its convex surface, and a group of branching trabeculae extend inward from the indented surface or hilum. Under the low power of the microscope it may be seen that the lymphocytes, which give the organ its dark color, are not evenly distributed. In the peripheral portion or cortex appear dense aggregations of lymphocytes known as nodules. When lymphocyte production is active, the primary nodule has at its center a light area, the secondary nodule or germinal center (Fig. 10-2). In the medulla of the lymph node the lymphocytes are collected in uneven clumps with no germinal centers. Between these central masses (medullary cords) are areas of reticular tissue that are almost entirely free from lymphocytes. These are the medullary sinuses through which the lymph flows. Each sinus intervenes between a medullary cord on the one hand and a trabecula on the other. In a similar fashion one may see that there is a sinus interposed between the capsule and the cortex and that this peripheral sinus courses down along the trabeculae to join the system of anastomosing medullary sinuses. The cortical nodules are not sharply separated from each other or from the cords at the border of the medulla.

Afferent lymph vessels approach the convex surface of the node and pierce the

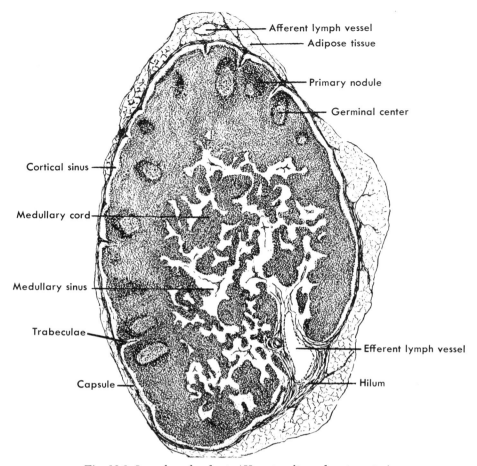

Fig. 10-1. Lymph node of cat. (Hematoxylin and eosin stain.)

capsule, opening into the cortical sinuses. From there the lymph passes to the medullary sinuses and is eventually collected at the hilum in the efferent vessels. Valves in both sets of vessels prevent the lymph from reversing its direction. Arteries enter the node at the hilum, run for varying distances in the trabeculae, and give off branches, which break up into capillaries in the reticular tissue of the node, thus supplying nutriment to the organ. Veins return in the trabeculae and leave at the hilum. The organization of the lymph node is illustrated in Fig. 10-3.

The basic structure of the node consists of a meshwork of reticular fibers that makes up the framework in which free cells occur. The cells are predominantly lymphocytes and may be either small, medium, or large in size (Fig. 10-4). The small lymphocytes are the most numerous types in germinal centers. In lymphoid tissue, they have an appearance somewhat different from that observed in blood or following entrance into connective tissue. In lymphoid tissue the nucleus of small lymphocytes contains clumps of chromatin that result in a mottled nuclear staining. In blood, the nucleus appears more uniformly stained. The medium-sized lymphocytes are less numerous than the small variety and may be observed among clusters of small lymphocytes. The nuclei of medium-sized lymphocytes contain small

Capsule

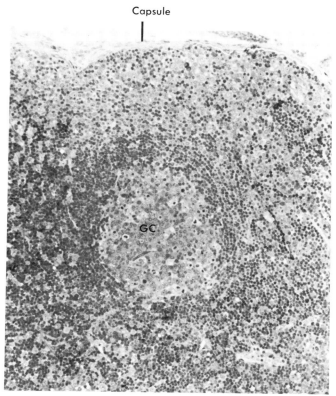

Fig. 10-2. Photomicrograph (plastic section) of the cortex of a cat lymph node showing germinal center, *GC*. (×160.)

particles of chromatin. They exhibit a small amount of basophilic cytoplasm and typically one or two nucleoli. Occasionally these cells may be observed in mitosis. Large lymphocytes are least numerous and are widely scattered throughout the node. They are spherical, measure up to 15 to 20 μ in diameter, and have a clear pale nucleus with distinct nucleoli. The cytoplasm of these cells is more abundant than in the other lymphocytes and is basophilic. Large lymphocytes can be found throughout the lymph node including the medullary cords, but their numbers vary with the functional state of the node and they may be absent entirely.

The basic cells of the lymphoid tissue meshwork are the reticular cells (Fig. 10-4). There are two types: (1) primitive reticular cells and (2) phagocytic fixed macrophages. The primitive reticular cells are members of the reticuloendothelial system. They have large, vesicular, irregularly shaped nuclei and cytoplasm with numerous cellular extensions. They may on occasion become free macrophages.

Other cells occasionally seen in lymph nodes are plasma cells and blood cells.

Cortex

Capsule and trabeculae. The capsule and trabeculae are composed of dense white fibrous tissue with occasional elastic and smooth muscle fibers. In the capsule one may usually see the afferent lymph vessels, while the trabeculae contain small blood vessels.

Cortical sinuses. The peripheral sinus and those that course inward along the

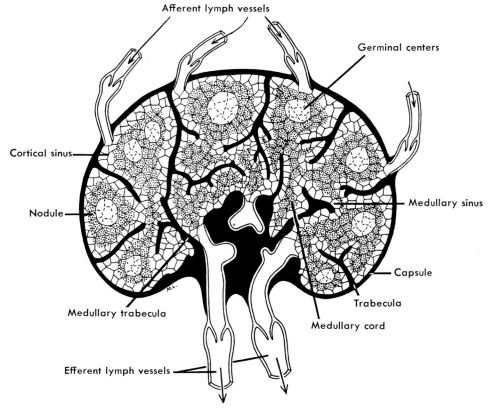

Fig. 10-3. Diagram showing relation of lymph node to lymphatic vessels. This diagram does not indicate arterial and venous supply of lymph node. (Redrawn from Maximow and Bloom.)

sides of the cortical trabeculae are not definite vessels enclosed in an endothelium. They are merely open spaces in the reticular framework of the node containing primitive reticular cells and macrophages but relatively few lymphocytes. The lymph seeps through the meshes of the reticular tissue in the sinuses.

Nodules. The nodules have a groundwork of reticular tissue like that of the sinuses. If secondary nodules (germinal centers) are present, they appear as regions of closely packed pale cells.

Blood vessels. Besides the vessels already mentioned as located in the trabeculae, the substance of the cortex contains numerous capillaries. These are so small that they do not form a prominent feature of the cortex.

Medulla

Medullary cords. The medullary cords, like the cortical nodules, have a great number of lymphocytes present in them (Fig. 10-5). They differ from nodules, however, in their irregular shape and in the fact that they do not at any time possess germinal centers. They are accompanied and surrounded by medullary sinuses.

Medullary sinuses. Medullary sinuses are like the peripheral sinus in structure and lie between the cords and the trabeculae of the medulla (Fig. 10-6).

Medullary trabeculae. Medullary trabeculae are composed chiefly of dense collagenous fibrous tissue and form a branching system radiating from the hilum, which is part of the framework of the gland. Like

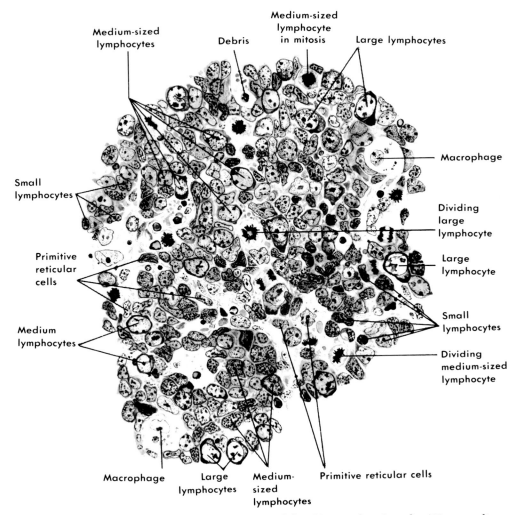

Fig. 10-4. Portion of actively lymphocytopoietic nodule of human lymph node. (Hematoxylin-eosin-azure II; ×750.) (From Bloom and Fawcett: A textbook of histology, ed. 9, Philadelphia, 1968, W. B. Saunders Co.)

the trabeculae of the cortex, they include blood vessels. Efferent lymph vessels are prominent in the connective tissue of the hilum.

The lymph node has a dual function. It is a site for the production of lymphocytes and a phagocytic organ in which particulate material in the lymph is removed ("a biologic filter"). Lymphocyte production occurs in the cortex of the node while "filtration" is performed by the fixed mac-rophages of the lymphoid sinuses and reticular stroma of the medulla. It has also been shown that the lymph node functions in immunologic reactions, especially in the production of antibodies to antigens.

SPLEEN

The spleen is the largest of the lymphoid organs. It is a mass of lymphoid tissue that in man is from 5 to 6 inches long and 4 inches wide. It has been shown

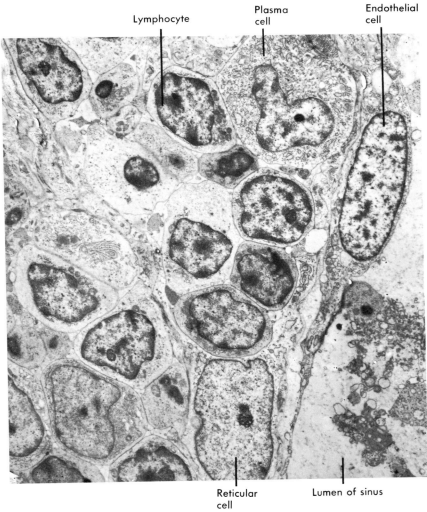

Fig. 10-5. Electron micrograph of part of medullary cord of lymph node of a cat in region of medullary sinus. (×4,800.)

that the lymph node consists essentially of a mass of lymphoid tissue placed in the path of one or more lymph vessels, serving as a filter for lymph. In a similar manner the spleen is interposed in the blood vascular system to remove impurities from the blood. Under low microscopic power the greater part of a section of spleen is seen to be reddish in color when stained with hematoxylin and eosin. Scattered through this reddish tissue or pulp are areas of tissue stained a deep purple. This is the white pulp, which contains nodules. There is no regular arrangement of nodules about the periphery of the organ and no division into cortex and medulla (Fig. 10-7). The nodules are pierced by small arteries and lack germinal centers in adult man. The general arrangement of capsule and trabeculae is like that in the lymph node; that is, a series of trabeculae run in from the surrounding capsule on the convex surface, and a system of strands of connective tissue radiates inward from the hilum.

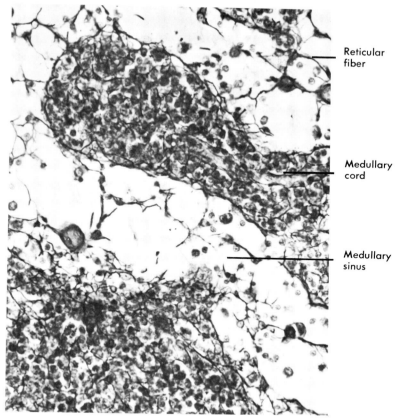

Reticular fiber

Medullary cord

Medullary sinus

Fig. 10-6. Photomicrograph of part of medulla of lymph node of dog stained to show reticular fibers. (×400.)

Since sections of the spleen are usually prepared from small pieces of the organ, this arrangement of trabeculae is not seen in them.

Blood enters the spleen at the hilum, and the arteries run in the trabeculae for some distance. They enter the pulp, however, while they still have the coats common to small arteries: intima, media, and adventitia. In the pulp the vessels ramify, and it is usually at the point of branching that the nodules are to be found. After passing through the nodules, the arteries emerge into the red pulp as the penicilli, in which three parts may be distinguished. The first part (arteriole of the pulp) is of fine caliber and the longest division of the penicillus. This divides into a number of vessels called the sheathed arteries, and these, in turn, divide into two or three branches exhibiting the structure of arterial capillaries, which may connect with the venous sinuses of the red pulp (Fig. 10-8).

Several theories exist concerning the course of the blood after it passes through the arterial capillaries. According to one view it goes directly into the reticular meshwork of the red pulp rather than passing by way of a continuous endothelial tubule to the venules. This is the "open circulation" theory. Other workers believe that no such "dumping" of corpuscles into the reticulum occurs and that the arterial capillaries lead to capillaries that, in turn, connect with the venules. This is the "closed circulation" theory. The third view

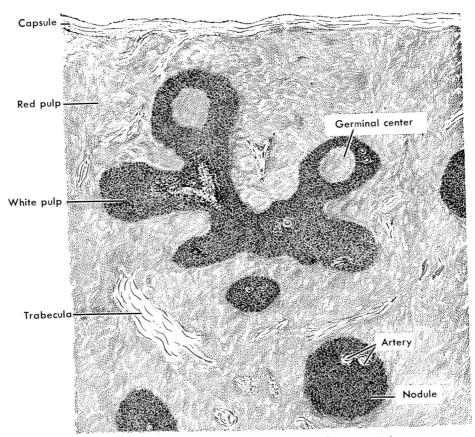

Capsule

Red pulp

Germinal center

White pulp

Trabecula

Artery

Nodule

Fig. 10-7. Spleen of monkey. (Hematoxylin and eosin stain.)

is that some arterioles open directly into the pulp whereas others connect with venules through capillaries.

The venous circulation begins with the splenic sinus, which is composed of an openwork endothelium through which corpuscles may pass readily. From the splenic sinuses, venules lead away and join each other, running back to the trabeculae. Blood leaves at the hilum. The circulation of the blood in the spleen is diagrammed in Fig. 10-8. Under the high power of the microscope the details of structure that may be seen are the capsule and trabeculae, red pulp, and white pulp.

Capsule and trabeculae. The capsule and trabeculae consist of dense, white connective tissue with a few scattered elastic fibers and smooth muscle much like the

corresponding structure in the lymph node. The capsule of the spleen, however, since the organ borders on the body cavity, is covered by mesothelium, which appears as a layer of squamous epithelium. This is often destroyed in preparing the specimen.

Red pulp. The framework of the red pulp is reticular tissue. It contains all types of blood cells, which have passed into it either from the open ends of the arterioles or through the walls of the sinuses. The numerous erythrocytes that are present give this part of the organ its red color in both fresh and stained specimens (Fig. 10-7).

Among the reticular cells and corpuscles will be found free macrophages. These cells have vesicular nuclei and stain readily with eosin. They ingest fragments of worn-

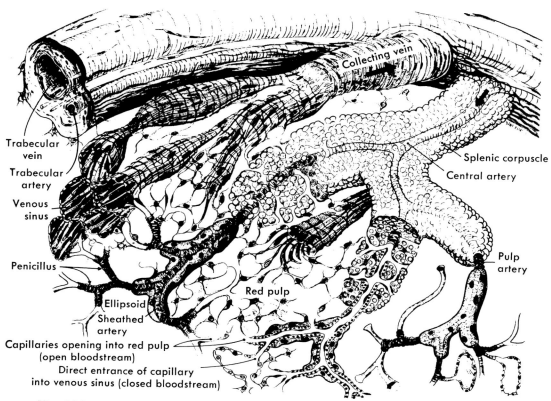

Fig. 10-8. Stereogram of the spleen, illustrating concepts of open and closed circulation. (From Elias and Pauly: Human microanatomy, ed. 3, Philadelphia, 1966, F. A. Davis Co.)

out erythrocytes, which may be seen in their cytoplasm. The macrophages are distributed throughout the red pulp. Two kinds of blood vessels in the red pulp are of unusual structure. The more prominent of these are the splenic sinuses (Fig. 10-9). These vessels are the beginning of the venous system. They may be recognized as small spaces in the pulp surrounded by a ring of endothelial-like cells whose nuclei project into the lumina of the vessels. Ordinarily endothelial cells are closely joined and their nuclei are flattened so as to project only slightly into the lumen of the vessels that they surround. In the splenic sinus these cells, known as reticular cells, are loosely grouped and the lack of tension of the cytoplasm permit the nuclei to extend into the vessel. These cells are sur-

rounded by a loose arrangement of reticular tissue forming a latticework through which the corpuscles may pass (Fig. 10-10). They are phagocytic and belong to the reticuloendothelial system.

The other type of blood vessel peculiar to the red pulp is the sheathed artery (second portion of the pencillus). Sheathed arteries are of capillary diameter and consist of endothelium plus a thin covering of concentrically placed cells, which are probably reticular. The vessels are inconspicuous elements of the red pulp in human beings and require special stains for adequate demonstration.

White pulp. The white pulp, like the red, has a groundwork of reticular tissue but differs from it in containing large numbers of lymphocytes, as well as monocytes

Endothelial cells   Basement membrane

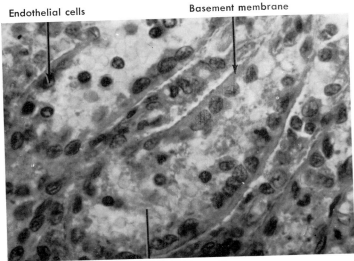

Lumen of sinus containing cells
undergoing phagocytosis

Fig. 10-9. Section of spleen showing splenic sinuses. (×640.)

and plasma cells. It thus resembles the medullary cords of a lymph node. It surrounds the arteries from the point where they leave the trabeculae to their division into penicilli, actually invading and replacing the adventitial connective tissue of the vessels. Elastic fibers belonging to the walls of the arteries are scattered through the white pulp. At various points, particularly where the vessels branch, the white pulp contains nodules, which form extensions of its substance, asymmetrically placed with respect to the artery. In fetal life and childhood the nodules contain germinal centers, and these persist into adult life in some animals but not in man.

It will be remembered that all kinds of red and white blood cells are formed in the spleen during embryonic life. One would, therefore, find in embryonic spleens the precursors of the corpuscles, including giant cells. These, like the germinal centers of the nodules, may persist into adult life in some forms.

Function of the spleen. The spleen is known to have four functions. (1) It is of importance in the metabolism and distribution of the erythrocytes. It acts as a storehouse for healthy corpuscles, retaining

varying numbers of them according to the demands of the body as a whole. The free macrophages of the red pulp ingest fragments of worn-out red blood cells, and the iron in the hemoglobin set free by the disintegration of corpuscles is stored in reticular cells. (2) It purifies the blood, since its phagocytes destroy infective agents. (3) It produces new blood cells during infancy and childhood. (4) It produces antibodies that are derived from plasma cells and are concerned with immunologic processes.

TONSILS
Palatine tonsil

The tonsils are masses of lymphoid tissue embedded in the lining of the throat between the arches of the palate. Three groups—the pharyngeal, palatine, and lingual tonsils—form a ring of tissue surrounding the pharynx. Their arrangement is best understood by reference to the structure of the wall of the pharynx. This consists of a layer of stratified squamous epithelium resting on a tunica propria of reticular or fine areolar tissue (Fig. 10-11). Beneath this lies the submucosa of coarser areolar tissue, which contains scattered

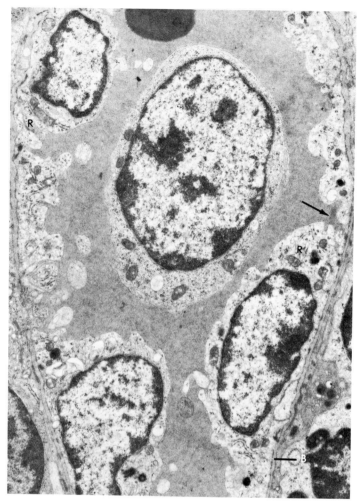

Fig. 10-10. Electron micrograph of longitudinal section of splenic sinus of mouse. The reticular (endothelial) cells, *R*, that line the sinus are elongated and are loosely applied one to the other. They rest upon a basement membrane, *B*, which is interrupted at intervals (arrow). (×10,000.)

mucous glands. The tonsil develops between the tunica propria and the submucosa. As it enlarges it elevates the former and depresses the latter. The epithelium of the mucosa does not go smoothly over the surface of the tonsil but dips down in numerous deep pits or fossae. Under the low power of the microscope the tonsil appears as a mass of lymphoid tissue, bordered on one side by stratified squamous epithelium and surrounded on the other sides by areolar tissue, which forms a tough capsule immediately around it. The mucous glands sometimes found in the areolar tissue outside the capsule are not part of the tonsil but belong to the pharyngeal wall. Noticeable features of the organ are its deep pits lined with stratified squamous epithelium and the presence of numerous germinal centers. The latter are usually grouped around the pits, but there is no division into cortex and medulla.

The pits (crypts) surrounded by lym-

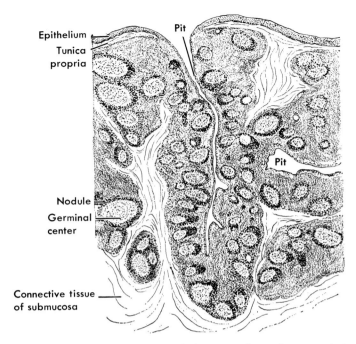

Epithelium
Tunica propria
Pit
Pit
Nodule
Germinal center
Connective tissue of submucosa

Fig. 10-11. Human palatine tonsil. (Hematoxylin and eosin stain.)

phatic tissue are partially separated from each other by connective tissue derived from the capsule. Lymphocytes, mast cells, and plasma cells occur in this connective tissue; also heterophilic leukocytes may be present, which indicates a mild inflammatory condition. In the deeper regions of the crypts an infiltration of lymphocytes displaces the epithelium of the crypts to a considerable degree. Some of these cells pass through the epithelium and are eventually found in the saliva as the salivary corpuscles.

The lumina of the crypts often contain accumulations of living and degenerating lymphocytes, desquamated epithelial cells, detritrus, and microorganisms. These last are said to cause inflammation and suppuration.

Pharyngeal tonsil

The pharyngeal tonsil is a median aggregation of lymphoid tissue that lies in the wall of the nasopharynx. In this region the epithelium, as is characteristic of the nasopharynx, is chiefly of the pseudostrati-

fied, ciliated, columnar variety. Patches of stratified squamous epithelium also occur and become more numerous in the adult. The lymphoid tissue is similar to that of the palatine tonsil. The capsule of this organ is thin and contains many fine elastic fibers, which radiate into the core of the folds.

Lingual tonsil

The lingual tonsil is located in the root of the tongue. The surface epithelium is of the stratified squamous variety and forms the covering of the numerous crypts that occur in this tonsil. The lymphoid tissue is similar to that found in the other tonsils except that the lymph nodules may contain germinal centers.

The tonsils generally reach their highest state of development in childhood and then usually undergo involution. Unlike the lymph nodes, the tonsils do not possess lymphatic sinuses, and hence lymph is not filtered through them. They do, however, possess lymph capillaries, which end blindly about the outer surface of the ton-

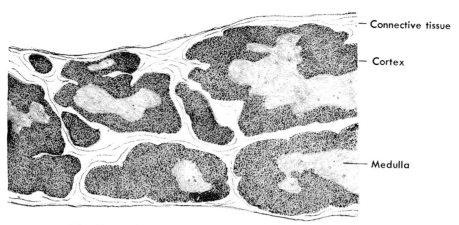

Connective tissue

Cortex

Medulla

Fig. 10-12. Thymus of monkey. (Hematoxylin and eosin stain.)

sil. The only established function of the tonsils is the formation of lymphocytes.

THYMUS

The thymus develops as an outgrowth from the pharyngeal wall of the embryo and has as a groundwork cells of epithelial (endodermal) rather than connective tissue (mesenchymal) origin. In later development the groundwork is infiltrated with cells that closely resemble lymphocytes in appearance and are probably derived from mesenchyme. It is claimed by some investigators that these small, darkly staining cells develop from the cells of the supporting framework and are, therefore, also endodermal in origin.

The fully developed thymus (Fig. 10-12) resembles the other members of the lymphoid group with which it is here placed in having a groundwork of relatively large, branching cells infiltrated with small, deeply staining elements. It differs from them in that it contains neither sinuses nor germinal centers, so that there is no morphologic evidence that it serves either as a filter. It does, however, produce new lymphocytes.

Under the low power of the microscope the thymus appears as a mass of purple and reddish tissue embedded in a loose investment of connective tissue. The capsule and trabeculae are less definitely organized than are those of the lymph node

and spleen. The organ is much lobulated and is divided into a cortex and a medulla (Fig. 10-13). Of these, the former is the more dense and is a deeper purple than the medulla, which is pink when stained with hematoxylin and eosin. The medullary substance extends from a central core into each lobule. Often a lobule is so cut that the connection of its medullary substance with the central core is not apparent, and it seems as if a mass of the lighter tissue were completely surrounded by cortical substance. If the lobule is small, it may look like a nodule with a germinal center, an appearance that is deceptive, since there are no centers in the thymus.

The cells found in the medulla consist of several epithelial cells, which are in intimate contact with lymphocytes and are more numerous than in the cortex. The epithelial cells, sometimes referred to as reticular cells, appear branched or stellate and maintain contact with one another by slender cytoplasmic processes. At the optical level, they appear as large, light, clear cells. In the electron microscope, they exhibit tonofibrils, desmosomes, and prominent cytoplasmic vesicles, as well as other organelles common to most cells. Other cells that are less numerous than those mentioned here and that also occur in the cortex are macrophages (either free or within vessels), fat cells, and mast cells (usually found in the septa). Scattered

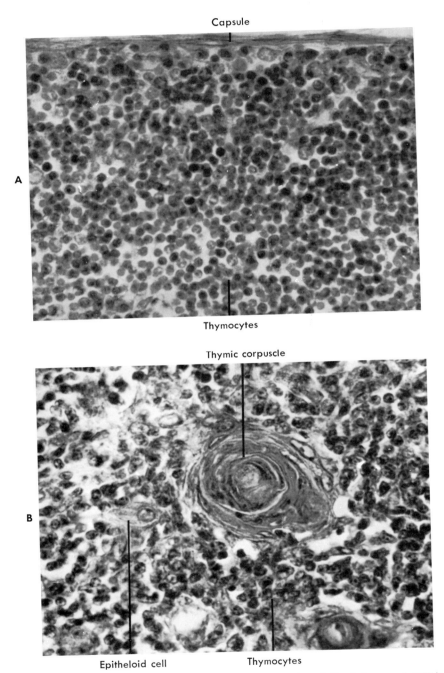

Fig. 10-13. A, Section of cortex of thymus. **B,** Section of medulla of thymus. (×640.)

plasma cells also occur throughout the thymus. The interstices between the epithelial cells are closely packed with lymphocytes of various sizes. Also present are many blood vessels from which reticular fibers associated with fibroblasts radiate between the epithelial cells. In addition, eosinophils and pigment cells may occur in the proximity of the blood vessels.

Another feature of the medulla of the thymus is the thymic corpuscle (Hassall's corpuscle) (Fig. 10-13, *B*). This is a group of cells ranging from 12 to 180 μ in diameter. These corpuscles have a hyaline center staining red with eosin, which seems to be derived from degenerating cells, since it may contain several pyknotic nuclei. Around this center are compressed cells concentrically arranged in a sort of whorl. Except for the hyaline center with its degenerating nuclei, the corpuscle somewhat resembles the small arteries that ramify through the thymic medulla. The cortex of the thymus consists of epithelial cells and thymocytes, but in this region the latter are so concentrated that they obscure the former (Fig. 10-13, *A*).

The thymus continues to grow in the child until the period of puberty. It then begins to degenerate in the majority of instances and is replaced by adipose tissue in adults. It has been found to persist in cases of infantilism (delayed sexual maturity) and in castrated animals.

The thymus has been suspected of being an endocrine gland for some time. It is only recently, however, that evidence, at least in the mouse, has shown that this is probably true. Very small amounts of a humoral substance released by the cells of the gland are conveyed to other lymphoid organs, such as the spleen, which, in turn, are stimulated to produced lymphocytes. A second important function now attributed to the thymus is a key role in directing the establishment of normal immunologic functions and also in restoring these functions in the event of loss or damage to them.

SUMMARY AND COMPARISON OF THE LYMPHOID ORGANS

Lymph node. The lymph node consists of a cortex and a medulla. The cortex contains nodules that may have germinal centers, a peripheral sinus, and sinuses beside the trabeculae. The medulla is composed of cords, sinuses, and trabeculae. The capsule and trabeculae are of dense connective tissue, with scattered fibers of smooth muscle in the former. The lymph node filters lymph, produces new lymphocytes, has a phagocytic action, removing impurities from the lymph, and is also involved in immunologic reactions.

Spleen. The spleen is composed of red and white pulp but not a cortex and medulla. The red pulp contains all types of blood cells and venous sinuses. The white pulp surrounds arteries and includes nodules that have no germinal centers in adult man. The spleen is phagocytic, forms new lymphocytes, and influences the metabolism and distribution of the erythrocytes.

Tonsil. The tonsils are masses of lymphoid tissue embedded in the wall of the pharynx. They are covered by stratified squamous epithelium, which dips into the substance of the organ, forming the pits. Lymph nodules with germinal centers are grouped around the pits. There are no sinuses. The tonsils form lymphocytes.

Thymus. The thymus is divided into cortex and medulla and is composed chiefly of epithelial cells and thymocytes, which resemble lymphocytes. The medulla contains thymic corpuscles. The cortex is a dense mass of thymocytes and epithelial tissue.

The thymus produces a humoral agent (hormone) that is effective in stimulating the production of lymphocytes in lymphoid organs. It is also responsible for establishing and regulating immunologic reactions.

11

Glands

In the following chapters glands become a prominent feature of each of the several organs to be considered. Accordingly, a general survey and orientation of typical characteristics of glands will be discussed at this juncture.

Glands are composed of epithelial cells, which perform the highly specialized function of producing *secretions*. These cells remove raw materials from tissue fluid or lymph and from them synthesize substances that ordinarily are not utilized by the gland cell itself to any great degree. The secretory products are released upon free surfaces or into the blood-lymphatic complex of vessels for distribution to sites where the secretion products are utilized. Some glandular secretions are stored until the demands of the organism require the substance involved. In others, the secretions are elaborated and released either continually or intermittently.

Excretion, sometimes used interchangeably with secretion, is a process by which the end products of carbohydrate, fat, protein, and mineral metabolism are removed from the internal medium of the organism. Thus liver cells can remove decomposition products of hemoglobin from the blood and convert them into bile salts and bile pigments, which are then passed into the bile system and eventually into the small intestine. Bile salts utilized in lipid absorption and digestion are resorbed and reutilized several times. Bile salts may accordingly be considered to be secretion products. By contrast, the bile pigments not utilized in the body are eliminated with the fecal mass. These pigments may be considered to be excretions produced by a secretory mechanism. Certain cells in kidney tubules are capable of adding substances to urine by secretory processes. The sweat glands secrete a modified tissue fluid that serves several functions, at least one of them being excretory in function. Even the salivary glands are partially excretory by virtue of their ability to remove salts, thiocyanate ion, and urea from the body fluid. *Elimination* is the process by which excretions, secretions, and undigested food residue are expelled by the organism.

ENDOCRINE GLANDS

The endocrine glands, or glands of internal secretion, may have ducts in the embryonic state, but in the adult ducts are absent and are accordingly classed as ductless glands. The secretions of endocrine glands may be stored or carried directly into blood capillaries, and it is by means of the latter that they are transported throughout the body to so-called target organs. The secretions of endocrine cells are called *hormones*, and in concert with the nervous system they regulate and coordinate the activities of all the cells in the body. Some hormones stimulate or suppress the activities of one or more specific glands or organs. Others, such as thyroxin, regulate the activities of most cells of the body.

Hormones have a varied chemical composition. Some are proteins (insulin), some modified amino acids (thyroxin), while others are modified sterols (cortisone-like substances, estrogens, androgens). Some endocrine glands have a dual function. The

136

pancreas, for example, elaborates the hormones insulin and glucagon as well as pancreatic fluid, which contains a mixture of enzymes and sodium bicarbonate, and is accordingly classed as one of the *mixed glands* (that is, both endocrine and exocrine in function).

In glands with known endocrine function there are three major cell arrangements: clumps, follicles, and cords.

Clumps. In the clump type of arrangement, secretion and utilization are of approximately the same magnitude. The secretion is stored within the epithelioid cells themselves and is released upon demand into the abundant capillary network that permeates the clump. Examples of this type are the islets of Langerhans in the pancreas and the so-called interstitial cells in the testes. Clumps may be composed of small or large groups of irregularly shaped cells, but they do not form hollow spheres or tubes.

Follicles. A follicle consists of a cylinder or sphere of cells enclosing a cavity containing the stored secretion product. In the thyroid (for example, see Fig. 20-2), which consists of many follicles, the cells are usually cuboidal and exhibit a deeply staining secretion in the lumen called the colloid substance. Increased demand for the secretion results in a transfer of a hormone from the lumen to the abundant capillary network surrounding each follicle. Depletion of the colloid reserves results in collapse of the follicle followed by a crowding of the cells, which appear columnar in transverse section. (See Fig. 20-2.) Since it is thought that a depleted reserve results in active secretory activity by the cells, the columnar form is associated with the active or secretory phase of these glands. In the embryo the follicles originate as clumps of epithelioid cells. These cells produce more secretion than can be either utilized or stored within the cells. The secretion is accordingly stored in cavities formed between the cells and thus gives rise to the space known as the "lumen" of the follicle.

Cords. In the cord the epithelioid cells are arranged in rows. The liver cords consist of two rows of cells closely aligned,

whereas the adrenal cortex exhibits many subparallel rows of cells. Secretions are stored within the cells and transferred to the abundant capillary network as required.

Epithelioid cells. By definition epithelia line cavities. With the exception of the follicular arrangement, endocrine gland cells do not line cavities. Prominent cuboidal or polygonal cells may occur in small or large irregular masses or in cords but invariably lack a cavity. (See Figs. 19-6, 20-8, and 20-11.) For this special situation the term *epithelioid* (epithelium-like) was introduced. When epithelioid cells occur, one is led to suspect an endocrine function; however, physiologic demonstration of endocrine activity is necessary before an endocrine role can be definitely ascribed to these cells.

EXOCRINE GLANDS

Exocrine glands, or glands of external secretion, retain connections with surfaces. Unicellular glands, for example, mucous cells, discharge their secretions directly on a free surface. Multicellular glands, for example, the salivary glands, discharge via a system of simple or branching ducts.

Ducts

There are several types of ducts: secretory, excretory, and intercalated.

Secretory ducts. One kind of secretory duct is lined by the glandular cells that produce the secretion. (See Figs. 11-1, *C* to *E*, and 12-6.) In the salivary glands another type of secretory duct is found, and it contains glandular cells supplying additional substances to the secretion produced at some distance from the main gland cells. Special techniques demonstrate the presence of basal striations in these cells, and, hence, they are frequently called *striated ducts.*

Excretory ducts. Excretory ducts, formed of simple epithelium, presumably conduct secretions without taking part in the elaboration of major secretory components. (See Figs. 11-1, *D, F* to *H,* and 15-1.)

Intercalated ducts. Intercalated ducts are interposed between the glandular units and their conducting portions (for exam-

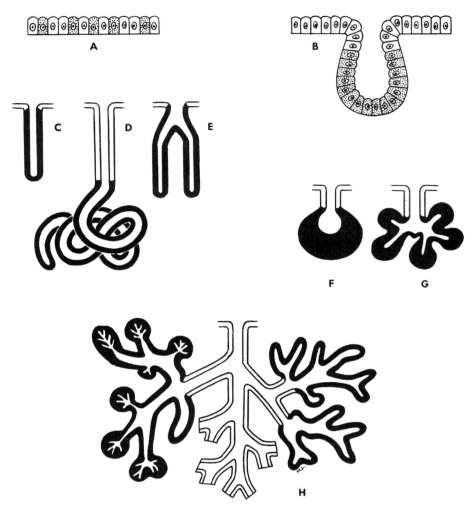

Fig. 11-1. Diagram showing different types of arrangement of glandular tissue. **A,** Glandular cells (granular) scattered among common epithelium cells (clear); **B,** glandular cells forming saclike invagination into underlying tissue; **C,** simple tubular gland; **D,** simple tubular gland coiled; **E,** simple branched tubular gland; **F,** simple alveolar gland; **G,** simple branched alveolar gland; **H,** compound gland. (Redrawn from Maximow and Bloom.)

ple, striated or excretory ducts). (See Fig. 15-1.) The intercalated ducts are lined with flattened cells, which presumably do not produce a secretion. The latter are found only in the larger glands (for example, pancreas and salivary glands).

Classification

The simplest glandular unit is the unicellular gland, which consists of a cell that forms part of a lining epithelium and also elaborates a secretion. The goblet cells scattered along the lining of the intestine and respiratory tract are of this type.

The next simplest type is the intraepithelial gland, which consists of a strip of consecutive glandular cells forming a slight thickening or pocket entirely within the limits of the epithelium. The lining epithelium of the gut contains fingerlike or tubular projections of glandular cells, which are below the level of the epithelium in the underlying connective tissue and which maintains their connection to the surface by means of a duct. (See Figs. 11-1, *B*, *C*, and *E*, and 14-5 to 14-22.)

Another means of classifying glands is by the manner and degree to which branching of the excretory or striated ducts occurs. If the ducts are absent (Fig. 11-1, *C* and *E*) or unbranched (Fig. 11-1, *D*, *E*, and *G*), the glands are termed *simple*. If the ducts branch (Fig. 11-1, *H*), the glands are called *compound*.

Simple and compound glands are subdivided according to whether the shapes of the secreting portions are tubular, alveolar (acinar), or tubuloalveolar. The name tubular is self-explanatory; an alveolar gland has secreting portions, which are spherical or flask shaped, whereas the tubuloalveolar variety may exhibit glandular portions intermediate between the two types already mentioned (Fig. 11-1, *H*, left side). Another variety of tubuloalveolar gland consists of tubular units and alveolar units attached to the same excretory duct. The simple tubular gland is further differentiated into tubular, coiled tubular, or branching tubular (Fig. 11-1, *C* to *E*). Also illustrated in Fig. 11-1, *G*, is the branching alveolar (compare Fig. 12-6, sebaceous glands). Other kinds of glands have been described such as those in the eyelid, but because of their highly specialized function and limited distribution they will not be discussed here. Other classifications depend on the mode of secretion (holocrine, merocrine, apocrine) and on the product of secretion (mucous, serous, mixed, zymogenic).

Secretions

The secretions of exocrine glands are varied, but at present none of these has been identified as a hormone. (The case for parotin has not been confirmed as yet.) Mucigen, for example, is an inadequately characterized mixture of carbohydrate and protein; zymogen (a precursor of enzymes) is in part protein and forms an important component of many serous secretions; se-

bum and cerumen contain protein, carbohydrate, and much lipid; in addition, secretions produced by the sweat, lacrimal, and lactating glands are extremely varied and complex. Glands such as the testes and ovaries and lymphoid and myeloid tissues are usually classed as *cytogenous*, since their chief activity is the production of living cells.

As indicated previously, the modes of secretion are utilized in classifying certain glands. In the case of *holocrine* secretion, the secretory product is stored in the gland cell, and the entire gland cell is extruded and destroyed in the process of secretion. The sebaceous glands are of this type. In *apocrine* secretion, the secretion accumulates in one or more large vacuoles below the free surface of the cell. During secretion a thin film of surface cytoplasm is removed with the secretory globules; the cell itself, however, is not usually destroyed in the process. In *merocrine* secretion, there is a cyclic increase and decrease of the secretory product, which is more or less continually released into the lumen of the gland without, however, destroying the cell or depleting the cytoplasm. Typical of this variety are the glands of the oral cavity and digestive tract.

Unicellular glands

The simplest glands are composed of one cell, and the most common respresentative of this group is the mucous or *goblet cell*. These cells are found in profusion in the digestive tract and in parts of the respiratory system. They are initially observed as tall columnar cells with elongate elliptical nuclei, distinguishable from their neighbors only by the absence of cilia or striated border. In the supranuclear position, minute granules appear, then droplets of mucigen, which migrate and accumulate at the free border of the cell. As more mucigen droplets accumulate in the cell the nucleus is forced toward the base, with concomitant changes in form from elliptical to a round and deeply staining conical form, until finally it appears as a flattened disk near the base of the cell. In addition, the apex of the cell expands laterally and distorts the neighboring epithelial cells. At this stage the cell looks like a goblet, with a narrow stem containing the nucleus and an expanded goblet-bell containing the nonstaining mucigen droplets in what appears to be a large cavity. In many instances the mucigen droplets nearest the surface are gradually released and dispersed in modified tissue fluid to form the viscid fluid known as *mucus.* In other instances the mucigen globules are released en masse; the goblet then collapses and appears as an irregularly outlined, tall columnar cell consisting of a narrow strip of cytoplasm containing a deeply staining, incredibly thin nucleus. The process of secretion is cyclic and may be repeated a number of times before the cell is replaced.

The presence of a large mass of nonstaining mucigen in hematoxylin and eosin preparations gives the impression of a large vacuole in cells filled with secretion. The principal ingredient of mucigen is a polysaccharide-containing protein called *mucin.* Aside from its adhesive properties, it has the ability to combine with, and coagulate in the presence of, acids to form a protective coating on surfaces. The PAS reaction

demonstrates the polysaccharide moiety as a red to purplish red staining region. Certain aluminum-containing stain mixtures (mucicarmine, mucihematin) stain mucigen droplets a vivid red or blue.

Multicellular glands

The usual example used to illustrate the multicellular variety of glands is the salivary glands. In these and similar glands the cells are grouped into *secretory units* of three types: mucous, serous, and seromucous, or mixed, units (Fig. 11-2). They are usually arranged in alveoli (acini) and branched or straight tubules.

Mucous units are composed of a type of cuboidal epithelium, which is so disposed about a small lumen that the cells take on the form of truncated pyramids and are accordingly called pyramidal cells. At the beginning of a secretory cycle the nuclei tend to be round or ovoid and occupy a position nearer to the base of the cell rather than the center. As the mucigen globules accumulate near the lumen of the gland, the nuclei are displaced toward the base and are compressed to such an extent that they appear as flattened, darkly staining rods in contact with the cell boundary. Some authors maintain that mucous units with rounded nuclei secrete thin mucus, but in view of their cyclic activity this contention would be difficult to verify. Since the mucigen takes up so much of the volume of the cytoplasm and does not stain with hematoxylin and eosin, the cytoplasm of these cells does not appear eosinophilic and may on occasion even exhibit a pale bluish color. In certain of the salivary glands, the mucous units are easily detected under low power of the microscope as very pale areas. With PAS the mucigen stains such a deep purplish red that all cellular detail may be obscured. Although these cells exhibit cyclic activity, the release of secretion is gradual and typical of the merocrine type of secretion.

Serous units are also composed of pyramidal cells but differ in that their nuclei are always centrally disposed in the cell. Their secretion granules are either slightly or extremely acidophilic and are primarily

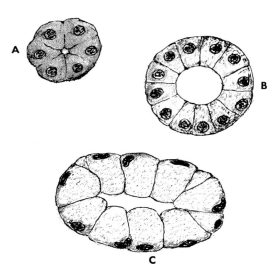

Fig. 11-2. Types of serous and mucus-secreting epithelium. **A,** Serous alveolus; **B,** alveolus secreting thick mucus; **C,** alveolus secreting thin mucus.

protein in character. Since these cells frequently elaborate enzymes (which are all partly protein), the secretion droplets within the cell all called *zymogen granules.* In many instances the granules are so small and so widely dispersed that the entire apex of the cell appears intensely acidophilic, while in other situations the granules are quite large and evenly distributed throughout the entire cell (Paneth cells). These cells produce an inactive precursor of the enzyme (zymogen). Zymogens are sometimes transported for a considerable distance before being activated. Since these cells are actively engaged in protein synthesis, the presence of large amounts of RNA or basophil substance in the perinuclear and subnuclear positions correlates well with their function. The serous cells of the pancreatic acini in well-stained hematoxylin and eosin preparations exhibit acidophilic apices and basophilic bases. The serous units of the salivary glands may be distinguished from the mucous units by the more central position of their nuclei and much greater affinity for dyes.

Mixed units are composed of both mucous and serous cells. The most easily demonstrated mixed units are found in the submaxillary glands of man. In one type of mixed unit the mucous cells form a tubular portion joining the duct, while the terminal portion consists of the more deeply staining serous cells. On occasion the mucous cells are so numerous that they crowd the serous cells away from the lumen and form a crescentic cap of deeply staining cells or *demilune.* Occasionally, a mucous cell is also extruded into the *demilune* complex. In section, it is not always possible to distinguish between a "pure" mucous unit and the tubular portion of a mixed unit. A "pure" serous unit exhibits a small but distinct lumen in its center. In favorable sections through the terminal part of a mixed unit the serous cells are separated from the lumen by mucous cells. In tangential sections of a demilune one may observe serous cells only; a central lumen is usually lacking, however. The student should be careful to distinguish between the mixed unit and the *mixed gland,* the latter being composed of both mucous and serous glands, and sometimes mixed units as well. Mixed glands of the type discussed here are also known as mucoserous or seromucous glands. The term *mixed gland* is also applied to glands that perform both an endocrine and exocrine function. (Compare pancreas, ovary and so on.)

Occasionally certain stellate contractile cells may be found between the secretory unit and its basement membrane. These cells are called basket or myoepithelial cells and contain thin, prominent, dark-staining cresentic nuclei. They are said to propel secretions into gland ducts as a result of their contraction.

A number of serous or albuminous cells of certain oral glands are slightly PAS-positive and from a histochemical point of view are termed mucoserous cells. They are not, however, morphologically distinguishable from serous cells and are accordingly classed with them.

Glands that are neither serous nor mucous do not, as a matter of fact, form a group united by similarities of function or morphology. They are mentioned here merely to point out that many glandular organs exist that are not to be classified as serous or mucous. They are so varied that no general statement regarding them can be made, and they will be discussed individually in later chapters.

12

Integument

The skin consists of an epidermal and a dermal layer (corium) and rests upon the subdermal connective tissue. The epidermis is a stratified squamous epithelium, modified in some portions of the body by the addition of a thick cuticular layer and in others by the development of the hair and nails. The corium is a layer of dense connective tissue in which are located the various glands of the skin and the hair follicles. The subdermal or subcutaneous tissue is also fibrous, but it is more loosely arranged than the corium and generally contains adipose tissue.

HAIRLESS SKIN

No hair grows on the palms of the hands or the soles of the feet. They are covered with thick skin consisting of epidermis and corium (Fig. 12-1).

Epidermis

Stratum corneum. The outer layer of the epidermis, or the stratum corneum, makes up about three fourths of the thickness of the epidermis. It consists of cornified nonnucleated cells, the outer layers of which are detached from the surface in ragged patches (desquamation). The inner layers of the stratum corneum are compact and the outlines of individual cells are visible (Figs. 12-2 to 12-4).

Stratum lucidum. Beneath the stratum corneum is the stratum lucidum, which consists of several rows of flattened nonnucleated cells. They form a hyaline, highly refractile band that appears homogeneous and stains deeply with eosin.

Stratum granulosum. The cells nearest the stratum lucidum are spindle shaped, with their long axes parallel to the surface of the skin. There are from two to five layers of cells in which the cytoplasm is full of granules that stain deeply with hematoxylin. These layers make up the stratum granulosum, which is prominent because of its color. On closer examination it may be seen that the stratum granulosum differs from other epithelia in the arrangement of its cells. Rather than being closely applied to each other, they are separated by narrow spaces so that each is surrounded by a light line (in section). This is demonstrable in ordinary preparations. In exceptionally good preparations and under high magnification, it may be seen that the polygonal cells below the stratum granulosum are also separated by clefts and that the spaces are traversed by minute cytoplasmic bridges, uniting each cell to its neighbors. The name prickle cells is sometimes given to the polygonal cells and those of the stratum granulosum because of these protoplasmic strands (Fig. 12-3).

Stratum spinosum. The stratum spinosum layer of the epidermis (Fig. 12-2) is several cells in thickness and is composed of polyhedral cells, which are irregular in shape and noticeably separated from each other. In the surface layers, the cells tend to flatten. The surface of these cells exhibits protoplasmic processes (Fig. 12-3), which appear to meet with similar processes from adjacent cells to form "intercellular bridges." These processes do not indicate protoplasmic continuity between these cells, which are sometimes referred to as "prickle" cells. Electron microscope studies have shown that

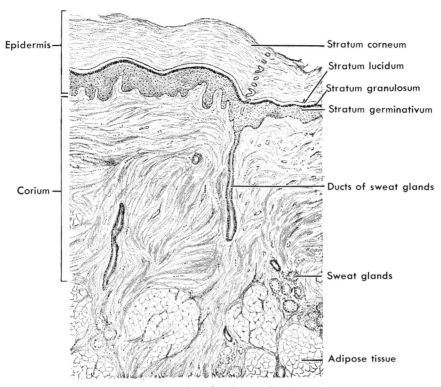

Epidermis —

Corium —

Stratum corneum
Stratum lucidum
Stratum granulosum
Stratum germinativum

Ducts of sweat glands

Sweat glands

Adipose tissue

Fig. 12-1. Hairless skin from palm of hand.

the processes contain tonofibrils and make intimate contact at a desmosome; accordingly, the cells are independent structures. (See Figs. 2-1 and 2-2.)

Stratum germinativum. The stratum germinativum (basale) consists of a single layer of modified columnar cells with deeply staining cytoplasm and indistinct cell boundaries. The boundary between the epidermis and the corium is irregular because of the great number of papillae formed by the corium. Granules of pigment (melanin) are present in this layer. They are derived from melanoblasts, which lie directly beneath this layer. (See Fig. 2-3.)

Corium

The corium, or dermis, is a compact layer of connective tissue containing numerous collagenous and elastic fibers. It varies in thickness from less than 0.5 mm. on the eyelid and prepuce to 3 mm. or

more on the palms and soles. The upper surface in contact with the epidermis is usually thrown into wavelike extensions called *papillae* that project into corresponding grooves at the base of the epidermis. The connective tissue within these papillae is richly vascular and contains delicate, loosely woven collagenous bundles in addition to a rich network of sensory nerve endings. It is more cellular than the deeper parts of the dermis. The layers of the dermis beneath the papillae (called the reticular layer) are composed of densely packed bundles of connective tissue running roughly along lines of strain in the skin.

The secretory coils of the sweat glands and the bases of the hair follicles (to be described later) are embedded in the dermis. Elastic fibers occurring in the reticular layer entwine around the sweat glands and the hair follicles, both of which

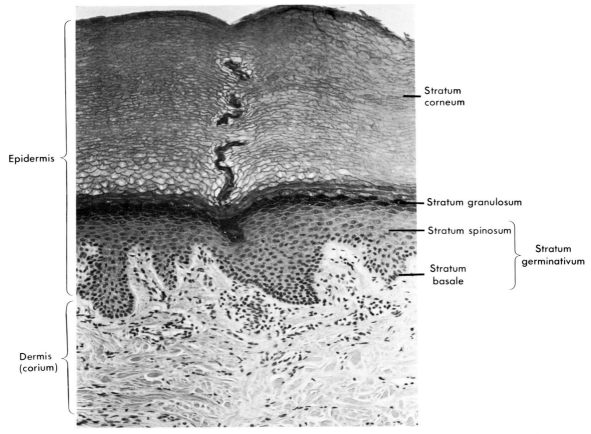

Epidermis

Dermis
(corium)

Stratum
corneum

Stratum granulosum

Stratum spinosum

Stratum
basale

Stratum
germinativum

Fig. 12-2. Section of thick skin of human showing duct of sweat gland in epidermis. (×160.)

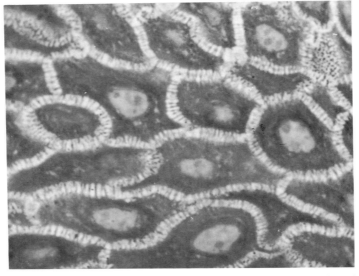

Fig. 12-3. Photomicrograph of part of the stratum spinosum of human gingival epithelium showing intercellular bridges. (×1,200.)

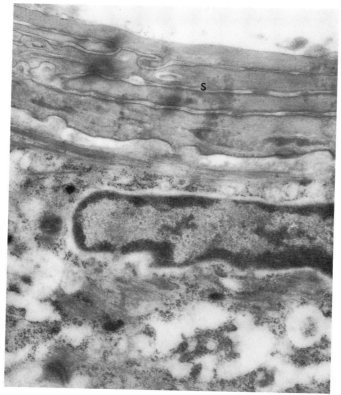

Fig. 12-4. Electron micrograph of surface of monkey lip. S, Cells of stratum corneum. (×29,000).

are originally derived from downward extensions of the epidermis. The basal portion of the reticular layer sometimes contains networks of smooth muscle fibers that may cause the surface to be thrown into folds (for example, in the areolae of the nipples, the perineum, the scrotum, and the penis). Bundles of smooth muscle (the *erector pili* muscles) are also attached to the hair follicles. In the skin of the face, bands of skeletal muscle (the facial musculature) are present in the dermis.

The subcutaneous layer *(hypodermis)*, which is a looser variety of the dermis, lies beneath the reticular layer. Where the skin is firmly attached to underlying muscle or bone, this layer is composed of tightly woven collagenous fibers continuous with those of the dermis. In areas where the skin is more loosely attached to underlying structures, the fibers of the hypo-

dermis are accordingly more loosely arranged. Frequently sheets of fat cells occur in the subcutaneous layer, for example, in the heel and in breast tissue. The subcutaneous layer is richly supplied with blood vessels and nerves.

HAIRY SKIN

In the skin of the greater part of the body, the stratum germinativum of the epidermis extends into the corium to form hair follicles (Figs. 12-5 to 12-7). These are most extensively developed in the scalp, which may be used as an example of hairy skin (Fig. 12-6). In this locality protection is afforded by the hair, and the cornified layer is much thinner than it is on the hands and feet. In some cases, it is reduced to less than one half the thickness of the basal and spinosum layers; the stratum lucidum is much reduced or en-

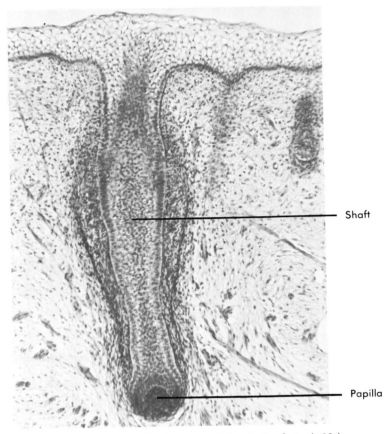

Shaft

Papilla

Fig. 12-5. Longitudinal section of developing hair. (×60.)

tirely lacking, and there are few granular cells.

A hair follicle has two layers. The outer layer is a poorly defined connective tissue sheath; the inner is a continuation of the germinative layer of the epidermis. At the base of the follicle the connective tissue forms a papilla, which projects into the epithelium, and at this point also the epithelium is continuous with the hair shaft. This part of the follicle is enlarged to form the bulb (Fig. 12-7).

A sebaceous gland and a strand of smooth muscle are associated with the hair follicle. The axis of the latter is never exactly perpendicular to the surface of the scalp, and the muscle and gland lie in the wider angle of the two, which the follicle

makes with the surface. The hair itself is epithelial and under high magnification may be seen to consist of the following layers:

1. Cuticula of transparent overlapping scales
2. Cortex of flattened cornified cells containing pigment
3. Medulla of cuboidal cells, usually in two rows

The follicle is composed of two sheaths, the outer of which is connective tissue, the inner, epithelium. The former is divided into three layers:

1. An outside layer of loose connective tissue containing blood vessels. The fibers of this sheath, some of which are elastic, run longitudinally.

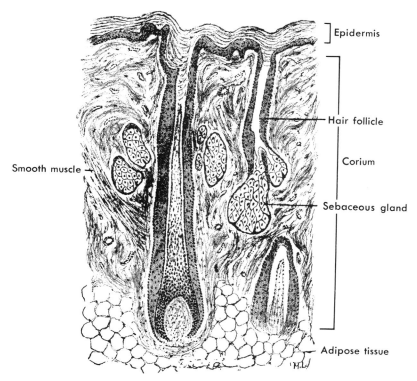

Fig. 12-6. Human scalp.

2. A middle layer consisting of white fibrous tissue in which the fibers are circularly arranged.
3. An innermost, hyaline layer sometimes containing white fibers longitudinally disposed (membrana vitrea).

The epithelial sheath consists of two parts:

1. An outer epithelial sheath, which is an impocketing of the skin that grows thinner as it nears the bulb of the hair.
2. An inner epithelial sheath, which is still further divided as follows:
   a. Henle's layer, located outside Huxley's layer, is composed of flattened or cuboidal cells having a clear cytoplasm. The cytoplasm contains longitudinal fibrils, and nuclei are present only in those cells lying deep in the follicle.
   b. Huxley's layer lies outside the root sheath and is composed of several

rows of elongated cells containing eleidin. Near the surface the nuclei of these cells are lacking or rudimentary.

Next to the hair is a cuticle of nonnucleated cornified cells, the cuticula of the sheath.

GLANDS OF THE SKIN

The glands of the skin are of two kinds, the sweat glands and the sebaceous glands.

Sweat glands

Sweat glands are distributed over most of the surface of the body. They are simple tubular glands with convoluted secreting portions. The latter may lie in the subcutaneous tissue or in the deeper portion of the corium and are lined with cuboidal or columnar epithelium. The cytoplasm contains secretory granules or droplets (Fig. 12-8).

The ducts of the sweat glands are lined

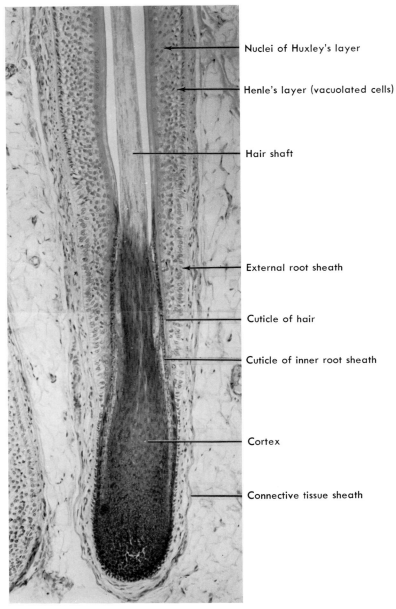

Nuclei of Huxley's layer

Henle's layer (vacuolated cells)

Hair shaft

External root sheath

Cuticle of hair

Cuticle of inner root sheath

Cortex

Connective tissue sheath

Fig. 12-7. Parasagittal section of human hair. (×160.)

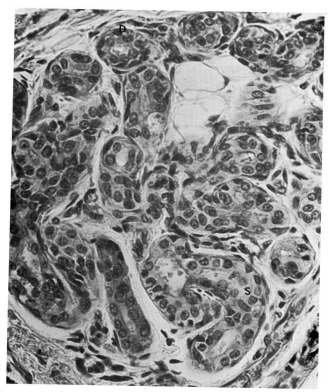

Fig. 12-8. Section of part of human sweat gland. *D,* Duct; *S,* secretory tubule. (×400.)

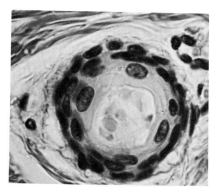

Fig. 12-9. Transverse section of duct of sweat gland of an infant. Note two layers of cells. (×400.)

with a double layer of stratified cuboidal cells resting upon a thin basement membrane (Fig. 12-9). The inner layer exhibits a homogeneous dark-staining cytoplasm, and the surface of the cells is refractile. In the epidermis, the cellular constituents disappear and the duct consists of a noncellular channel.

In some regions of the body such as the axilla, the mammary areolae, and the circumanal region, the sweat glands are much larger than those located in the palms and other areas. These glands are of the apocrine type producing thicker secretions than the sweat formed by the smaller (merocrine) glands. Also included in this group of larger glands are the wax-secreting *ceruminous* glands located in the external auditory canal and the margin of the eyelid. The secretion of the glands is carried to the lower border of the epi-

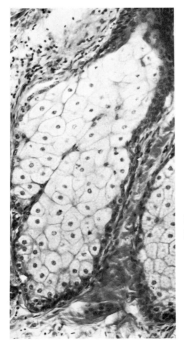

Fig. 12-10. Section of part of human sebaceous gland. (×160.)

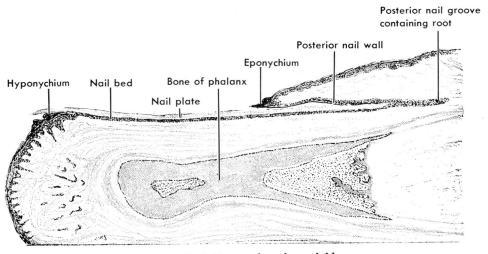

Fig. 12-11. Finger of newborn child.

dermis, where it passes into a coiled channel through the tissues to emerge on the surface by way of a minute pore.

Sebaceous glands

Sebaceous glands are almost always associated with hair follicles, opening through ducts into the spaces between the follicles and the hair shafts. Structurally they are different from any other glands thus far described. Their secreting portions are not composed of a single layer of cells grouped around a lumen but are rounded masses of cells. At the periphery of each mass the cells are cuboidal; in the center they are polygonal. The central cells are filled with vacuoles, so that their appearance is somewhat like that of developing adipose tissue cells (Fig. 12-10). The secretion of the sebaceous glands is accompanied by the breaking down of the central cells, and their remains are poured out with the oily accumulation into the hair follicle. The cells thus destroyed are replaced from the peripheral layer.

NAILS

The nails (Fig. 12-11), which are modifications of the epidermis, are composed of the body, wall, and bed.

The body with its free edge is composed of several layers of clear, flattened cells, which differ from the stratum corium of the skin in that they are harder and also possess shrunken nuclei. The proximal part of the nail body lying under the fold of skin is called the root.

The nail wall is the fold around the proximal and lateral borders of the nail, marked off from the latter by the nail groove. The wall consists of skin that has all the layers of other parts of the skin except, sometimes, the stratum lucidum. The stratum corneum of the wall at the proximal part of the fold extends out over the body of the nail (eponychium).

The nail bed is the skin under the body of the nail. It lacks the stratum corneum and stratum lucidum and consists of the stratum germinativum only. Under the proximal part of the nail, in the region called the lunula, the germinativum thickens. It is from this region, the matrix, that growth of the nail takes place, the superficial cells of the matrix being transformed into nail cells. The corium of the nail bed has its connective tissue fibers arranged in two groups: (1) a group running in the long axis of the nail and (2) a group running vertically to the periosteum of the underlying bone. The dermal papillae of the nail bed form ridges, which run in the long axis of the nail.

13
Oral cavity

LIPS

The lips are muscular organs covered on the outside by skin and on the inside by the mucous membrane of the mouth. The muscles of the lips are striated and consist of the orbicularis oris, the compressor labii, and the mimetic. The lip is usually sectioned vertically in prepartion for microscopic study and when so cut presents as a type of core the cross sections of the orbicularis oris, with a relatively small number of strands of the mimetic and compressor labii muscles cut longitudinally (Fig. 13-1).

The skin covering the outside of the lip is like that of the greater part of the body. It consists of stratified squamous epithelium, which is cornified at the surface and rests upon a layer of connective tissue. In the latter are sweat glands, sebaceous glands, and the bases of hair follicles. In the region transitional between skin and oral mucosa, hair follicles and glands disappear and the epithelium is somewhat modified. Its basal layer follows a very irregular course so that tall projections of the underlying connective tissue extend toward the surface of the lip. These cells are not pigmented but are well supplied with blood vessels, giving this part of the lip a brighter color than that of the surrounding skin.

On the oral surface the epithelium changes again. The height of the connective tissue papillae gradually diminishes, as does the cornification of the surface, and at the base of the lip on the inside the mucous membrane is like that lining other soft parts of the oral cavity. In this region there are seromucous glands lying in the connective tissue between the epithelium and the muscle.

LINING OF THE ORAL CAVITY

The epithelium lining the oral cavity is of the stratified squamous variety. It rests on a tunica propria of reticular or fine areolar tissue, which blends in most parts of the cavity with a submucosal layer of areolar tissue. Beneath the submucosa lie tissues that vary in different parts of the mouth. In the cheeks and lips, for example, the mucosa and submucosa lie against muscle, making a soft and somewhat elastic wall of the oral cavity (Fig. 13-2). In the hard palate and the gingivae, on the other hand, the layers in question lie directly against bone. Modifications of the mucous membrane are correlated with these differences in the tissue it covers.

Lips and cheeks

The inner surface of the lip is a good example of conditions in parts of the mouth that are bounded by muscle. The epithelium is not cornified. It has a surface layer of flattened cells that slough off in patches. Connective tissue papillae are low; the tunica propria blends without demarcation with the submucosa. The latter is fairly thick and in some regions contains glands, the ducts of which penetrate the mucosa and open into the oral cavity.

Gingivae and hard palate

Where the mucosa and submucosa lie over bony tissue, as in the gingivae and hard palate (Figs. 13-3 and 13-4), modifi-

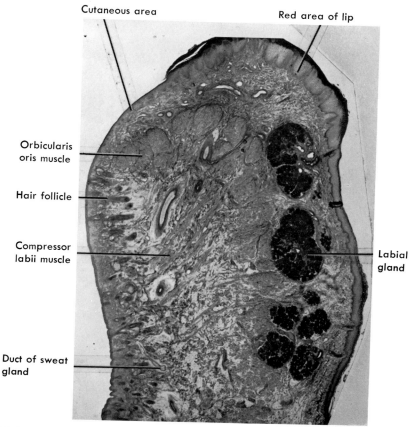

Cutaneous area

Red area of lip

Orbicularis oris muscle

Hair follicle

Compressor labii muscle

Labial gland

Duct of sweat gland

Fig. 13-1. Parasagittal section of human lip in newborn infant. (×14.) (Courtesy Dr. S. Bernick, Los Angeles, Calif.)

cations of arrangement are to be observed. In the gingival region the connective tissue papillae of the tunica propria are long and slender and close together. The submucosa blends with the periosteum of the underlying bone. In the region immediately surrounding each tooth, fibers are present, which are specialized as part of the apparatus by which the tooth is held in its socket. No glands exist in this portion of the oral mucosa.

In the hard palate the papillae of the tunica propria are well developed, and there is a layer of elastic fibers, which forms a line of demarcation between the mucosa and submucosa. The latter coat blends here, as in the gingivae, with the periosteum of the underlying bone. There

are glands in the submucosa of the palatal region.

TEETH

The human dentition consists of twenty deciduous and thirty-two permanent teeth. The teeth vary among themselves as to size, shape and number of cusps and roots; each particular tooth, however, has its own unique morphologic characteristics.

The teeth are divided into two parts: (1) the crown, covered by enamel, is the part of the tooth that is ordinarily visible and extends beyond the margin of the gingivae; (2) the root is the part of the tooth that lies deep to the gingivae and is implanted within the socket. The term *cervix*, or neck, is sometimes used to designate a

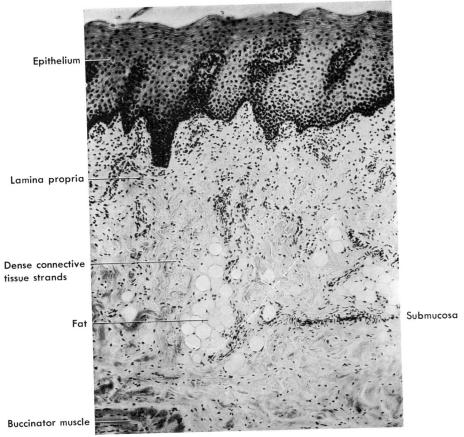

Epithelium

Lamina propria

Dense connective
tissue strands

Fat

Submucosa

Buccinator muscle

Fig. 13-2. Section through mucous membrane of cheek. Note the strands of dense connective tissue attaching the mucous membrane to the buccinator muscle. (From Sicher and Bhaskar, editors: Orban's oral histology and embryology, ed. 7, St. Louis, 1972, The C. V. Mosby Co.)

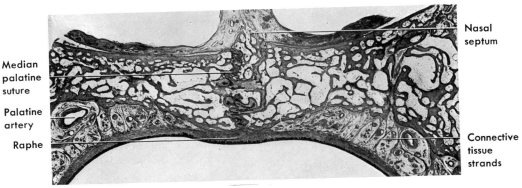

Median
palatine
suture

Palatine
artery

Raphe

Nasal
septum

Connective
tissue
strands

Fig. 13-3. Transverse section through hard palate. Palatine raphe; fibrous strands connecting mucosa and periosteum; palatine vessels. (From Pendleton.)

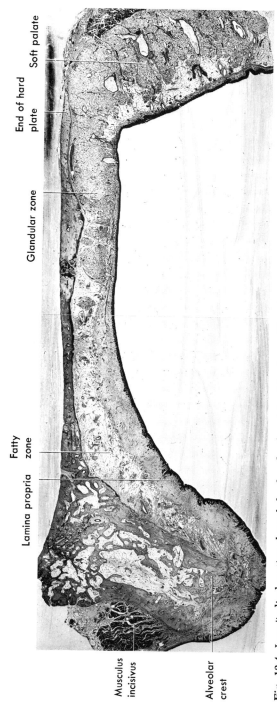

Fig. 13-4. Longitudinal section through hard and soft palates lateral to midline. Fatty and glandular zones of hard palate. (From Sicher and Bhaskar, editors: Orban's oral histology and embryology, ed. 7, St. Louis, 1972, The C. V. Mosby Co.)

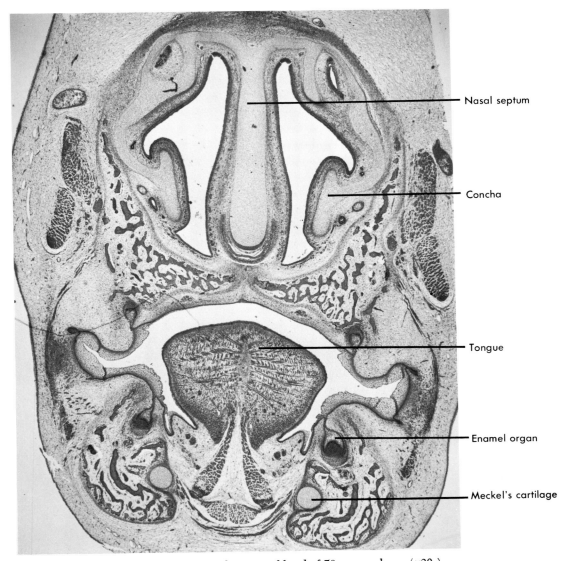

Nasal septum

Concha

Tongue

Enamel organ

Meckel's cartilage

Fig. 13-5. Frontal section of head of 70-mm. embryo. (×20.)

slight constriction at the junction of the crown and root.

The tooth consists of enamel, dentin, and cementum, which are calcified tissues. In addition, each tooth has a vascular connective tissue component, the pulp, located within the pulp cavity.

Early development

The teeth are derived from two embryonic tissues: (1) ectoderm, which gives rise to the enamel, and (2) mesoderm, which gives rise to the dentin, cementum, and pulp and also the supporting tissues.

The dental lamina appears in the human embryo at approximately the sixth week of the gestation period. This lamina is derived from the oral epithelium. It consists of a band of cells that proliferate from the epithelium and extends into the underlying mesenchyme. Taken as a whole, the lamina is U-shaped, following the shape of the jaw

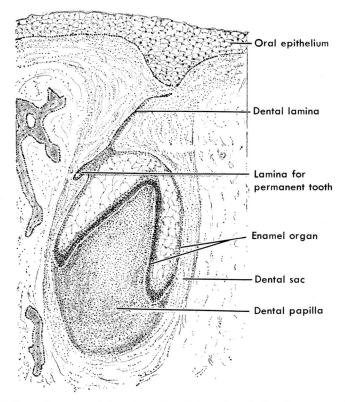

Oral epithelium

Dental lamina

Lamina for
permanent tooth

Enamel organ

Dental sac

Dental papilla

Fig. 13-6. Enamel organ and dental papilla of pig embryo before formation of dentin.

and foreshadowing the shape of the dental arch. There is one labiodental lamina in each jaw (Fig. 13-5).

Soon after the dental lamina is differentiated, one can observe that it is made up of two parts; one part consists of the original lamina, the other of an outgrowth that is inclined away from the tongue and is known as the gingival lamina. Later this lamina hollows out from the oral surface. The tissue located labially gives rise to the inside of the lip, and the tissue located lingually gives rise to the epithelium of the gums; the cavity between the two becomes the vestibule (Fig. 13-5).

Development of enamel organ

In each of the two dental laminae localized proliferations of tissue occur in the region where the future teeth are to form. There are ten of these outgrowths in each jaw; they are known as tooth buds or

germs. These buds lie some distance removed from the oral epithelium and are connected with it by a narrow strand of the dental lamina. The tooth buds are at first rounded and solid. They gradually become invaginated on their distal surface by the invasion of the subjacent mesenchyme. The mesenchyme continues to proliferate, and, eventually, this leads to a rearrangement of the epithelial part of the tooth germ from a solid organ to one that is hollow and goblet shaped. While the change in the external configuration takes place, a differentiation of the tissues in this structure now known as the enamel organ also occurs. The rearrangement and differentiation result in the reestablishment of four distinct parts of the enamel organ: the outer enamel epithelium, the stellate reticulum, the stratum intermedium, and the inner enamel epithelium (Fig. 13-6).

In this stage of development in the

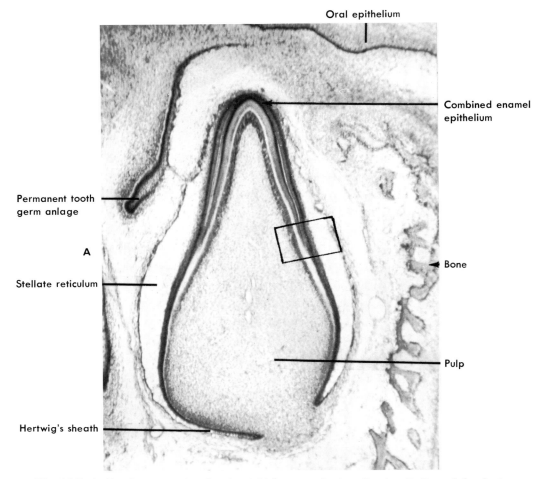

Oral epithelium

Combined enamel epithelium

Permanent tooth germ anlage

A

Bone

Stellate reticulum

Pulp

Hertwig's sheath

Fig. 13-7. A, Developing canine showing initial stages of mineralization. **B,** Part of developing tooth indicated by box in **A,** showing early stages of dentin formation. (×160.)

human being (about 12 weeks), the portion of the dental lamina connecting the enamel organ and the oral epithelium becomes reduced in size and begins to disintegrate. Its distal portion, however, now appears as a small projection on the lingual aspect of the enamel organ and later develops into the anlage for the permanent tooth. Enamel organs of permanent teeth that do not have deciduous predecessors are derived from the original dental lamina in the same manner as the deciduous enamel organs, but at a later time.

Enamel formation. In the fifth to sixth

month of intrauterine life, shortly after dentin has begun to form on the crown of the developing tooth, enamel formation begins (Figs. 13-7 and 13-8). Before this occurs the several layers of cells that comprise the enamel organ come together to form the combined enamel epithelium, which is closely applied to the tip of the crown. The cells that compose the innermost layer, the inner enamel epithelium, have by this time differentiated into tall columnar cells with prominent nuclei, which are located peripheral to the surface that is in contact with the dentin. These

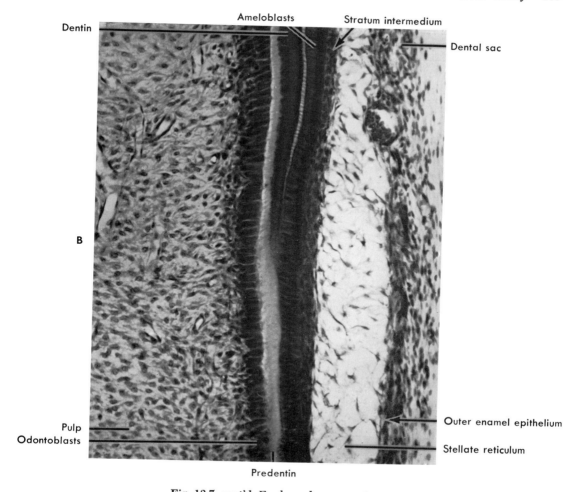

Fig. 13-7, cont'd. For legend see opposite page.

cells, known as ameloblasts, elaborate a rather wide protoplasmic process from the free surface of the cell, Tomes' enamel process, which comes in contact with the dentin. This is the region of the future dentinoenamel junction. In the process of enamel formation this tissue is first laid down at the periphery of dentin and, as more enamel is deposited, the ameloblasts move outward, in a direct opposite to that toward which the odontoblasts move in dentin formation.

The space formerly occupied by Tomes' processes gradually become impregnated with mineral salts; this eventually leads to the production of the fully calcified enamel rod (Fig. 13-9). Between the rods are fine interstices, which also contain calcified material and are known as the interprismatic areas. The process of enamel formation continues until the crown is completely formed. By the time the tooth erupts, the ameloblasts and the other enamel epithelia in the coronal region degenerate, leaving only the enamel cuticle covering the crown.

Mature enamel. Enamel is the hardest tissue in the body. It is approximately 98%

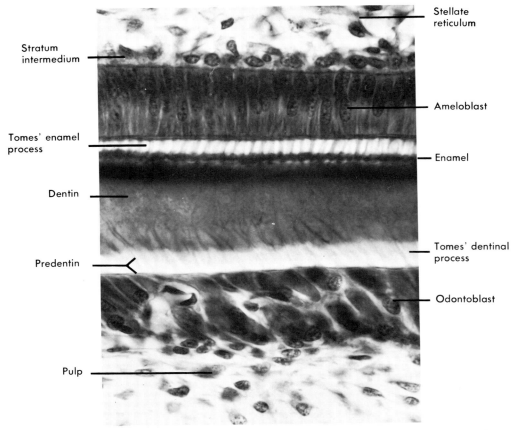

Stellate reticulum

Stratum intermedium

Ameloblast

Tomes' enamel process

Enamel

Dentin

Tomes' dentinal process

Predentin

Odontoblast

Pulp

Fig. 13-8. Section of developing tooth showing formation of dentin and enamel. (×420.)

calcified. It also contains small amounts of keratin and moisture. Enamel covers the crown of the tooth and is whitish in color. It is in contact with dentin, cementum, and the gingiva.

Enamel consists of highly calcified rods or prisms, which are separated by minute amounts of interprismatic substance (Figs. 13-10 and 13-11). The enamel rods extend from the periphery of the dentin to the free surface of the crown. Their direction generally is radial in the region of the tip or the cusp; toward the cervix of the crown, they sometimes form a slight angle with reference to the dentinal tubules. In certain parts of the crown the rods frequently intertwine. When viewed in longitudinal section this enamel appears gnarled. The shape of the enamel rod in cross section varies (Fig. 13-12). It is sometimes hexagonal. Frequently, however, one side may be concave or convex.

Imbrication lines, known as the striae of Retzius, are frequently observed in sections of enamel. They represent modification or change in the degree or rate of mineralization occurring during the formative period of the tooth. These striae originate at the dentinoenamel junction and extend to the free surface of the crown in an arc paralleling the surface of the dentin. In transverse sections of the crown the striae appear concentrically arranged.

Organic material in the form of keratin appears in enamel of most teeth as strands or tufts that originate at the dentino-

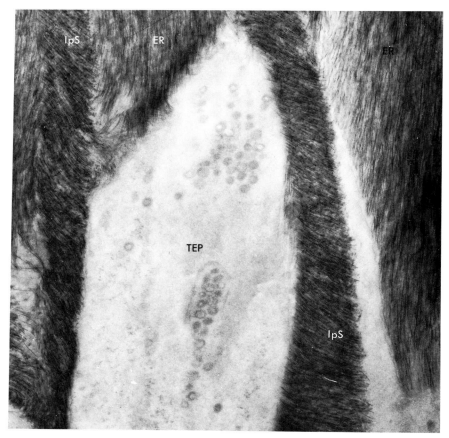

Fig. 13-9. Electron micrograph of developing enamel. *ER,* Enamel rod; *IpS,* interprismatic substance; *TEP,* Tomes' enamel process. (×15,000.) (From Bevelander: Atlas of oral histology and embryology, Philadelphia, 1967, Lea & Febiger.)

enamel junction. This organic component is most readily observed in transverse sections of the crown.

Development of dentin. Dentin is laid down in the developing deciduous tooth just before the appearance of enamel.

The first step in the development of this tissue consists of the formation of reticular fibers, which radiate from the pulp to the distal surface of the inner enamel epithelium. This tissue and other elements incorporated into dentin are derived from the mesenchyme or the primitive pulp. The reticular fibers become arranged radially, first at the tip of the crown and later toward the apex of the developing tooth.

These radially arranged reticular fibers undergo two important changes during the development of dentin: (1) they come to lie within the calcified tissue more or less parallel to the contour lines of the tooth; and (2) they change from reticular to collagenous fibers.

Dentin is first differentiated at the tip of the crown; then it gradually envelops the entire pulp cavity. When dentin is first formed, certain cells, which align themselves along the periphery of the pulp cavity, gradually differentiate into special columnar cells known as odontoblasts. The odontoblasts have a dark-staining, rounded basal nucleus and relatively clear cyto-

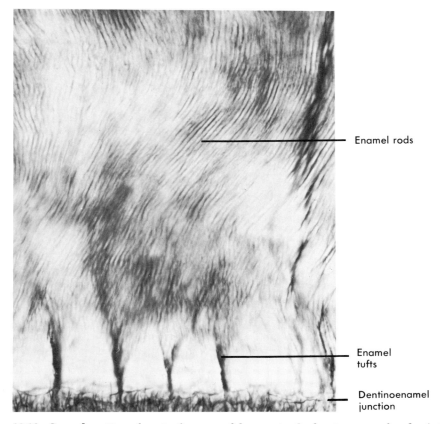

Enamel rods

Enamel tufts

Dentinoenamel junction

Fig. 13-10. Ground section of part of crown of human tooth showing enamel rods. (×420.)

plasm, which stains intensely with eosin. A protoplasmic extension known as Tomes' dentinal process, which comes to occupy a space in the dentin, is elaborated at the free surface of the cell. The basal surface of these cells frequently ends in a blunt tapering projection. In the tip of the crown the layer of odontoblasts is several cells deep. Approaching the apex, the cells thin out until eventually they are arranged in a single epithelioid layer. It is in such an area that they may be most advantageously studied in sections of the developing tooth (Figs. 13-7 and 13-8).

The first dentin, which can be observed in hematoxylin and eosin preparations, appears as a relatively narrow zone of tissue peripheral to the pulp cavity in the coronal region of the tooth. It takes the eosin stain,

and one may observe Tomes' dentinal fibrils occupying a radial position within this tissue. In this, the uncalcified state, it is known as predentin.

After the initial zone of predentin has been established, examination of a slightly later stage in tooth development reveals that a new zone of predentin has formed on the pulpal side of the first increment. During this process the odontoblasts retreat pulpward, retaining meanwhile their connection with the dentin by means of the dentinal fibrils, which lie embedded in the dentin.

While the second zone of predentin forms, the initial, or peripheral, zone undergoes partial calcification. In this process small droplets of bluish staining material appear, which come together to form cal-

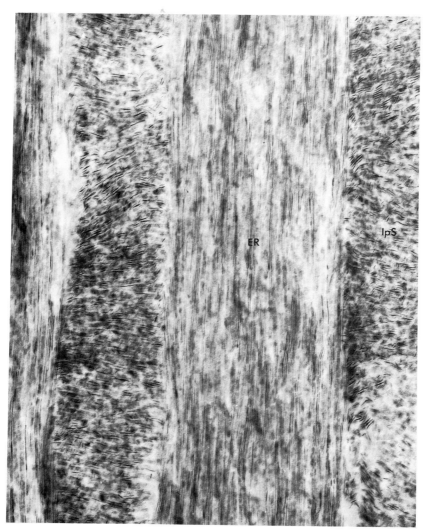

Fig. 13-11. Electron micrograph of longitudinal section of enamel. *ER,* Enamel rod; *IpS,* inter-prismatic substance. (×28,000.) (From Bevelander: Atlas of oral histology and embryology, Philadelphia, 1967, Lea & Febiger.)

Interrod substance Matrix of prism Prism sheath

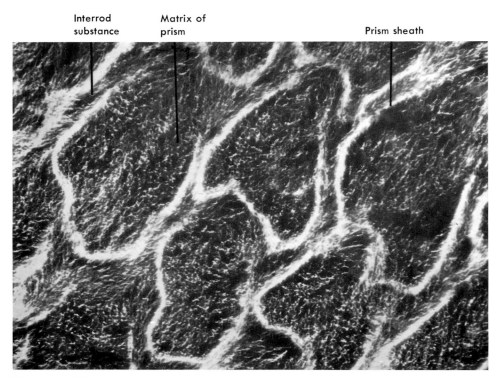

Fig. 13-12. Electron photomicrograph of cross section of demineralized enamel. (×10,000.) (Courtesy Dr. D. Scott, Cleveland, Ohio.)

coglobules. This gives a fairly characteristic globular appearance to calcifying dentin. In the later stages of development the globules usually coalesce to form a tissue that is fairly uniform in appearance.

The dentinal fibrils meanwhile do not calcify. They occupy spaces within the calcified tissue that are known as dentinal tubules (Fig. 13-13).

In comparing the development of enamel with that of dentin, it should be emphasized that enamel is a solid, nontubular tissue, which grows peripherally with reference to the dentin. Unlike dentin, which retains vital connections by means of Tomes' dentinal processes, enamel loses all contact with vital tissues when the tooth erupts. This has an important bearing on the metabolism of these tissues in the erupted tooth.

Mature dentin. Mature dentin is a translucent, compressible tissue consisting of a calcified component (apatite) and an organic component, which is chiefly collagen. It also contains moisture. Examination of a ground section of this tissue reveals a relatively homogeneous translucent calcified tissue (Fig. 13-14). The collagenous fibers that are embedded within this calcified tissue are not visible except in specially prepared sections. Dentin is traversed by numerous tubules, which extend from the pulp to the periphery of the dentin. In the living state these tubules contain Tomes' dentinal processes and tissue fluid. The tubules are arranged in the form of the letter S in the crown. In the root they are relatively straight. Before they terminate, the tubules branch dichotomously into from two to four branches. As the tubules traverse the dentin, they also give off many lateral side branches known as tubuli; some of these later connect with tubuli or adjacent tubules. The

Peritubular dentin   Matrix   Dentinal tubule

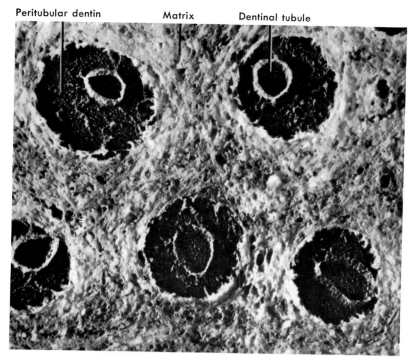

Fig. 13-13. Electron photomicrograph of demineralized section of dentin. (×5,000.) (Courtesy Dr. D. Scott, Cleveland, Ohio.)

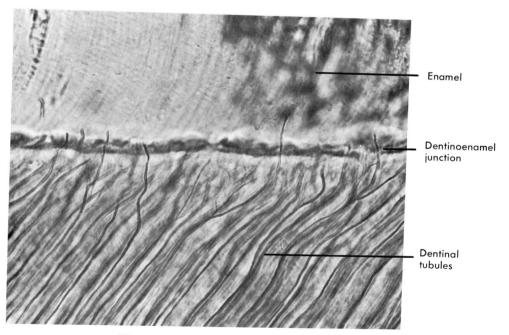

Enamel

Dentinoenamel junction

Dentinal tubules

Fig. 13-14. Ground section of human dentin. (×640.)

tubiculi are best shown in ground sections stained with silver nitrate. In decalcified sections stained with hematoxylin and eosin, a dark zone surrounds the dentinal tubules, called Neumann's sheath.

Variations. On the periphery of the root, one may observe in ground sections of a tooth an imperfectly calcified zone of dentin, which, because of its characteristic appearance, is known as Tomes' granular layer. Imbrication lines, also known as the lines of Owen, are also frequently observed in dentin. They are rather wide bands of dentin, which follow the contour of the tooth and have a less dense appearance in section. They probably indicate disturbances in metabolism during the formation of dentin.

More extensive variations in the appearance of dentin may also be observed in many teeth that have developed under conditions of faulty mineral metabolism. These areas in the dentin are readily seen in ground sections of teeth and are most commonly observed in the crown just below the dentinoenamel junction. This tissue is known as interglobular dentin and represents areas practically devoid of calcified materials. The scallop-edged areas appear black in ground section.

Abrasion of tooth surfaces and caries also produce variations in the histologic appearance of dentin. In the former situation the dentin in contact with an abraded area usually becomes nonvital or sclerosed, and in both of these situations an irregular variety of the tissue known as secondary dentin may be deposited on the margin of the pulp cavity in an apparent attempt to protect pulp tissues.

Cementum

Cementum is a calcified tissue that forms a thin shell around the periphery of the root. In origin, appearance, and composition it closely resembles bone. It is first formed in the cervical part of the tooth; gradually it encloses the entire root.

There are two varieties of cementum: (1) primary, or cell free, which appears hyaline in ground sections and usually occurs on the coronal part of the root (Fig. 13-15); and (2) secondary, or cellular, which is deposited later than primary cementum and occupies a position on the periphery of the apical third of the root. In ground sections of the tooth, one observes a hyaline calcified tissue in which scattered cells, cementoblasts, occupy a space within lacunae—much as in sections of bone. The fibers of the peridental membrane, which suspend the tooth in the socket, are firmly anchored to the root of the tooth by means of cementum.

Pulp

Pulp is essentially a connective tissue organ. In ordinary sections the pulp in the young tooth is extremely cellular. The appearance of the pulp cells is similar to that of fibroblasts. Histiocytes also have been described as being present in the pulp. As the tooth increases in age the character of the pulp changes: the relative number of cells decreases, and the fibers increase.

Odontoblasts, previously referred to, occupy a position on the periphery of the pulp. These cells constantly retreat pulpward as dentin is slowly deposited throughout the life of the tooth. In the mature tooth the region just below the odontoblasts may have fewer cells than other parts of the pulp, and it is known as the cell-poor zone of Weil.

The pulp tissue contains an abundant nerve and vascular supply.

Gingiva

The gingiva is the modified part of the oral mucous membrane that covers the surface of the alveolus (Fig. 13-16). It is attached to the tooth at the level at which the tooth is inserted into the oral cavity. It consists of two parts: (1) dense connective tissue, the lamina propria, and (2) a covering of stratified squamous epithelium.

The tissues that make up the gingivae are normally attached to the alveolus and to the tooth surfaces. The undersurface of the epithelium is frequently thrown into folds or pegs. The outer surface usually shows a slight degree of cornification. The chief function of this tissue is protective.

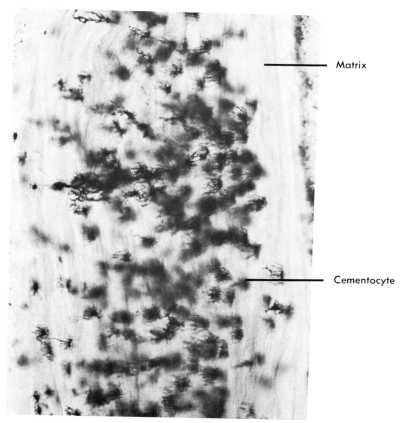

Matrix

Cementocyte

Fig. 13-15. Ground section of human cementum. (×420.)

The following parts of the gingivae are usually recognizable in sections: (1) the outer border of the gingiva, known as the gingival margin; (2) the gingival crevice, a space of variable size between the tooth surface and the gingiva; (3) the epithelial attachment, a strip of stratified squamous epithelium, which originates at the approximate level of the cementoenamel junction. It is attached to the tooth at this level and continues up to the free margin of the gingiva. For some considerable distance, it is in intimate contact with the cervical part of the crown. With advancing age this tissue migrates rootward.

PERIDENTAL LIGAMENT

Peridental ligament is a term used to designate a group of collagenous fibers that suspend the tooth in the socket and support the gingivae. The fibers occupy a space between the bony socket or alveolus, on the one hand, and the periphery of the root, on the other. Above the level of the alveolus, the fibers run up to the gingiva. They also connect the cervical parts of adjacent teeth.

The fibers concerned with the suspension of the tooth and support of the gingivae are known as principal fibers. They are relatively short fibers that, in the region of the root, are arranged horizontally or obliquely with reference to the long axis of the tooth.

Other fibers, known as interstitial fibers, occur in the peridental space as isolated islands of connective tissue in which one may observe in section the vessels and

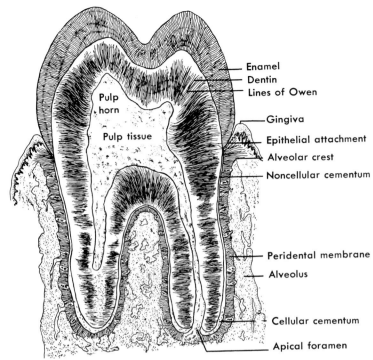

Enamel
Dentin
Lines of Owen

Pulp horn

Gingiva
Epithelial attachment
Alveolar crest
Noncellular cementum

Pulp tissue

Peridental membrane
Alveolus

Cellular cementum

Apical foramen

Fig. 13-16. Section of human maxillary molar cut buccolingually to show general relationships of tooth and surrounding tissues.

nerves that supply this tissue. Clusters of dark-staining cells, the epithelial rests, may frequently be seen in the peridental ligament. They are remnants of the enamel epithelium.

ALVEOLUS

The alveolus, or socket, is the bony crypt in which the tooth is suspended (Fig. 13-16). The alveolus proper consists of a thin lamina of bone, which surrounds the root just peripheral to the peridental ligament. This plate is made up of compact bone. The distal ends of the fibers of the peridental ligament are firmly cemented into this tissue. Between the compact bone making up the alveolus and the external parts of the jaw are numerous trabeculae of supporting bone, which are advantageously arranged to take up the stresses that the teeth transmit to the bone surrounding them.

TONGUE

The tongue is primarily a muscular organ. It is covered with a mucous membrane (Fig. 13-17), parts of which are modified to conform to its function as an organ of mastication and of taste.

The muscles of the tongue are in three main groups: longitudinal, transverse, and sagittal fibers, arranged in interlacing groups and embedded in areolar and adipose tissue.

The mucosa covering the dorsal surface of the tongue is modified to form a great number of elevations, or papillae. It should be noted that these papillae are different from the projections of connective tissue of the epithelium, which have been mentioned in descriptions of the parts of the oral mucosa. The papillae of the tongue are elevations of both connective tissue and epithelium. Within each of them there also may be projections of the tunica

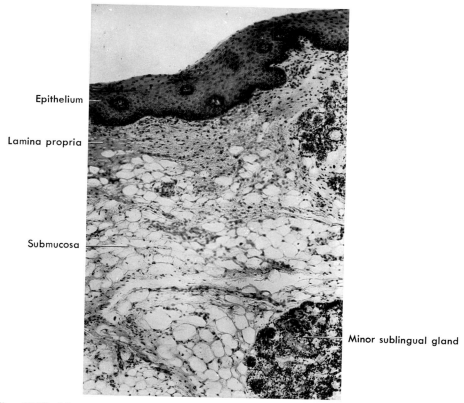

Epithelium

Lamina propria

Submucosa

Minor sublingual gland

Fig. 13-17. Mucous membrane from floor of mouth. (From Sicher and Bhaskar, editors: Orban's oral histology and embryology, ed. 7, St. Louis, 1972, The C. V. Mosby Co.)

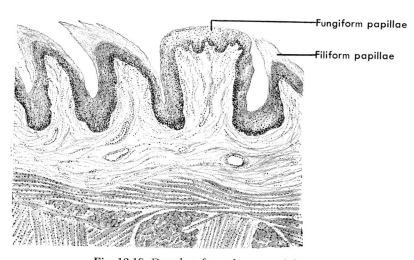

Fungiform papillae

Filiform papillae

Fig. 13-18. Dorsal surface of tongue of dog.

propria into the epithelium, which are termed secondary papillae. The distribution and characteristic forms of the papillae of the tongue are filiform, fungiform, foliate, and vallate.

Filiform papillae

Filiform papillae are the most numerous of the papillae and are distributed over the entire dorsal surface of the tongue. Each consists of a conical elevation of the tunica propria and stratified squamous epithelium. The whole papilla is inclined in an anteroposterior direction. Its surface epithelium is cornified, the cornification extending in strands, which gives this type of papilla its name (threadlike) (Fig. 13-18).

Fungiform papillae

Fungiform papillae are distributed unevenly among the filiform papillae on the dorsal surface of the tongue, being most numerous near the margin of the organ but never as numerous as the filiform variety. They are club shaped, with flattened free surfaces, and have a diameter somewhat greater than that of the basal portion of a filiform papilla. The epithelium covering them shows little, if any, cornification and is relatively thin. This, combined with the fact that they have a rich blood supply, gives them a red color in the living state. Their secondary papillae are a characteristic feature of these structures (Fig. 13-18). Taste buds are sometimes visible on

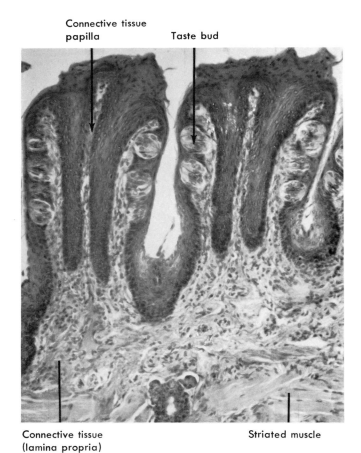

Connective tissue papilla   Taste bud

Connective tissue (lamina propria)   Striated muscle

Fig. 13-19. Foliate papilla of rabbit tongue showing taste buds. (×160.)

the free surfaces of fungiform papillae but are small and not always noticeable.

Foliate papillae

Foliate papillae are well developed on the tongues of certain rodents but are rudimentary in man. When fully developed they have some features in common with fungiform papillae, being club shaped with flat tops. The types are readily distinguishable, however, by the following facts: (1) the foliate papillae occur in groups along the lateral margins of the tongue and are not intermingled with filiform papillae; (2) they have numerous prominent taste buds set close together along their sides; and (3) they are characterized by the presence of the secondary connective tissue papillae, which occupy approximately three fourth of the depth of the primary papilla. Lingual glands occur in the same part of the tongue as do the filate papillae (Figs. 13-19 and 13-20).

Vallate (circumvallate) papillae

Vallate (circumvallate) papillae are the largest papillae of the tongue and the least numerous. There are only twenty to thirty of them, arranged along the sulcus terminalis, and they are so large that they are macroscopically visible. Each projects but a short distance above the surface of the tongue but is, as the name implies, surrounded by a deep groove (Fig. 13-21). Their secondary papillae are short and usually occur only on the surface. The outstanding characteristics, aside from their size and positions, are: (1) the walls of the grooves surrounding them are beset with large taste buds and (2) the grooves serve as the point of exit for the ducts of conspicuous serous glands, which are present in this part of the tongue (Ebner's glands).

The taste buds are composed of two kinds of cells: the specialized taste cells and the supporting cells. In ordinary sections the two kinds may be distinguished

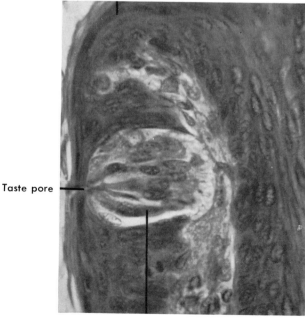

Stratified squamous epithelium

Taste pore

Cell in taste bud

Fig. 13-20. Taste bud showing pore. (×640.)

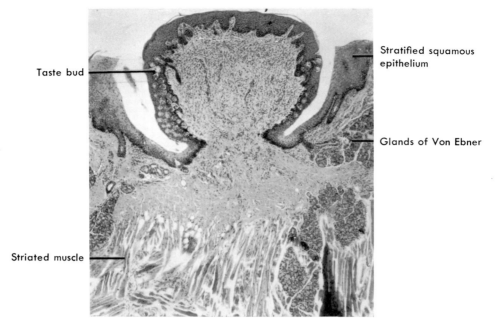

Taste bud

Stratified squamous
epithelium

Glands of Von Ebner

Striated muscle

Fig. 13-21. Section through circumvallate papilla. (×40.)

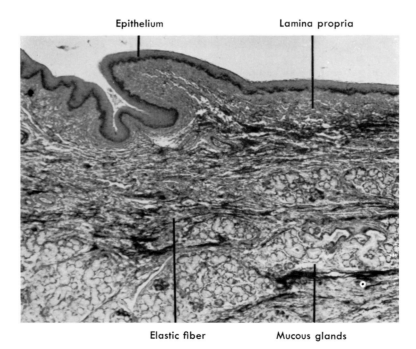

Epithelium

Lamina propria

Elastic fiber

Mucous glands

Fig. 13-22. Longitudinal section of laryngeal portion of pharynx of dog. (×16.)

by their nuclei, those of the taste cells being dark and spindle shaped and those of the supporting cells pale and round or oval. The taste bud as a whole is a flask-shaped structure lying in the epithelium and opening onto the surface through a minute circular pore (Fig. 13-20). In specimens treated with silver nitrate, nerve fibers may be traced into the center of the buds.

The ventral surface of the tongue is covered by mucous membrane not unlike that lining the lips and cheeks (Fig. 13-17). In all parts of the organ the interlacing bands of striated muscle are a characteristic feature. In regions where glands occur, their secreting portions lie in the connective tissue, which forms a stroma around the muscles, producing an arrangement of glandular and muscular tissue not often seen in other organs. It may be said that the tongue has no submucosa, this layer being replaced by a mixture of connective tissue, muscle, and glands.

GLANDS OF THE ORAL CAVITY

Saliva, the fluid in the oral cavity, is secreted principally by three large glands, the parotid, the submaxillary, and the sublingual, which lie outside the lining of the cavity and communicate with it by means of large ducts. Contributions to the saliva are also made by numerous smaller glands that are situated in the submucosa of some parts of the wall of the oral cavity and among the muscles of the tongue. They are of three kinds, serous, mucous, and seromucous, and are located as follows:

1. The serous glands are located in the tongue, in the region of the vallate papillae (Ebner's).
2. The mucous glands are located on the anterior surface of the soft palate (palatine), on the hard palate, on the borders near the foliate papillae (lingual) of the tongue, and on the root of the tongue.
3. The seromucous glands are located on the anterior portion (anterior lingual) of the tongue and on the lips (labial).

Posterior to the sulcus terminalis there are no papillae on the dorsal surface of the tongue. It is covered by stratified squamous epithelium like that lining the remainder of the cavity at this point. The tunica propria consists of reticular tissue and contains condensations of lymphoid tissue and the palatine and lingual tonsils described in Chapter 8. Mucous glands are present in the submucosa of the fauces.

PHARYNX

The oral cavity opens through the *fauces* into the oropharynx. This region is only partly separated from the upper respiratory region or *nasopharynx* by the soft palate and the uvula. The latter abuts on the *pharyngeal tonsils* (adenoids). At the level of the hyoid bone the oropharynx merges into the *laryngeal pharynx*, which in turn leads to the epiglottis of the respiratory system and the esophagus of the digestive system.

The pharynx is thus the meeting place for the nasal passages, oral cavity, larynx, and esophagus. Histologically the pharynx takes on the mixed characteristics of all these structures (Fig. 13-22).

The nasopharynx has a lining characteristic of the respiratory tract, that is, a pseudostratified epithelium and a tunica propria that is separated from the submucosa by an elastic membrane. This region will be described in Chapter 16.

The oropharynx and laryngopharynx are intermediate in composition, as they are in position between the oral cavity and the esophagus. They are lined with nonkeratinized stratified squamous epithelium and have a lamina propria containing numerous elastic fibers, some of which form an incomplete membrane at the border of the mucosa. Branches of this elastic lamina also extend between groups of muscle bundles (Fig. 13-22).

In the superior lateral regions of the pharynx the submucosa may be of considerable extent and contain the secreting portions of mucous glands. In some parts of the pharynx, however, the elastic membrane of the mucosa rests immediately on the muscular layer, in which situation the glands occupy a position between the strands of muscle, similar to the pattern found in the tongue. The arrangement described has given rise to the statement that the pharynx has no submucosa. It is obvious, however, that in a transitional region such as the pharynx different conditions obtain at different levels of the organ. Sections of the laryngopharynx are, in fact, difficult to distinguish from sections of the upper part of the esophagus, especially since the elastic lamina is thoroughly dispersed in this region.

The muscular layer of the pharyngeal wall consists of bundles of striated muscle obliquely arranged to form a constrictor. The bundles interlace and form irregular layers.

14

Digestive tract

The digestive tract is a hollow tube running from the oral civity to the anus, modified in its various parts but consisting throughout of four coats or layers: mucosa, submucosa, muscularis, and adventitia or serosa (Fig. 14-1).

Mucosa. The mucosa is made up of (1) an epithelial lining that borders on the lumen of the tract and rests upon (2) a lamina propria of reticular or fine areolar tissue. The lamina propria may contain glands, scattered fibers of smooth muscle, and lymph nodules. The nodules are often quite large, extending below the mucosa into the adjacent coat of the tract. Fine capillaries and lymphatics are present in the lamina propria. In the greater part of the digestive tube the mucosa includes a third layer, (3) the muscularis mucosae, which is a thin coat of smooth muscle fibers.

Submucosa. The second coat of the wall is the submucosa. This is composed of areolar tissue, which contains a plexus of small blood vessels known as Heller's plexus. It also includes numerous lymphatics and a plexus of nerves (Meissner's plexus). In the esophagus and the duodenum the submucosa contains the end pieces of mucous glands. In other parts of

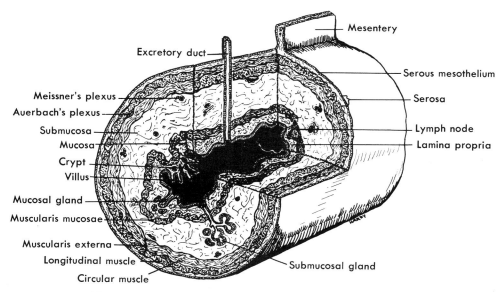

Fig. 14-1. Stereogram of general plan of gastrointestinal tract.

175

the tube, lymphoid tissue extends from the mucosa into the submucosa.

Muscularis. The muscularis is composed of two layers of muscle. The fibers of the inner coat are arranged circularly about the tube, whereas those of the outer coat lie in its long axis. This arrangement is followed throughout the tract, but in the stomach there is a third oblique layer, next to the submucosa. Thickenings of the circular layer form sphincters at various points of the tract. In the upper end of the esophagus and the lower end of the rectum the muscle is striated; elsewhere it is smooth. The two layers of muscle are separated by a thin layer of connective tissue in which may be seen the myenteric (Auerbach's) plexus of nerves.

Adventitia or serosa. The adventitia or serosa, the fourth layer of the tract, is composed of loose areolar tissue frequently containing adipose tissue. Where the tract borders on the body cavity the areolar tissue is covered by the mesothelium and is called the serosa. Elsewhere it blends with the surrounding fascia and is called the adventitia.

The coats of the digestive tract are summarized as follows:

1. Mucosa
   a. Epithelium
   b. Lamina propria containing:
      Glands°
      Lymphoid tissue
      Scattered muscle fibers
      Capillaries and small lymphatics
      Muscularis mucosae
2. Submucosa
   a. Areolar tissue containing:
      Glands
      Lymphoid tissue
      Heller's plexus of blood vessels
      Meissner's plexus of nerves
      Lymphatics
3. Muscularis
   a. *Oblique layer*
   b. Circular layer
   c. Connective tissue containing Auerbach's plexus of nerves
   d. Longitudinal layer
4. Adventitia or serosa
   a. Areolar tissue containing:

°Italics indicate the structures present in some but not all divisions of the digestive tract.

Lamina propria   Lumen   Muscularis mucosae

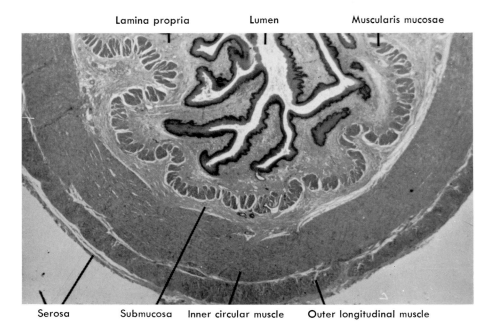

Serosa   Submucosa   Inner circular muscle   Outer longitudinal muscle

Fig. 14-2. Transverse section of esophagus of dog. (×16.)

Adipose tissue
Blood vessels
Mesothelial covering

ESOPHAGUS

Mucosa. The esophageal region of the mucosa of the digestive tract is distinguished from the remainder by the fact that it is lined with stratified squamous epithelium, which rests upon a fairly thick lamina propria (Fig. 14-3). In many mammals the epithelium is cornified at its surface. Two narrow zones of glands are present in the mucosa of the esophagus, one at its junction with the stomach and the other at the level of the cricoid cartilage. These glands, called superficial glands (cardiac), are shallow branching tubules that secrete mucus into the lumen of the organ. The mucosa also contains small lymph nodules and scattered lymphoid tissue.

The muscularis mucosae is absent in the upper part of the esophagus, its place being taken by a rather indefinite elastic membrane, which separates the mucosa from the submucosa (Fig. 14-2). Smooth muscle first appears about one fourth of the way down the tube in the form of scattered bundles longitudinally arranged. Farther down the tract these are consolidated in a complete layer. Unique features of the muscularis mucosa of the esophagus are that it is thicker than in any other part of the digestive tract and that the fibers run in only one direction.

Submucosa. The submucosa of the esophagus is generally described as a layer of areolar tissue containing throughout its length blood vessels, nerves, and the secreting portion of mucous glands, the ducts of which run through the mucosa to open onto the epithelial surface. As a matter of fact the glands are not constant in their distribution, and some animals (for example, the monkey) have only a few in this layer.

Muscularis. In the upper half of the esophagus the muscle is striated like that of the tongue. It is not, however, under voluntary control. In the lower half of the esophagus the muscle changes to the

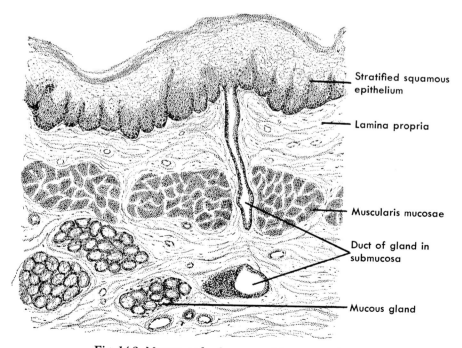

Stratified squamous epithelium

Lamina propria

Muscularis mucosae

Duct of gland in submucosa

Mucous gland

Fig. 14-3. Mucosa and submucosa of human esophagus.

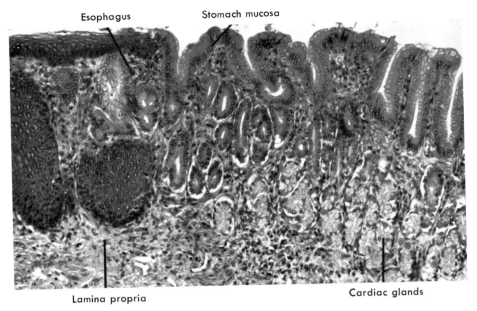

Fig. 14-4. Gastroesophageal junction in dog. (×160.)

smooth variety; in the middle portion the two kinds may be found intermingled. The arrangement of the muscular coats of the esophagus is less regular than that of other parts of the digestive tract. Two coats are present, but both may have the fibers obliquely placed so that the typical orientation in any inner circular and outer longitudinal layer may not be apparent. This is particularly true in the esophagus of the dog.

The mucosa and submucosa of the esophagus are illustrated in Figs. 14-2 and 14-3. Particular attention is called to the wide lumina of the ducts, which lead from the glands of the submucosa to the surface.

STOMACH

Mucosa. At the junction of the esophagus and stomach the lining epithelium changes abruptly from stratified squamous to simple columnar (Fig. 14-4), the cells of which secrete mucus. The epithelium of the stomach, unlike that of the small intestine, does not have a cuticular border. The surface of the mucosa is thrown into folds (rugae), the height and number of which

depend on the degree of distention of the organ. In addition to the rugae the surface of the mucosa is marked by closely set pits, which are lined with the same type of epithelium (Fig. 14-5). Beneath the epithelium there is a lamina propria of reticular or fine areolar tissue, and below the level of the pits this layer contains glands. The shape and proportionate depth of the pits and the characteristics of the glands are different in different parts of the stomach. At the junction of the esophagus and stomach the pits are shallow, and the glands, which are lined with a simple cuboidal epithelium, have wide lumina and secrete thin mucus (Fig. 14-6).

In the fundic region (Fig. 14-7) the mucosa is much deeper than in the zone immediately below the esophagus and it contains a greater number of glands. The lamina propria is reduced to a fine interglandular stroma in its deeper portion, and the pits extend only about one fourth of the distance from the surface to the muscularis mucosae. The glands are called fundic glands, or, since they are found in all parts of the organ except the cardiac and pyloric

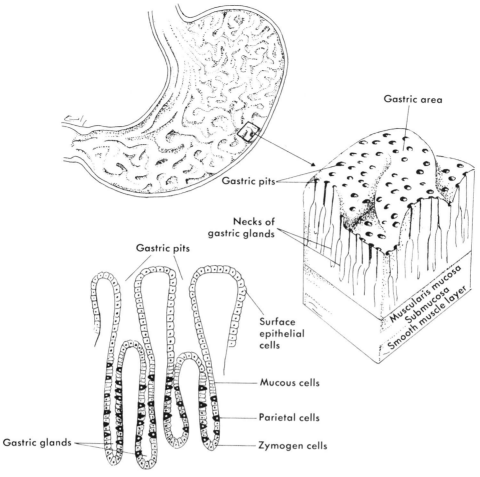

Gastric area

Gastric pits

Necks of
gastric glands

Muscularis mucosa
Submucosa
Smooth muscle layer

Gastric pits

Surface
epithelial
cells

Mucous cells

Parietal cells

Gastric glands

Zymogen cells

Fig. 14-5. Diagram showing folding of stomach mucosa and detail of a gastric area and gastric pits. A section through a gastric gland is shown on the lower left. (Drawing by Emily Craig.)

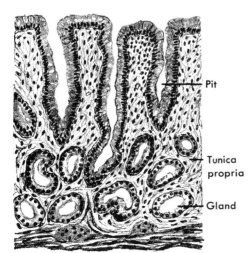

Pit

Tunica
propria

Gland

Fig. 14-6. Mucosa of cardiac region of stomach of monkey.

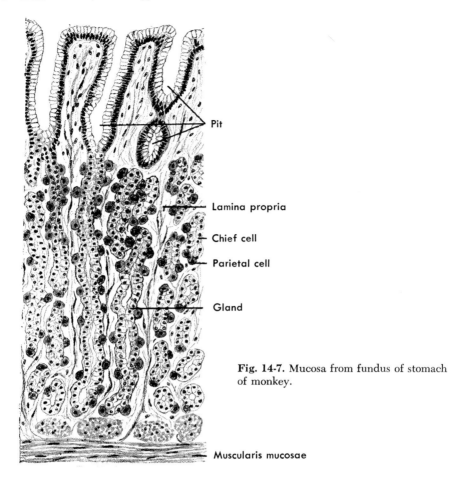

Pit

Lamina propria

Chief cell

Parietal cell

Gland

Muscularis mucosae

Fig. 14-7. Mucosa from fundus of stomach of monkey.

zones, they may be called gastric glands.

The surface mucous cells cover the entire surface and line the pits. They are columnar cells with nuclei located in the basal region. With routine preparations the apical cytoplasm stains faintly and has a foamy appearance. The electron microscope shows dense elliptical secretory granules in the apical part of the cell (Fig. 14-8). Each gastric gland is composed of four kinds of cells: (1) chief (peptic) cells, (2) parietal or oxyntic cells, (3) neck mucous cells, and (4) argentaffin cells.

The chief cells (Fig. 14-9) line the lower part of the gastric glands. They are of the low columnar variety and have the appearance of typical serous cells. These cells con-

tain abundant striated basophilic material corresponding to the cisternae of the endoplasmic reticulum. They also exhibit numerous mitochondria and secretory granules containing the precursor of pepsin.

The parietal cells are relatively large and intensely acidophilic. They are most numerous at the neck of the gland. They do not border directly on the lumen but are crowded away from it by the chief cells. The parietal cells appear somewhat oval, with the narrow end directed toward the lumen. These cells elaborate the antecedent of hydrochloric acid and are believed to elaborate the *intrinsic* factor in humans. At the electron microscope level, it has been shown that the cytoplasm contains numer-

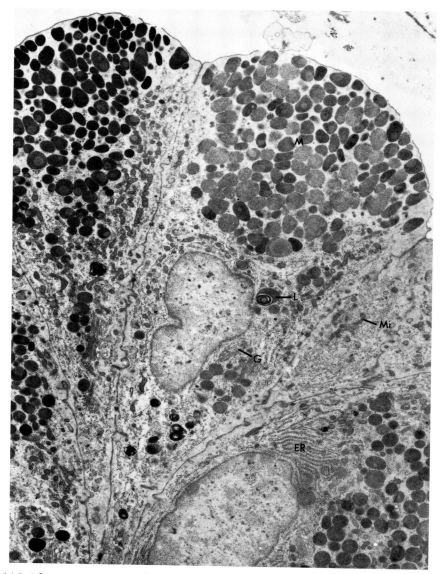

Fig. 14-8. Electron micrograph of surface cells of stomach of mouse. These cells are columnar and contain numerous mucinogen granules, *M*, at the distal surface. *ER,* Endoplasmic reticulum; *G,* Golgi apparatus; *L,* lysosomes; *Mi,* mitochondrion. (×9,000.)

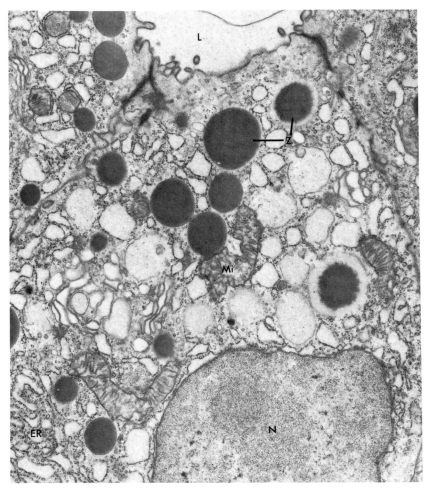

Fig. 14-9. Electron micrograph of apical part of a chief (zymogen) cell of gastric gland of mouse. *ER*, Rough endoplasmic reticulum; *L*, lumen; *Mi*, mitochondrion; *N*, nucleus; *Z*, zymogen granule. (×16,000.)

ous mitochondria and surface indentations, the secretory canaliculi (Fig. 14-10). The surfaces of the canaliculi are lined with microvilli.

The neck mucous cells are relatively few in number, have a wide base, and taper in the apical region. They are smaller than the surface cells and exhibit a considerable amount of basophilia. The mucous droplets in these cells, as shown by the electron microscope, are larger and less dense than those of the surface cells, and they are distributed deep in the cell as well as in the apical region.

The argentaffin cells are few and are scattered between the basement membrane and the chief cells. They contain characteristic granules, which are clearly shown in electron micrographs (Fig. 14-11). The granules are believed to contain serotonin, a vasoconstrictor that stimulates the contraction of smooth muscle. The nucleus is markedly infolded.

In the pyloric region the pits are relatively deep, extending at least halfway to the muscularis mucosae (Fig. 14-12). They are V shaped, tapering off into the glands that open into them. The glands in this

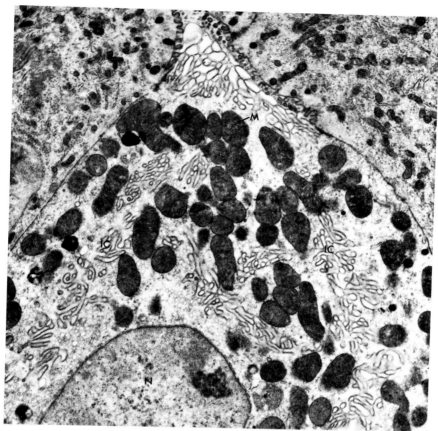

Fig. 14-10. Electron micrograph of a parietal cell of mouse gastric mucosa. The extensive intracellular secretory canaliculae, *IC*, within the cell exhibit numerous irregularly oriented microvilli. *N*, Nucleus; *M*, mitochondrion. (×15,000.) (Courtesy Dr. S. Luse, New York, N. Y.)

portion of the stomach are composed of large mucus-secreting cells and have wide lumina. No parietal cells exist in the pyloric glands except in the transition zone, where they merge with glands of the gastric type.

The muscularis mucosae of all parts of the stomach is a complete layer of smooth muscle, which includes both the circular and the longitudinal fibers.

Submucosa. The submucosa is composed of areolar tissue and does not contain glands in any part of the stomach. In a section of the junction of the esophagus and stomach some of the end pieces of

deep mucous glands may extend into the submucosa of the stomach, but, since their ducts open into the esophagus, they should be considered as part of the wall of the latter organ. Small arteries, veins, and lymphatics may easily be seen in the submucosa. Meissner's plexus of nerves and ganglia is less conspicuous.

Muscularis. In the stomach the muscular coat consists of two complete layers (inner circular and outer longitudinal), with an incomplete layer of obliquely arranged fibers between the circular layer and the submucosa. The circular layer is by far

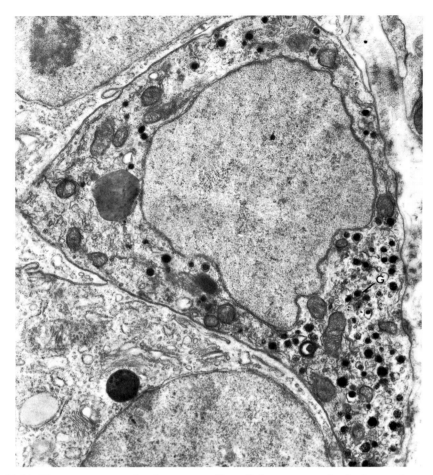

Fig. 14-11. Electron micrograph of an argentaffin cell from gastric gland of mouse's intestine. The argentaffin cell contains numerous dense spherical granules, G, enclosed by a membrane. (×15,000.) (Courtesy Dr. S. Luse, New York, N. Y.)

the thickest of the three coats. The arrangement of fibers is somewhat irregular, and it may be difficult to distinguish the three coats of the muscularis in a microscopic section of this region. Auerbach's plexus is present between the circular and longitudinal fibers.

Serosa. The greater part of the stomach is covered with a layer of mesothelium located outside the loose connective tissue that invests the muscle layers. This is, however, usually destroyed in the preparation of the piece of tissue for sectioning, so that all that is seen of the serosa is a coating of areolar tissue containing blood vessels, adipose tissue, and occasional nerve trunks.

SMALL INTESTINE

The small intestine extends from the pyloric part of the stomach to the large intestine. Its inner surface may be seen, on gross examination, to be marked by the presence of ridges that are circularly disposed and that extend into the lumen throughout this part of the tract. These ridges are the plicae circulares. Each consists of a projection of the connective tissue of the submucosa covered by the mucosa.

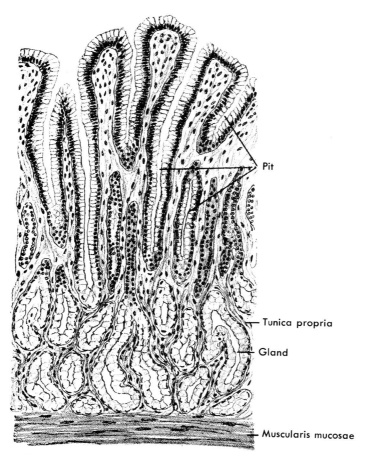

Pit

Tunica propria

Gland

Muscularis mucosae

Fig. 14-12. Mucosa from pyloric region of stomach of monkey.

The plicae circulares provide a greater surface for the absorption of food.

Mucosa. The mucosal surface is still further increased by the presence of minute fingerlike projections of epithelium and lamina propria, which cover the surface of each plica. These villi are hardly visible to the naked eye (Fig. 14-13).

Villi. Under the microscope each villus is seen to consist of a projection of the lamina propria covered by simple columnar epithelium and scattered goblet cells. The lamina propria is reticular tissue and contains capillaries, lymphatics, and scattered muscle fibers. In an injected specimen, it is apparent that the vessels have a definite plan of distribution. In each villus is a central lymphatic called a lacteal (Figs. 14-14 and 14-15), into which certain lipids from the tract are absorbed. An arteriole enters the villus at one side and breaks up into capillaries at the distal end. Blood is collected from the capillaries by a venule, which passes out along the side opposite that occupied by the arteriole. Villi occur in all parts of the small intestine and are its most characteristic feature. In the duodenum, they are leafshaped; in the jejunum, tall and somewhat enlarged or forked at their distal ends. The ileum has shorter, club-shaped villi. Other parts of the tract have projections that at first sight might be mistaken for villi. In the stomach, for instance, the tissue between two pits

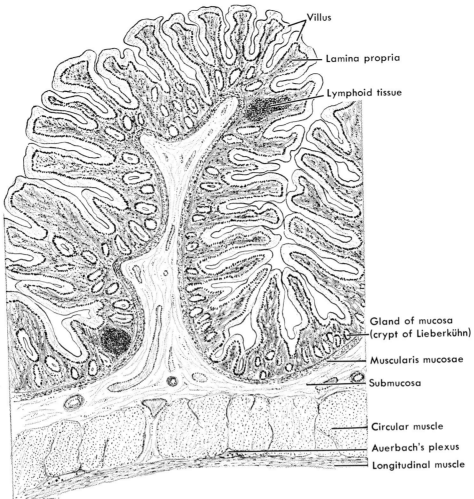

Fig. 14-13. Longitudinal section of jejunum of monkey showing a plica circularis.

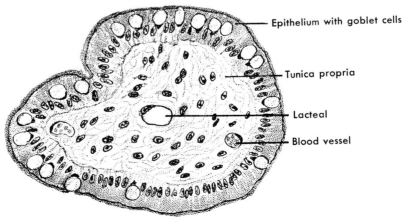

Fig. 14-14. Transverse section of a villus.

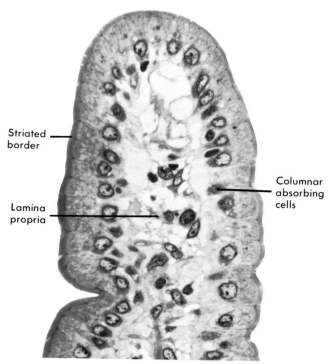

Striated border

Lamina propria

Columnar absorbing cells

Fig. 14-15. Photomicrograph of a villus from the small intestine of a mouse. Striated border on surface of epithelium is typical of absorbing cells. (×640.)

has somewhat the same form as a villus and consists of a mass of reticular tissue covered by columnar epithelium. Closer examination reveals, however, that the organization of vessels that is characteristic of a villus is lacking in the stomach.

The lining cells of the small intestine are of the tall columnar variety, having round or oval nuclei located in the basal part of the cell. With the light microscope (Fig. 14-15), it is possible to observe a striated border at the free surface, which has been shown to consist of minute fingerlike extensions, the microvilli, arranged in parallel arrays (Fig. 14-16). This specialization increases the surface and is characteristic of absorptive cells. At or near the free surface are terminal bars. Also present are the Golgi apparatus and numerous mitochondria. The endoplasmic reticulum is abundant and of the smooth variety.

Glands. Between the bases of the villi, glands extend into the lower part of the

mucosa (Fig. 14-17). These are the intestinal glands (crypts of Lieberkühn). At the base of each gland is a group of cells, the cells of Paneth, which are somewhat larger than the surrounding cells and have paler nuclei (Figs. 14-18 and 14-19). Their cytoplasm is sometimes darker, sometimes lighter, than that of the surrounding cells. Cells similar to the Paneth cells have been found in other parts of the digestive tract, but it is in the small intestine that they are most numerous and therefore most easily found.

It has long been assumed that Paneth cells secrete enzymes. It appears that cell secretion is related in some way to amino acid and protein metabolism since in children with severe protein nutrition (kwashiorkor) Paneth cells are markedly reduced or absent. These cells reappear when nutrition is restored to normal. There is at present no evidence that Paneth cells do secrete digestive enzymes, and in fact the

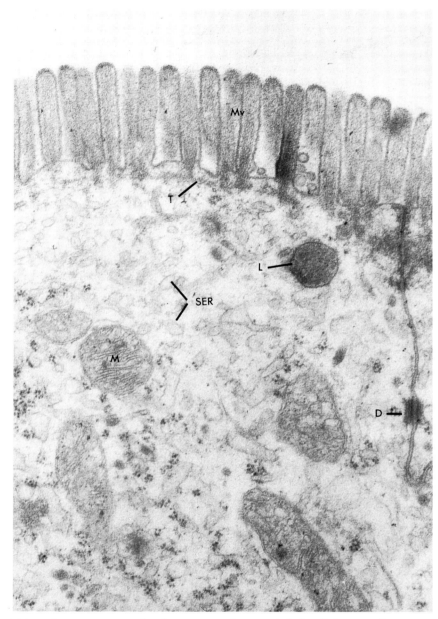

Fig. 14-16. Electron micrograph of a portion of an epithelial cell from small intestine of a mouse. *D*, Desmosome; *L*, lysosome; *M*, mitochondrion; *Mv*, microvilli; *SER*, smooth endoplasmic reticulum; *T*, terminal web. (×48,000.)

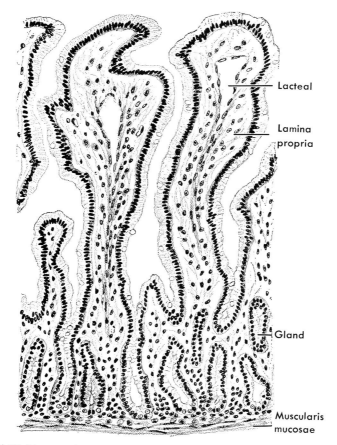

Fig. 14-17. Mucosa of jejunum of monkey showing villi and crypts of Lieberkühn.

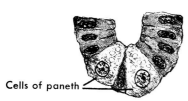

Fig. 14-18. Epithelium at base of a crypt of Lieberkühn.

burden of information suggests that the cells may be involved in some other aspect of digestion. They are more numerous in the ileum than in the upper parts of the small intestine.

The rest of the crypt is lined with columnar epithelium somewhat resembling that which covers the villi. Its cells, however, are not quite as tall as those covering the villi, and fewer of them are goblet cells. Special stains bring out the fact that some of the lining cells have an affinity for silver stains, but this type (argentaffin cells) is not distinguishable when stained with hematoxylin and eosin. Like the cells of Paneth, argentaffin cells occur in other parts of the gut as well as in the small intestine. The cells of the crypts provide new cells for the villi surfaces to replace those shed into the lumen. It has been estimated that the villus surface is renewed every few days in humans.

Lymphoid tissue. Lymphoid tissue is widely distributed throughout the mucosa

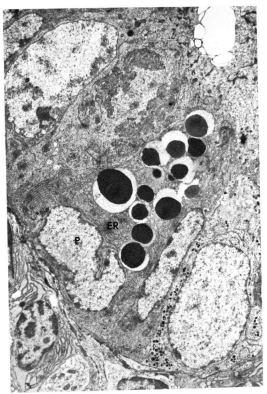

Fig. 14-19. Electron micrograph of several cells at the base of an intestinal gland of the mouse. Cell with prominent dark granules. *P*, Paneth cell; *ER*, endoplasmic reticulum. (×6,700.)

of the small intestine. In the ileum the nodules are gathered into groups (Peyer's patches) and fill not only the mucosa but also the submucosa. These groups of nodules will be further described later in this discussion.

Muscularis mucosae. The muscularis mucosae consists of two thin layers of smooth muscle, an inner circular and an outer longitudinal layer. It thus repeats in miniature the arrangement of the muscularis coat.

Submucosa. The submucosa of the intestinal wall is different in the three divisions of the small intestine. Its basis is the same throughout, a layer of areolar tissue containing the vessels and nerves of Heller's and Meissner's plexuses, respectively. In the duodenum the layer contains,

in addition, groups of mucous glands. These are duodenal glands of Brunner (Fig. 14-20). Their secretion, which is mucus like that formed in the cardiac glands of the stomach, enters the duodenum through ducts, which open on the surface between the crypts of Lieberkühn or into the crypts themselves. These glands are thought to secrete a fluid that aids in protecting the duodenal surface from the acidic contents of the stomach as they enter the duodenum. In adults, these glands do not extend much beyond the mouth of the duct of Wirsung, through which the pancreas empties its buffered secretions into the duodenum. In the ileum, groups of lymph nodules occupy both mucosa and submucosa (Fig. 14-21). Each group consists of from ten to sixty nodules with germinal centers, and the groups are so large that they are visible to the naked eye. They not only fill the submucosa and the mucosa but also extend a little into the lumen of the intestine, obliterating the villi. They are called Peyer's patches or the aggregate lymph nodules of the intestine. Similar aggregates may be present in the lower part of the jejunum, but the majority of the sections from this part of the tract have only a small amount of lymphoid tissue in them. Glands are never found in the submucosa of the jejunum. It is characterized by its exceptionally high branching plicae circulares and its long villi.

Muscularis. The muscularis of the small intestine consists, throughout its length, of an inner circular and an outer longitudinal layer of smooth muscle. Between these, as in other parts of the tract, lies Auerbach's plexus of nerves.

Serosa. As in the stomach, the serosa is a layer of connective tissue covered by mesothelium.

LARGE INTESTINE

In the large intestine the plicae circulares are replaced by the semilunar folds, which include not only the mucosa and submucosa but also the inner layer of the muscularis and are grossly visible on the outside, as well as on the inside, of the gut. As the name implies, they are crescentic in shape,

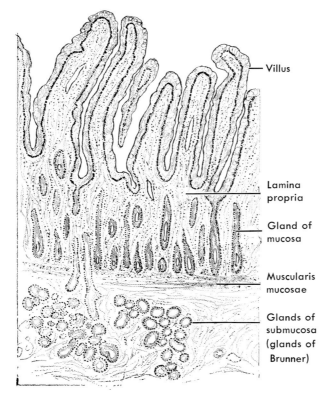

Villus

Lamina propria

Gland of mucosa

Muscularis mucosae

Glands of submucosa (glands of Brunner)

Fig. 14-20. Mucosa and submucosa of duodenum of monkey.

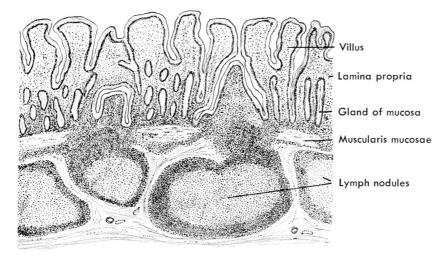

Villus

Lamina propria

Gland of mucosa

Muscularis mucosae

Lymph nodules

Fig. 14-21. Mucosa and submucosa of ileum showing Peyer's patches.

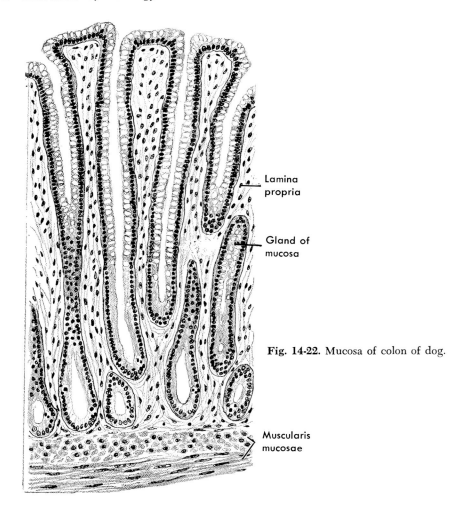

Lamina propria

Gland of mucosa

Fig. 14-22. Mucosa of colon of dog.

Muscularis mucosae

each one extending about one third of the way around the wall of the large intestine. Following is a description of the characteristics of the four coats of this region.

Mucosa (Fig. 14-22). Water is absorbed from the large intestine, and its lining is well supplied with mucus-secreting cells. It has no villi. In the embryo villi are present in the large intestine, but they disappear during late fetal life. The epithelium consists of simple columnar absorbing cells and numerous goblet cells. The lamina propria contains many glands. These are simple tubular glands, closely set, lined with epithelium like that which covers the surface of the mucosa. They have very few

cells of Paneth in them. The lamina propria contains blood and lymph capillaries, but these are not organized in definite units like those of the small intestine. Solitary lymph nodules are present and are often so large that they break through into the submucosa. The muscularis mucosae is composed of an inner circular and an outer longitudinal layer (Figs. 14-22 and 14-23), as in the small intestine.

Submucosa. The submucosa of the colon has no glands in it. Besides the areolar tissue with vessels and nerves, it contains only the solitary lymph nodules mentioned previously.

Muscularis. The inner circular layer of

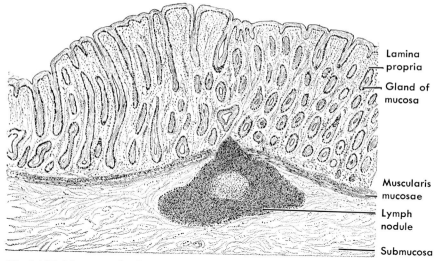

Fig. 14-23. Mucosa and submucosa of colon of dog showing a solitary lymph nodule.

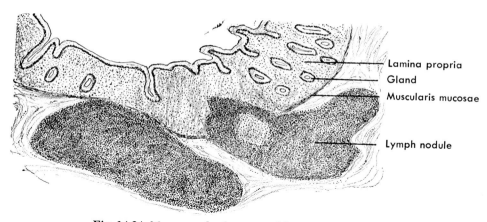

Fig. 14-24. Mucosa and submucosa of human appendix.

the muscularis is continuous around the wall and is thrown into folds with the mucosa and submucosa. The longitudinal layer is in the form of three bands, which run through the length of the large intestine. These are called the taeniae coli. When dissected away from the rest of the wall they are found to be considerably shorter than the wall, and this difference in length produces the semilunar fold in the longer parts. The effect of the taeniae is like that of a drawstring run through a piece of cloth.

Serosa. The serosa contains large deposits of adipose tissues, which protrude on the outer surface of the tube and are macroscopically visible as the appendices epiploicae.

VERMIFORM APPENDIX

The wall of the vermiform appendix resembles that of the colon but is thickened

Table 3. Peculiarities in parts of digestive tract

	Mucosa	Submucosa	Muscularis
Esophagus	Stratified squamous epithelium Glands confined to two narrow zones Muscularis mucosae lacking in upper part	Mucous glands	Striated in upper part
Stomach	Cardiac—Shallow pits 　　　　Mucous glands Fundus—Pits elongated 　　　　Fundic (gastric) 　　　　Glands prominent Pyloris—Pits relatively deep 　　　　Glands mucous type		Oblique layer of muscle inside circular layer
Duodenum	Villi; leaflike	Mucous glands; plicae are low	
Jejunum	Villi; tall	Tall branching plicae	
Ileum	Villi; club-shaped	Large groups of lymphoid nodules	
Colon	No pits or villi Many goblet cells in epithelium		Longitudinal muscle arranged in three bands
Appendix	No pits or villi; much lymphoid tissue	Much lymphoid tissue	
Rectum	Like colon; stratified squamous		
Anus	Noncornified, stratified squamous epithelium		Internal circular muscle forms internal sphincter

by accumulations of lymphoid tissue (Fig. 14-24).

Mucosa. The epithelium of the mucosa is simple columnar and in the normal appendix is highly folded. Extending from the surface are simple tubular glands containing numerous mucus-secreting and occasional Paneth cells. Argentaffin cells are a frequent occurrence in the middle third of the wall of the crypts. The lamina propria contains an accumulation of lymphoid follicles resembling those of the pharyngeal tonsils and, like the latter, may show inflammatory changes. In a condition of subacute inflammation of the appendix, the lumen may be narrowed or obliterated and the mucosa replaced in part by fibrous scar tissue and confluent nodules of lymphoid tissue. This condition will be seen rather frequently. The muscularis mucosae is interrupted by the lymph nodules and in places is reduced to only a few strands of muscle. The mucosa of the appendix is

basically arranged like that of the colon except that the glands are less numerous and the lymph nodules more prevalent in the appendix.

Submucosa. The submucosa is composed of areolar tissue with vessels, nerves, and lymphoid tissue.

Muscularis. The muscularis is composed of two complete layers, as in other parts of the tract.

Serosa. The serosa presents no exceptional features.

The peculiarities of the different parts of the digestive tract that may be used as diagnostic features in identifying sections are presented in Table 3.

RECTUM AND ANUS

The rectum is divided into an upper and a lower part. The upper part extends from the third sacral vertebra to the diaphragm of the pelvis. The mucosa of the upper part is similar to that of the colon. The crypts

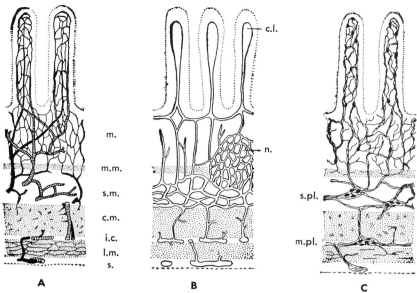

Fig. 14-25. A, Diagram of blood vessels of small intestine; the arteries appear as coarse black lines; the capillaries as fine ones; and the veins are shaded. (After Mall.) **B,** Diagram of lymphatic vessels. (After Mall.) **C,** Diagram of nerves based upon Golgi preparations. (After Cajal.) The layers of the intestine: *m,* mucosa; *mm,* muscularis mucosae; *sm,* submucosa; *cm,* circular muscle; *ic,* intermuscular connective tissue; *lm,* longitudinal muscle; *s,* serosa; *cl,* central lymphatic; *n,* nodule; *spl,* submucous plexus; *mpl,* myenteric plexus. (From Bremer and Weatherford: Text-book of histology, Philadelphia, 1948, The Blakiston Co.)

of Lieberkühn are, however, longer and contain many goblet cells. The muscularis mucosa, submucosa, and circularly arranged smooth muscle are also similar to those of the colon. The taeniae coli, however, spread out and form a continuous layer, which is much thickened in the dorsal and ventral surface of the gut wall.

The surface of the lower part of the rectum (anal canal) is thrown into several longitudinal folds known as the rectal columns (of Morgagni). At the lower termination these folds unite with one another to form the anal valves. At the level of the anal valves, the epithelium becomes stratified squamous of a noncornified variety. The noncornified epithelium extends nearly to the anal orifice, where it changes to stratified squamous, characteristic of the epidermis. At the level of the anal orifice, hairs, sweat glands, and sebaceous glands occur. The sweat glands are of two types. One type has the structure characteristic of glands found in various parts of the body, the second type (circumanal) is large and resembles the axillary sweat glands.

At the approximate level of the anal valves, the muscularis mucosae becomes much diminished and eventually is lacking entirely. The submucosa contains an abundant supply of arteries and veins. The inner circular layer of the muscularis of the anal canal is composed of smooth muscle, is relatively thick, and serves as the internal anal sphincter. The outer longitudinal layer of smooth muscle continues over the internal sphincter and attaches to connective tissue. Also present is an external sphincter composed of striated muscle lying internal to another sphincter, the levator ani.

BLOOD SUPPLY OF STOMACH AND INTESTINES

The arteries that supply the gut pass through the mesentery to reach the serosa where they branch into smaller vessels. The latter continue through the two coats of the muscularis to the submucosa, where they form an extensive plexus (Heller's plexus). From the plexus of the submucosa, blood passes to the mucosa and to the muscular coat of the gut (Fig. 14-25).

NERVE SUPPLY OF STOMACH AND INTESTINES

The nerve supply of the stomach and intestines consists chiefly of nonmedullated and medullated (preganglionic) fibers of the autonomic system. When the nerves reach the connective tissue between the two layers of the muscularis coat, they are associated with ganglion cells to form the plexus of Auerbach. From the plexus, fibers pass to the submucosa where they form another plexus, Meissner's plexus.

LYMPHOID TISSUE IN THE GUT MUCOSA

Few tissues have such a dense or diverse accumulation of lymphoid cells as the gut. These cell groups can be divided into three categories: lymphoid follicles, accumulations of plasma cells, and epithelial lymphoid cells (the theliolymphocytes). The lymphoid follicles occur in the mucosa or submucosa throughout the entire extent of the gut. They are most prominent, however, in the lower ileum (Peyer's patches),

the appendix, and the nasopharyngeal adenoid tissue. The theliolymphocytes can be observed between the epithelial cells in the basal third of the lining of the gut, especially in the small intestine. The lymphoid follicles and the theliolymphocytes (which are thought to be young lymphocytes returning to the lamina propria via the bloodstream) are said to be the equivalent of the bursa of Fabricius, a hindgut lymphoid organ present in birds that appears to be involved in the development of the immunoglobulin-producing system (*humoral immunity*). In contrast, the thymus is held responsible for controlling the development of *cell-mediated immunity*. Plasma cells are uniformly scattered in the lamina propria of the villi and between the glandular crypts as well, especially in the duodenum, jejunum, and colon. Most of the plasma cells produce immunoglobulin A (IgA) in contrast to cells of the lymph nodes and spleen, which produce mostly immunoglobulin G (IgG). It has been suggested that these plasma cells respond to local antigenic stimulation since IgA production is scant or lacking in germ-free animals, a situation that is reversed when animals are placed on a septic diet. The function of IgA is not well understood. There is, however, some suggestion that these molecules may be bactericidal.

15

Glands associated with the digestive tract

In addition to the glands situated in the wall of the digestive tract, large masses of glandular tissue lie outside the limits of the tube and pour their secretion into it through ducts. These are the salivary glands, the ducts of which open into the oral cavity, and the pancreas and liver, secretions of which go to the intestine. The pancreas resembles the salivary glands and is most conveniently studied in connection with them. The gallbladder will also be included in this discussion.

SALIVARY GLANDS AND PANCREAS

Because microscopically the tissues of the salivary glands closely resemble those of the pancreas, they are discussed in the same section of this chapter. Differentiation between the two is discussed on p. 211 and in Figs. 15-1 and 15-2.

Salivary glands

The salivary glands consist of several glandular structures that secrete a fluid known as *saliva.* Numerous small glands are located in the oral mucous membrane. The secretions of these glands serve to moisten and lubricate the membrane. In addition, three pairs of large glands are situated some distance from the oral cavity. These structures, usually known as the salivary glands proper, are the parotid, submaxillary (submandibular), and sublingual glands. In the human, the parotid gland has only serous alveoli; the submaxillary and sublingual glands have both serous

and mucous alveoli. Accordingly, the parotid glands are classified as serous, the palatine glands as mucous, and the submaxillary and sublingual glands as mixed.

Saliva assists in the process of chewing by dissolving readily soluble components of the food, initiating digestion of starch (via salivary amylase), softening the food mass, and coating the mass with a lubricant film. Saliva also contains substances (such as IgA) that discourage bacterial growth and thus may help to suppress tooth decay. Although the amount of antibodies in saliva is small, over 1,200 ml. of saliva is secreted per day, containing a total of about 250 mg. of immunoglobulin.

The salivary glands consist of the glandular tissue proper, also known as the *parenchyma,* and a supporting interstitial connective tissue framework, the *stroma.* The connective tissue septa divides the glands nective tissue septa divides the glands into units known as lobes and lobules. Collecting ducts and vascular and nerve elements are located in the septa.

PAROTID GLAND

As will be seen from Figs. 15-1 to 15-3, the parotid has excretory, secretory, and intercalated ducts, which lead out from serous alveoli. The arrangement of these elements in sequence is not as clear in sections as it is in Fig. 15-1. Numerous alveoli with intercalary and secretory ducts are crowded together to form a lobule. A fine connective tissue stroma, often contain-

197

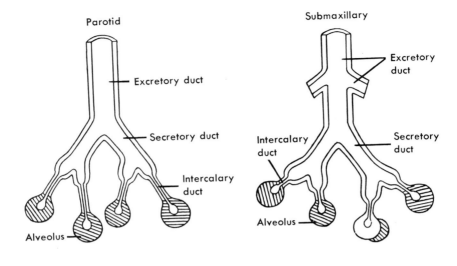

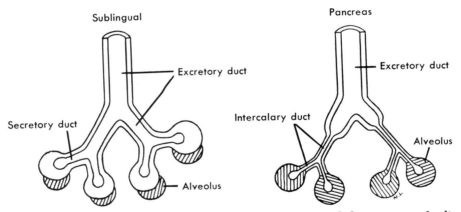

Fig. 15-1. Diagram to show composition of secreting portions and duct systems of salivary glands and pancreas. Alveoli and crescents that are shaded are serous cells; those unshaded are mucous cells.

ing fat cells, surrounds the alveoli, and a heavier sheath of the same tissue separates adjacent lobules. A group of lobules forms a lobe, which is, in turn, covered with a connective tissue sheath that mingles at the outer borders of the gland with the surrounding fascia. Within the lobule the alveoli and ducts are cut in various directions, and their connections are not always clear. One may, however, find a group of alveoli through which the plane of section has passed vertically, and in such a case the arrangement is visible.

Several alveoli open together into a fine duct called the intercalary duct. This tubule is composed of flattened cells. Several intercalary ducts open into a tubule lined with columnar epithelium, the secretory (striated) duct. The cells lining this branch of the duct system show, under special treatment, striations in the basal part of the cytoplasm, which are supposed to be indicative of secretory activity. These ducts open, in turn, into excretory ducts, which are lined with tall columnar epithelium. As one traces these ducts toward

Secretory duct

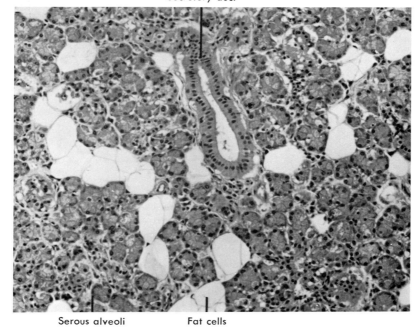

Serous alveoli   Fat cells

Fig. 15-2. Section of human parotid gland. (×160.)

Serous alveolus

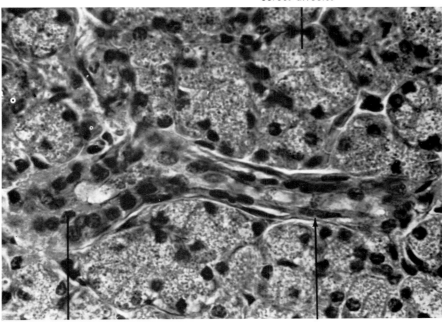

Secretory duct   Intercalary duct

Fig. 15-3. Human parotid. (×640.)

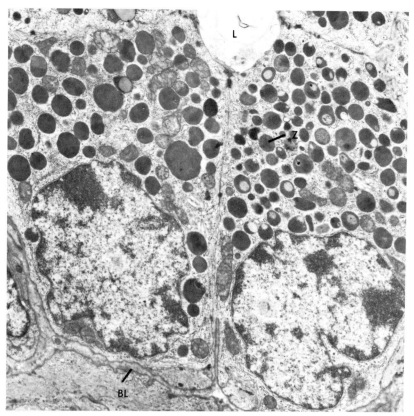

Fig. 15-4. Electron micrograph of two acinar cells of Rhesus parotid. *BL,* Basement lamina; *Z,* zymogen granules; *L,* lumen of acinus. (×9,400.)

the opening into the oral cavity, the epithelium is seen to change first to pseudostratified, then to columnar, and finally to stratified squamous.

The end pieces or alveoli are composed entirely of serous cells, which are wedge shaped and grouped about a small lumen. The cell boundaries are usually indistinct. The appearance of the cells varies considerably depending upon the state of activity. In the resting condition, numerous granules appear in the distal portion of the cell. After secretion, the number of granules is reduced while the number of vacuoles is increased. The fate of these vacuoles is uncertain since the membrane material does not appear to be recycled for use in new secretory granules. These granules, which are refractile, are known as *zymogen gran-*

ules and are concerned with the elaboration of the enzyme produced by the cell (Fig. 15-4).

In addition to mitochondria and a Golgi apparatus, which are common to secreting cells, a constituent of the cytoplasm known as the *chromatophilic material* (ergastoplasm), appearing as a group of membranes adjacent to the nuclei, is also an important cytologic component of the serous cells. The granules associated with the membranes are strongly basophilic, are composed of ribonucleoprotein, and are associated with the synthesis of proteins within the cells, such as zymogen granules.

With the aid of special techniques, delicate *intercellular secretory canaliculi* may be demonstrated in serous alveoli. These canaliculi appear to penetrate the cells themselves and are then known as the *intracellular secretory canaliculi*. They are common to serous alveoli. An additional element demonstrated by special methods is a peculiar stellate-shaped cell occupying a position between the secreting cells and the basement membrane. Closely associated with the secreting cells, their processes form a basketlike structure around the alveolus. The function of these *basket*, or myoepithelial, cells is not well established although they are thought to be contractile and to be involved in some way in secretion.

Fine structure of acinar cells. The parotid is a serous type of gland and the pyramid-shaped cells rest upon a well-defined basement lamina. The nucleus is prominent, irregularly shaped, and basally located. In favorable sections, a cytocentrum is observed in a supranuclear position and close to the Golgi apparatus. Profiles of rough endoplasmic reticulum cisternae are numerous and scattered throughout the cytoplasm. Mitochondria are few and are usually located in the distal part of the cell. The most prominent feature of the cytoplasm is the presence of numerous, large, spherical secretory granules containing the precursor of amylase, which is concerned with the digestion of carbohydrates. The cells lie in close apposition to one another, and desmosomes occasionally occur where the cells appose each other. The distal surface that forms the border of the lumen of the acinus subtends small microvilli (Fig. 15-4).

The process of secretion. Cells concerned with the elaboration of proteins released from the cell contain elaborate cellular machinery for secretion. Studies in pancreatic acinar cells have shown that synthesis of protein occurs on ribosomes associated with the endoplasmic reticulum. These proteins are transported to the Golgi apparatus. In cells such as liver cells that manufacture sugar-containing proteins (glycoproteins), the carbohydrate molecules are added sequentially as the protein passes to the Golgi apparatus. In the liver, for instance, N-acetyl glucosamine is incorporated while the nascent protein is still on the ribosomes. Mannose and galactose are added after the protein has left the ribosomes and is in passage to the Golgi apparatus. A main function of the Golgi complex is to produce secretory vesicles whose membranes resemble those of the plasma membrane. The Golgi membranes are usually stacked in a curved layer. At one surface of the stack (the maturing or distal face) there are developing secretory granules. At the opposite face there are collections of small vesicles that appear to be coalescing to form new Golgi membranes. The evidence suggests that the manufacture of protein secretions and the package that contains them (the secretory granule) takes place as an assembly line process. Details of the process vary, but all protein-secreting cells have a number of structural and functional features in common. Some final modification of the secretory product probably occurs in the secretory granules.

Secretion appears to occur by a process called *exocytosis* in which secretory granules fuse with the cell surface, open, and release their contents.

SUBMAXILLARY GLANDS

As in the parotid glands, there are excretory, secretory, and intercalary ducts in the submaxillary gland (Figs. 15-1 and 15-5), but the last named are short and difficult to find. The alveoli are of two kinds. Many are pure serous, like those of the parotid; others are mixed serous and mucous (Figs. 15-6 and 15-7). The mucous cells of a mixed alveolus are grouped around the lumen and are distinguished from the serous cells by their paler cytoplasm and their basal, flattened nuclei. The serous cells are arranged in the form of a cap outside the mucous cells. They do not border on the lumen of the alveolus but pour their secretion into it through minute channels between the mucous cells. Such groups of serous cells are often crescent shaped in sections and are called demilunes of Heidenhain. In the submaxillary gland, which has many purely serous alveoli, the demilunes of the mixed alveoli are small.

The mucous cells occurring in either the mixed or pure mucous alveoli are modi-

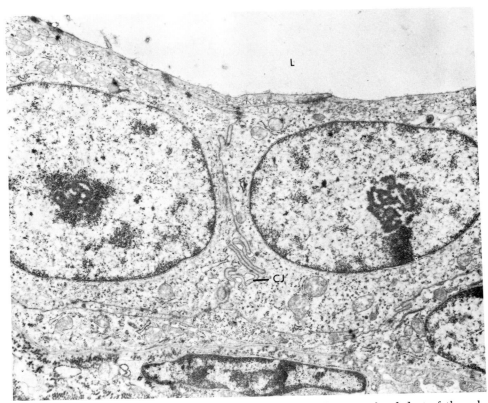

Fig. 15-5. Electron micrograph of part of the epithelium of the intercalated duct of the submaxillary gland of the cat. These cells are of the low cuboidal type, having large centrally placed nuclei and prominent cell junctions, *CJ;* lumen, *L.* (×12,000.)

fied cuboidal or low columnar cells and when stained with hematoxylin and eosin appear as follows: the cells rest upon a fine reticular basement membrane, and in this resting condition their nuclei appear flattened and occupy a position near the base of the cell. The cytoplasm appears pale blue in contrast to the deeper blue or purple coloration of the serous cells. The cytoplasm contains a basophilic network and numerous granules. In the active condition, the granules enlarge and become droplets, which may occupy a considerable portion of the cell. During secretion, the droplets of mucin are discharged and the cell returns to the resting state. Mitochondria and the Golgi apparatus are not prominent features of these cells, and intracellular canaliculi are lacking.

SUBLINGUAL GLANDS

The duct system of the sublingual glands differs from that of the other salivary glands in that the intercalary ducts are usually lacking entirely and the striated or salivary ducts are few in number (Figs. 15-8 and 15-9). The overall appearance of a section of this gland shows it to be a mixed gland, predominantly mucous in character (Figs. 15-9 and 15-10). The terminal alveoli are usually mucous. Pure serous alveoli are infrequently present. However, large serous cells in the form of demilunes surrounding mucous alveoli are numerous. This gland does not have a distinct capsule.

BLOOD AND NERVE SUPPLY

The salivary glands have a relatively rich blood supply consisting of arteries, veins,

Serous alveolus   Salivary duct

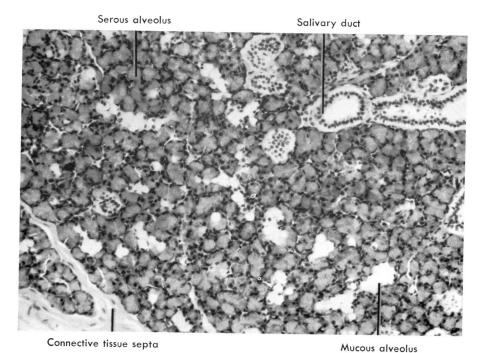

Connective tissue septa   Mucous alveolus

Fig. 15-6. Mixed salivary gland (submaxillary) of cat, serous type. (×40.)

Serous alveolus

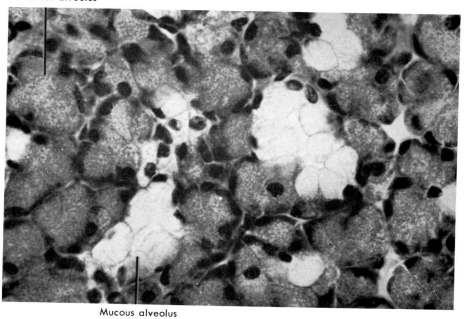

Mucous alveolus

Fig. 15-7. Mixed salivary gland (submaxillary) of cat, chiefly serous alveoli. (×640.)

Salivary duct

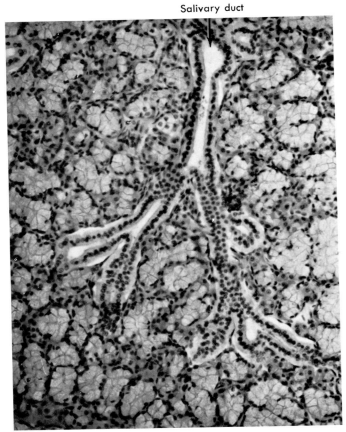

Fig. 15-8. Mixed salivary gland, sublingual, of dog, chiefly of mucous alveoli together with ducts in septa. (×200.)

and lymphatics, which run in the connective tissue septa along with the ducts. The arteries branch into capillary networks where they eventually surround the alveoli. The innervation of the salivary glands is complicated and involves fibers of the sympathetic and parasympathetic systems.

Physiology of salivation

The flow of saliva is regulated by nerves of the autonomic nervous system. Both sets of nerves, parasympathetic and sympathetic, are able to affect the secretory process, which occurs reflexly. The primary centers of secretion are the salivatory nuclei located in the medulla oblongata. Higher regions of the central nervous system can excite or inhibit the medullary reflexes as

shown by the classic studies of Pavlov on conditioning this reflex in dogs. Mechanical stimulation of the oral cavity and the presence of most types of food or highly seasoned substances evoke salivation reflexly. Since saliva can be secreted against pressure, it is now generally agreed that saliva formation is the result of some metabolic process. Electrolytes presumably are transported from the plasma to saliva by duct cells, and some ions are selectively resorbed along the ducts. Water, mucus, and protein are probably contributed by the acinar portions of the gland. The secretory process is very complex, and there is little evidence at this time that specific histologic cell types have selective functions.

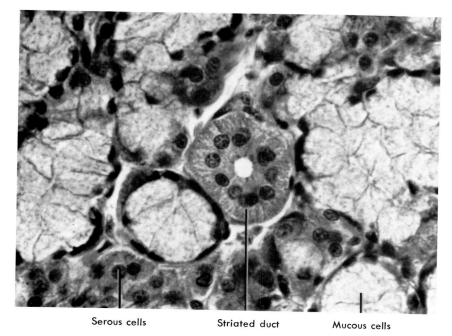

Serous cells   Striated duct   Mucous cells

Fig. 15-9. Mixed sublingual gland in dog. (×640.)

Pancreas

The pancreas is really a union of two organs having entirely different functions. These are the pancreatic tissue proper and the islands of Langerhans. If the entire pancreas is removed from an animal, diabetic symptoms occur, which indicate a disturbance of the carbohydrate metabolism. If, however, the pancreatic duct is ligated, the alveoli degenerate but the islands of Langerhans are unharmed. In this case there is no disturbance of carbohydrate metabolism. It is thus clear that the two kinds of tissue have entirely different functions. The alveoli compose a gland of external secretion, forming an alkaline fluid containing enzymes used in digestion (trypsin, amylase, lipase). The islands are glands of internal secretion (endocrine glands) producing hormones: insulin, glucagon, and gastrin.

The pancreas has long intercalary ducts, which lead directly into excretory ducts without the intervention of a secretory portion (Fig. 15-1). The alveoli are shorter and rounder than are those of the parotid and are composed of pyramidal cells resting upon a basement membrane. The basal portion of the cells appear basophilic, while the apical portion is characterized by the appearance of *zymogen granules,* their number depending upon the functional state of the cell (Fig. 15-11).

A peculiar feature of the pancreatic alveoli is the presence of one or more small epithelial cells lying in contact with the apices of the secreting cells. These are the *centroalveolar cells.* Although the function of these cells was previously unknown, it has now been established that they are a continuation of the epithelium of the intercalated duct, which is carried over into the acinus as a projection rather than directly into the lumen (Fig. 15-12).

FINE STRUCTURE OF THE ACINAR CELLS

In electron micrographs (Fig. 15-13) the well-delineated nucleus is bounded by a bilaminar membrane interrupted at intervals by pores. One or two nucleoli may be present and may exhibit a central portion of low density in stained preparations.

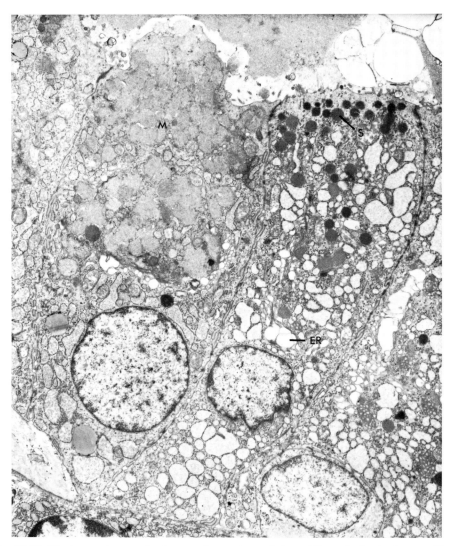

Fig. 15-10. Electron micrograph of part of an acinus of the sublingual gland of a cat. Shown on the left is a mucous cell with droplets of mucinogen, *M,* and on the right a serous cell exhibiting numerous dilated cisternae of the endoplasmic reticulum, *ER,* and distally, secretory granules, S. (×7,200.)

Zymogen granules

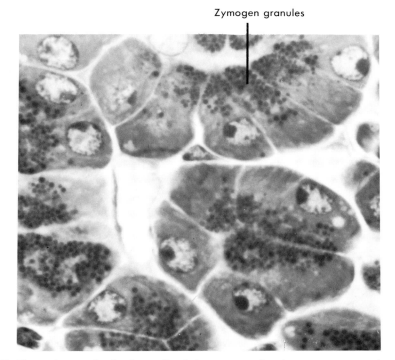

Fig. 15-11. Photomicrograph of acinar cells of the pancreas showing zymogen granules. (×800.)

Acinar cells   Intercalary duct

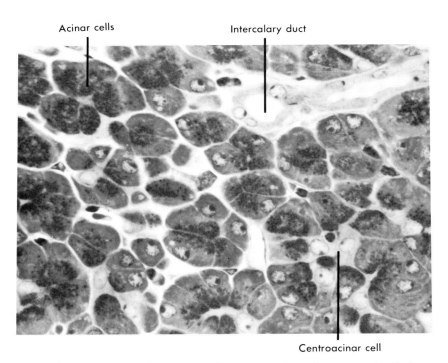

Centroacinar cell

Fig. 15-12. Photomicrograph of a section of pancreas of monkey. Note the dark secretory granules in the apical parts of the acinar cells. (×400.)

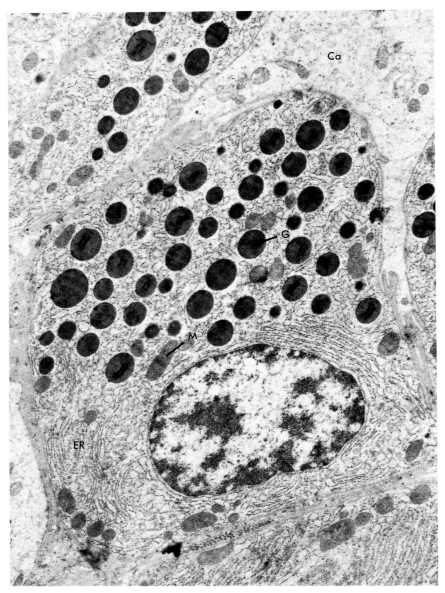

Fig. 15-13. Electron micrograph of a pancreatic acinar cell of a monkey. Characteristic of the cytoplasm is the prominent endoplasmic reticulum, *ER,* and the numerous dense zymogen granules, *G. M,* Mitochondrion; *Ca,* centroacinar cell.

Around this center is a dense network, the nucleolonema, comprising the basophilic part of the nucleolus. It consists of particles closely resembling ribosomes.

The basal portion of the cell contains an extensive endoplasmic reticular system exhibiting parallel cisternae studded with ribosomes. Ribosomes are also present in great numbers in the cytoplasm. The endoplasmic reticulum and free ribosomes correspond to the basophilic substance (ergastoplasm) observed in the basal part of the cell at the optic level. The mitochondria, although not numerous, are well defined and contain granules distributed in the matrix between the cristae. A prominent Golgi apparatus located in a supranuclear position consists of parallel arrays of membranes, vacuoles, and sinuses. Many of the vacuoles contain a dense homogeneous material representing the precursor of zymogen. The zymogen granules located in the distal region of the cell appear dense and are enclosed by a membrane.

ISLANDS OF LANGERHANS

The islands of Langerhans are collections of cells that arise as outgrowths from the walls of the ducts of the pancreas during embryonic life. Although they are thus connected developmentally with the ducts, they do not secrete into the tubules. They may become entirely detached from them or retain a connection through a cord of cells that has no lumen. They consist of coiled anastomosing cords of cells penetrated by a network of capillaries into which they secrete (Fig. 15-14, A).

In hematoxylin and eosin preparations, the islands appear as spheroidal masses of pale-staining cells arranged in the form of anastomosing cords. Interspersed between the cords of cells are numerous blood capillaries. The walls of these blood vessels are in intimate contact with the cells making up the cords, an arrangement that facilitates exchange of secretion between the cells and the vessels, which are surrounded by a thinner basement membrane than they are in the exocrine pancreas.

At least three cell types can be distinguished in the islets: the alpha (A) cell, the beta (B) cell, and the delta (D) cell. Some authors also recognize another cell type, the C cell that has a pale cytoplasm, few organelles, and no secretory granules.

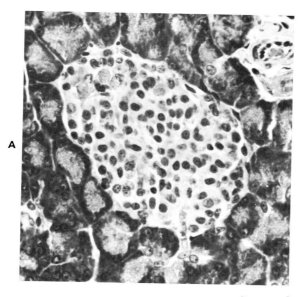

Continued.

Fig. 15-14. A, Photomicrograph of island of Langerhans of squirrel monkey surrounded by acinar cells. (×400.)

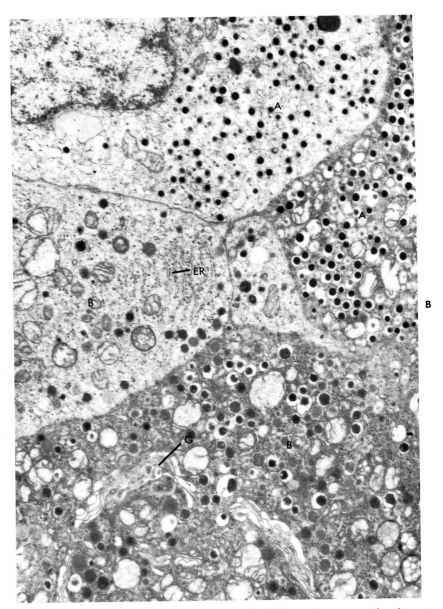

Fig. 15-14, cont'd. B, Electron micrograph of islet cells of Rhezus' pancreas. The character and size of the granules are the most important distinguishing features of these cells. *A,* Alpha cell; *B,* beta cell; *ER,* endoplasmic reticulum; *G,* Golgi apparatus. (×11,500.)

The alpha cells in man tend to be found in clusters at the edges of the islets but may also occur individually within the deeper parts of the cell mass. They cannot be readily distinguished from the beta or delta cells with routine hematoxylin and eosin staining, but special stains, such as chrome hematoxylin-phloxine, permit identification on the basis of the differential color reaction of the granules within the cells. With the chrome hematoxylin-phloxine stain, the granules of alpha cells appear as small, intensely red–staining bodies, while the granules of the more numerous beta cells are larger and stain dark blue. The most distinguishing ultrastructural feature of the alpha cells is the presence of dense spherical granules of uniform size, arranged primarily on the side of the cell facing the capillary bed (vascular pole). These granules are separated from a surrounding membrane by a clear space of low electron density. The cells contain mitochondria similar to those of beta cells although noticeably smaller, a Golgi complex smaller than that of the beta cells, and a few cisternal profiles of rough endoplasmic reticulum, as well as many free ribosomes. The nucleus is often indented or lobulated (Fig. 15-14, *B*). The alpha cells have been divided into two groups, one of which has an affinity for silver stains. The argyrophilic alpha$_1$ cells may secrete gastrin, a hormone that affects gastric secretion and the motility of gut muscle. The nonargyrophilic alpha$_2$ cells have been shown to produce glucagon, a hormone involved in maintaining body metabolism during fasting.

The beta (B) cells tend to occupy the middle of the islets. They are responsible for the secretion of insulin, a hormone concerned with controlling the utilization of nutrients shortly after a meal. Beta cells are very similar in appearance to alpha cells in both size and shape and can only be distinguished from alpha cells by special stains or by ultrastructural features. The beta cells show a wide species variation in the structure of the secretory granules. In man, the beta granules contain one or more elongate or polygonal crystals surrounded by a homogeneous matrix of relatively low density. The cells also contain another granule type that lacks a crystalline core. It has been suggested that these other granules are an immature form. Both granule types contain insulin. The beta cells have slightly larger mitochondria and a more extensive Golgi apparatus than do alpha cells. The endoplasmic reticulum is less prominent and the nucleus is of a fairly regular form.

The delta (D) cells have been described as having numerous membrane-bound granules of a somewhat larger size and lower density than alpha cell granules. The cell is often rounded in shape with a pale cytoplasm and a spherical or indented nucleus. Delta cells are usually found within alpha cell clusters and may represent a modified alpha cell type.

The C cells, which are without granules and virtually without cell organelles, have been called both precursor cells and degenerative, dying cells by various authors.

BLOOD AND NERVE SUPPLY

The blood supply to the pancreas is derived chiefly from the superior and inferior pancreaticoduodenal arteries and also from divisions of the splenic artery. As in the salivary glands, the arteries pass in the connective tissue septa to end in capillaries among the acini and islands of Langerhans. Corresponding veins return the blood to the superior mesenteric and portal veins. The nerves that supply the pancreas are derived from the splanchnic and the vagus nerves.

Summary

It is sometimes difficult for the student to distinguish the four glands just described (parotid, submaxillary, sublingual, and the pancreas), and to aid him in doing so the following facts may be emphasized. Of the four glands, two contain no mucous cells. These are the parotid and the pancreas, which are alike in that the cells of their alveoli are all serous. They are differentiated by the presence of islands of Langerhans and centroalveolar cells in the pancreas. In differentiating between the submaxillary and sublingual glands, one should look for purely serous alveoli in the former. It must be remembered, however, that the large serous crescents of the sublingual may be cut so that their relation to the mucous alveoli is not seen and they appear to be separate alveoli. Such instances are, however, isolated, and, if more than half the cells in a section are serous, it is quite certain that the section is from the submaxillary gland. Some specimens are difficult to identify, especially as the proportions of serous and mucous cells vary in different animals and even in different parts of the same gland.

LIVER

The liver develops embryologically as an outgrowth from the wall of the gut, lying in the pathway of the vitelline veins. It later intercepts the umbilical veins, and all four vessels are broken up by the glandular tissue (hepatocytes) into a multitude of small sinusoids. In the adult, blood is brought to the liver by two routes, the hepatic arteries from the celiac trunk and the hepatic portal circulation from the capillary beds of the gut (conducting blood laden with the absorbed products of digestion). After the blood has circulated through the sinusoids of the liver, it leaves the posterior surface via the hepatic veins to enter the inferior vena cava.

The liver is a complicated organ both structurally and functionally. It is a compound tubular exocrine gland producing a secretion called *bile* and also an endocrine gland elaborating secretions (such as blood proteins and glucose) that are released by the liver into the blood. In addition, it is an integral part of the reticuloendothelial system because of the fact that the sinusoids are lined in part by Kupffer cells (Fig. 15-19) that can remove particulate matter from the blood in the sinusoids by virtue of their phagocytic properties. The functioning liver thus has two cell types: the phagocytic Kupffer cells of the sinusoidal wall and the secretory hepatocytes, which secrete bile into a continuous duct system and also secrete various products into the blood.

The hepatocytes (secretory cells) are arranged in cords no more than two cells thick that lie between an interlacing network of sinusoids. Cords and sinusoids together are arranged into polygonal columns that are prismatic in shape, known as *lobules* (Fig. 15-22). This lobular arrangement is more pronounced in animals such as the pig (Fig. 15-15) than in man. The lobule is a continuous mass consisting of parenchymal cells penetrated by vessels through which venous blood passes on its way to the heart. Along the edges of each polygonal prism of cells is a drainage system consisting of the afferent blood vessels (portal circulation and hepatic arteries) and the biliary tree (draining bile from the liver lobule). Blood flows from the periphery of the lobule (the *limiting plate*) through the sinusoids toward the center of the lobule where it drains into the central vein. At points within the sinusoids and along the edge, more highly oxygenated blood from the hepatic arteries is mixed with the nutrient-laden venous blood from the portal veins. Blood in the central veins passes into the sublobular veins running beneath the lobule and is conveyed to the inferior vena cava.

At points where three or more structural units (lobules) join, there is usually present a more abundant accumulation of connective tissue together with a bile duct and one or more branches of the portal vein and hepatic arteries. This triangular-shaped zone is called the *portal canal* and the vessels and ducts contained within it, the *portal triad*. In certain liver diseases there may be considerable changes in the portal canal, including the multiplication of bile ducts.

Because the arrangement of cells into lobules is less clearly defined in man, attempts have been made to describe the functional unit of the human liver on the basis of blood supply. Rappaport has described the functional unit (the liver *acinus*) as an angular mass of parenchyma surrounding an axis containing the terminal branch of a portal vein, a hepatic artery, and a bile duct rather than a polygonal prism surrounded by a connective tissue

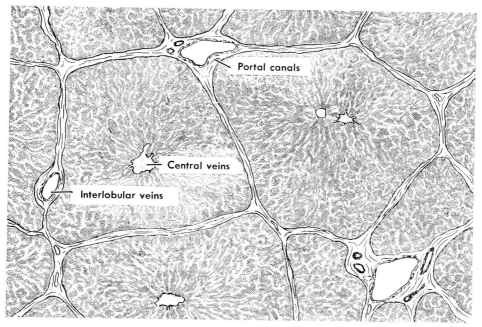

Fig. 15-15. Liver of pig, low magnification, showing relations of lobules to portal canals, central veins, and interlobular veins.

capsule (the classic liver lobule). This definition takes into account the territory of drainage of a branch of a portal vein and is based on the portal canal as a boundary. Functionally, cells closest to the edge of the parenchymal mass (where the venous blood and arterial blood enter the sinusoids) would be expected to have a richer blood supply than cells closest to the central vein.

The entire liver is surrounded by a connective tissue capsule, which contains a number of elastic fibers. At the point where the major incoming and outgoing vessels and the outgoing bile duct enter and leave the liver (the *porta hepatis*), the capsule surrounds the vessels and follows them into the gland, forming a connective tissue framework around each of the lobules that is continuous with the superficial covering of the whole liver. This framework is not very obvious in the human liver but in the pig it forms an easily identifiable sleeve around each lobule (Fig. 15-15). This surface sheet of connective tissue, called *Glisson's capsule*, is covered by an outer tunica serosa derived from the peritoneum.

Liver cells and sinusoids

The parenchyma of the liver is composed of large epithelial cells supported by reticular fibers (Fig. 15-17) and apparently arranged in irregular interconnecting plates known as the hepatic cords. The plates are arranged in a radiating fashion around the central vein (Fig. 15-16). The hepatic plates form the secretory part of the liver and are accordingly analogous to the secretory tubules of other glands. Special technique is required to demonstrate the capillaries by which the bile, secreted by the liver cells, is carried to the larger ducts in the portal canals. Each cell has, in the side adjacent to its neighboring cell, a minute groove. Two grooves fitting together form a duct known as the bile canaliculus (Fig. 15-18).

The hepatic cells are relatively large, are polyhedral in shape, and usually exhibit clear cell boundaries. The appearance of the cytoplasm is variable depending on the physiologic state of the cell. The usual cytologic components consist of a centrally placed nucleus with a prominent nucleolus. Occasionally the cells are binucleate. The

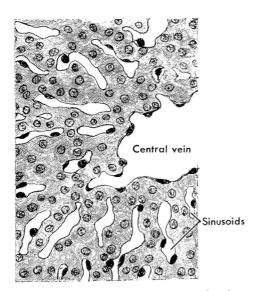

Fig. 15-16. Region of liver lobule immediately surrounding a central vein.

mitochondria are fairly numerous. The Golgi apparatus is situated adjacent to the bile canaliculus. Scattered basophilic material corresponding to rough endoplasmic reticulum or dispersed ribosomes is abundant (Fig. 15-18). The various kinds of observable granules are glycogen, lipid, and bile pigment. The cords of cells anastomose freely, forming a spongy network that radiates from the central vein. The meshes of the network of secreting cells contain the sinusoids, which are lined with an endothelium, part of which belongs to the reticuloendothelial system. In an ordinary preparation stained with hematoxylin and eosin, the lining of these vessels appears to be composed of cells that lie flat along the sides of the liver cells. The nuclei of these endothelial cells are small and dark, and their cytoplasm forms a thin film along the border of the sinusoid. Such cells are the undifferentiated lining cells. With special methods a second type of cell may be demonstrated, the stellate cell of Kupffer. When properly stained these cells

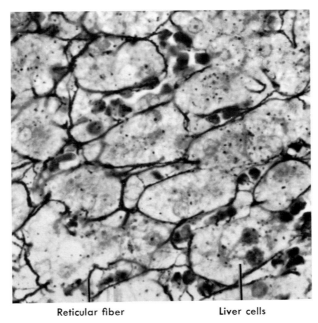

Fig. 15-17. Section of human liver showing reticular fibers. (Bielschowsky method; ×640.)

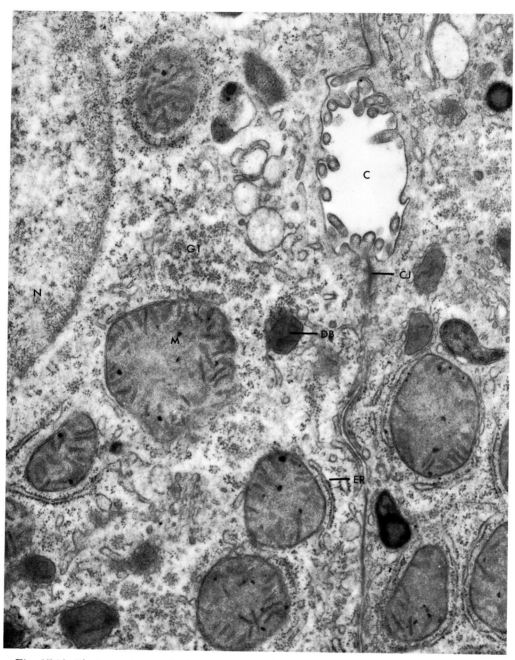

Fig. 15-18. Electron micrograph of parts of two adjacent cells of rat liver, showing bile canaliculus, *C. CJ,* Cell junction; *DB,* dense body; *ER,* rough endoplasmic reticulum; *Gl,* glycogen; *N,* nucleus; *M,* mitochondrion. (×15,000.) (Courtesy Dr. S. Luse, New York, N. Y.)

Hepatic cell | Macrophage (Kupffer) | Red blood corpuscles in hepatic sinusoid

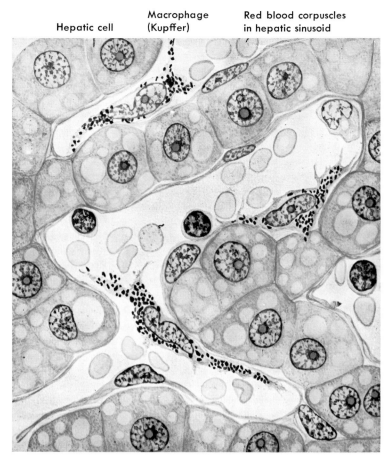

Fig. 15-19. Hepatic sinusoids showing endothelial cells and macrophages lining them. (×1,200.) (From Nonidez and Windle: Textbook of histology, New York, 1953, McGraw-Hill Book Co.)

appear to be in the bloodstream anchored to the wall of the sinusoid by cytoplasmic processes. Their reaction to vital dyes is that characteristic of other reticuloendothelial cells (Fig. 15-19).

Fine structure of hepatic cells

The nuclear membrane of hepatic cells is bilaminar and resembles the endoplasmic reticulum with which it is continuous. It also contains numerous pores. The cell surface is a single membrane about 75 Å in thickness; at high magnification it appears to be three layered (typical of unit membranes elsewhere) and shows specializations in certain regions. At the surface of

a sinusoidal blood space, the hepatic cell is separated from the margin of the vascular space by a narrow *perisinusoidal* area known as the *space of Disse*, and in this area the surface of the cell subtends many microvilli (Fig. 15-20). As is true for epithelia elsewhere, the cells are separated by a space of about 100 Å. In the region of the canaliculus the cell membranes and underlying cytoplasm become denser, giving rise to structures resembling terminal bars.

The mitochondria are typically round or elongate, exhibiting cristae and a matrix. Also present is an extensive endoplasmic reticulum of both the rough and smooth varieties as well as numerous ribosomes

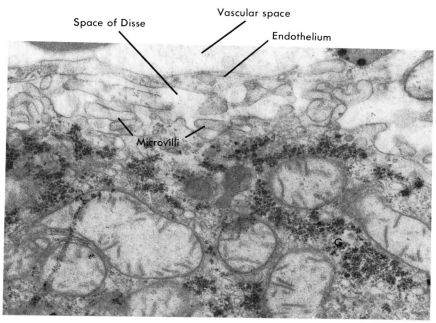

Fig. 15-20. Electron micrograph of sinusoidal surface of mouse liver cell showing relation of surface microvilli, the space of Disse, and the endothelial cells. *G*, Glycogen. (×27,000.)

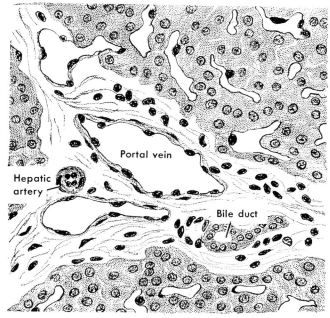

Fig. 15-21. Portal canal containing branch of portal vein. Notice in upper left a small vein opening into a sinusoid.

scattered throughout the cytoplasm. The Golgi apparatus, usually located near the bile canaliculus, consists of several smooth-walled lamellae and several associated vacuoles. In addition to glycogen and lipid granules, a prominent, dense, membrane-enclosed granule occurs in varying numbers. These bodies contain many hydro-lyzing enzymes and are known as lysosomes (Fig. 15-18).

Portal canal

The portal canal consists of an island of connective tissue, which is approximately triangular in shape. It contains a branch of the hepatic artery, a branch of the portal vein, and the bile duct. Of these the vein is by far the largest. The bile duct is readily distinguished from the blood vessels by its lining of columnar epithelium (Fig. 15-21).

Circulation

The circulation of the liver is peculiar in that it is derived from two sources: (1) arterial blood from branches of the hepatic artery and (2) venous blood by way of the portal vein (Fig. 15-22). The hepatic artery is chiefly concerned with nourishment of the liver tissue.

The portal vein carrying venous blood from the intestine and spleen, together with branches of the hepatic artery, enters the liver at the porta hepatis. These vessels divide and run through the connective tissue septa of the lobes as the interlobar vessels. The interlobar veins give off branches that run between the lobules and are known accordingly as interlobular veins. These vessels encircle the lobule, eventually penetrate it, and break up into fine capillaries, the hepatic sinusoids. The sinusoids empty into the central vein, which is considered to be the first part of the efferent system of the hepatic vessels. The central vein passes down through the lobule, collecting blood from many sinusoids, and eventually unites with other central veins that lead into the sublobular vein. Blood from these veins is eventually collected by the hepatic vein and is finally carried to the vena cava.

This circulatory arrangement enables the liver to perform one of its functions—the storage of glycogen. The blood of the portal vein comes from the intestine and is laden with nutrients. Through the arrangement of sinusoids, it easily reaches the liver cells, which store glycogen obtained from the blood. The same arrangement serves to return the nourishment to the circulation when it is needed.

Another function of the liver is the formation of bile for the digestion of food in the intestine. This substance is apparently secreted by the same cells that store the glycogen. The bile duct system consists of intrahepatic and extrahepatic portions. The interlobular ducts of the right and quadrate lobes form the right hepatic duct. Those of the left and caudate lobes form the left hepatic duct. The right and left ducts unite to form the common hepatic duct; this receives the cystic duct and then continues to the duodenum as the common bile duct.

In addition to the functions already mentioned, the liver also plays an important role in intermediary metabolism by serving as an organ in which various substances (lactate, glycerol, amino acids) can be converted into glucose (*gluconeogenesis*) during fasting. The liver also contains a readily releasable storage form of energy (glycogen) and is an important source of fats and water-soluble ketones for energy use during fasting. By virtue of its channels lined with phagocytic cells, it takes part in "filtering" the blood. It also contains numerous enzymes involved in the enzymatic degradation of toxic substances such as drugs, insecticides, and natural body products such as hormones. Finally, the liver is the site of manufacture of most blood proteins (except the immunoglobulins). Blood proteins are important in osmotic pressure of body fluids, are involved in blood clotting, can serve as an emergency source of nutrition during starvation, and serve as carriers for copper, calcium, lipids, hormones, and other materials that must be transported in blood.

Nerve supply

The nerves that supply the liver are chiefly nonmedullated fibers derived from

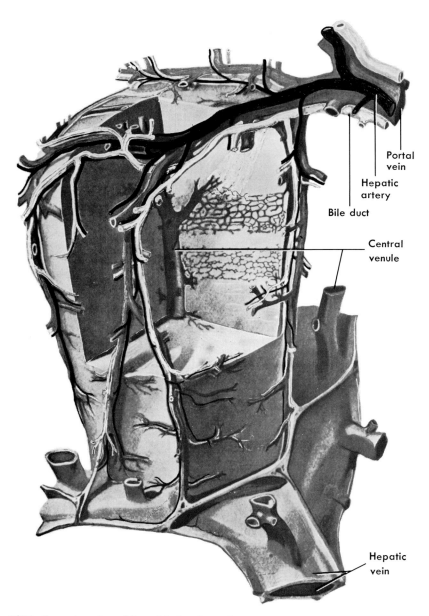

Portal
vein

Hepatic
artery

Bile duct

Central
venule

Hepatic
vein

Fig. 15-22. Reconstruction of liver lobule of pig showing relation of blood vessels and bile ducts to liver parenchyma. (Modified from Braus: Anatomie des Menschen, vol. 2, Berlin, 1924, Julius Springer; from Nonidez and Windle: Textbook of histology, New York, 1953, McGraw-Hill Book Co.)

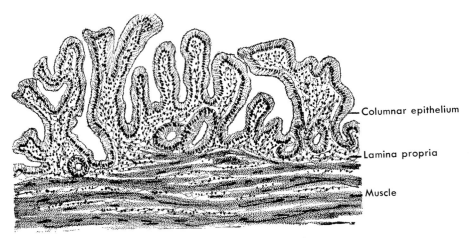

Fig. 15-23. Gallbladder of monkey.

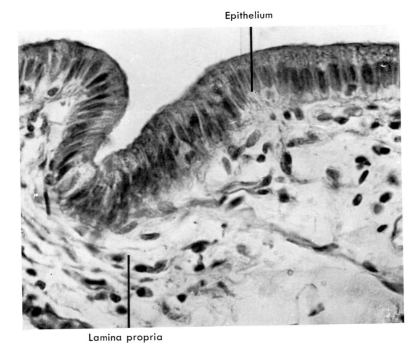

Fig. 15-24. Mucosa of gallbladder. (×640.)

the sympathetic system. They accompany the blood vessels and ducts, terminating in these structures and among the liver cells.

GALLBLADDER

The gallbladder is a hollow, pear-shaped organ closely adherent to the posterior surface of the liver. It consists of a blind end known as the fundus, a body, and a neck, which continues as the cystic duct.

The layers common to other parts of the digestive tract are poorly developed and are more or less intermingled in the gallbladder (Fig. 15-23). It is lined with a columnar epithelium in which the cell walls are distinct (Fig. 15-24). This epithelium rests on a connective tissue layer (lamina propria) that represents the lamina propria and submucosa of other parts of the tract. The connective tissue and epithelium are irregularly folded, forming numerous elevations and pockets. After the latter are tangentially cut, they appear as closed sacs, which look like glandular follicles. There is, however, no secretion in the gallbladder except that of a small group of mucous glands near its neck.

Outside the connective tissue there is a layer of smooth muscle, which consists of intermingled groups of circular, longitudinal, and oblique fibers. The muscular coat is thick and has much connective tissue combined with the muscle fibers. There is a fairly thick serosa of loose connective tissue covered by the mesothelium.

Blood and nerve supply

The gallbladder is supplied by the cystic artery, and the venous blood is collected by veins that empty into the cystic branch of the portal vein. The gallbladder is richly supplied by lymphatics, and many plexuses occur in this organ. Branches of both the vagus and splanchnic nerves supply the gallbladder.

16

Respiratory tract

Functionally, the respiratory tract can be divided into a *conducting portion,* consisting of cavities and tubes that convey air from outside the body into all parts of the lungs, and a *respiratory portion,* consisting of those divisions within the lung where exchange of gases between the air and the blood occur. Anatomically, the conducting passageways consist of structures outside the lung (nose, nasopharynx, larynx, trachea, and main bronchi) and inside the lung (smaller bronchi, bronchioles, terminal bronchioles) (Fig. 16-1). Each terminal bronchiole terminates in several respiratory bronchioles that mark the entrance into the respiratory division of the lung. Each respiratory bronchiole branches into a system of alveolar ducts and alveoli in which gaseous exchange takes place (Fig. 16-4).

Embryologically, the primordium of the respiratory tract arises as a small bud from the ventral wall of the foregut. This bud gives rise to a tube, the trachea, which soon loses all connection with the foregut except at the opening of the larynx. The trachea then begins to branch and at the time of birth seventeen subdivisions of the original tube have occurred, during which the bronchi, bronchioles, and terminal bronchioles are formed. With the beginning of breathing at birth, the ends of the terminal bronchioles (the smallest passageways in the conducting system) expand into alveolar ducts and alveoli and six more sets of branches are added. For the purpose of presentation, the respiratory tract will be divided into an upper part including the passageways above the larynx and a lower part beginning with the first derivative of the embryonic bud from the foregut wall, the trachea. The problems of wall construction in these two parts of the respiratory system are solved in different ways. Since air is moved through these passages by negative pressure, the air passages must resist collapse in order to function. Without the reinforcement of bone, the large masses of cartilage and dense fibrous tissue of the upper respiratory passages would collapse. In the tubes making up the lower passageways, rings and plates of cartilage gradually give way to layers of muscle and elastic fibers braided around the air passageways (Fig. 16-4). Breathing stretches the lung and holds these slender passageways open; reinforcement of the walls is then no longer necessary. Instead provision is made to permit greater elasticity and ability to adjust in both diameter and length with the changes in lung size. The muscle also participates in adjusting the volume of the airways or "respiratory dead space." Muscle tone is controlled by the parasympathetic nervous system, and changes in tone during coughing or cold weather act as a protective device for the lung passageways.

Aside from its respiratory function (which involves the exchange of gases between the tissue fluids, plasma, and air spaces in the lung), the air in the respiratory system must be moistened, filtered, and warmed to permit proper functioning of the component parts. The mucus supplied by goblet cells in pseudostratified columnar epithelium and by the submucosal glands serves to entrap dust particles and bacteria

222

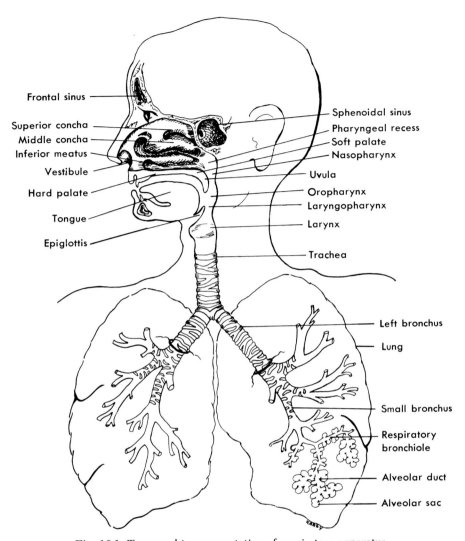

Frontal sinus

Superior concha
Middle concha
Inferior meatus
Vestibule

Hard palate

Tongue

Epiglottis

Sphenoidal sinus
Pharyngeal recess
Soft palate
Nasopharynx

Uvula
Oropharynx
Laryngopharynx

Larynx

Trachea

Left bronchus

Lung

Small bronchus

Respiratory
bronchiole

Alveolar duct

Alveolar sac

Fig. 16-1. Topographic representation of respiratory apparatus.

and also to supply enzymes that lyse certain bacteria. The same secretion serves to moisten the air and also dissolves certain molecules, which are perceived as odors, with the aid of the olfactory organ in the nasal passages. The coordinated beating of cilia on cell surfaces moves the secretions from the nasal passages through the nasopharynx to the oropharynx, while similar activity of ciliated cells located in the bronchioles, bronchi, and trachea propels mucus to the glottis. From this locus the secretions are either expectorated or pass into the esophagus. An abundant supply of venous blood vessels in the submucosal tissues of the nasal passages warm the air. Several of the functions mentioned are facilitated by an abundant surface area in each nasal passage occurring in (1) four accessory sinuses (frontal, ethmoidal, sphenoidal, and maxillary, named for the bones that enclose them) and (2) the presence of three conchae containing the tortuously twisted turbinate bones. Certain phagocytic cells called "dust cells" are located in the lung tissues. They remove and store foreign particles that enter the lungs. The olfactory organ serves to warn the organism of the presence of noxious substances in the air. The specialized respiratory epithelium of the lung alveoli is admirably suited for its function of gas exchange. The conducting tubules are constructed so that open passageways for gases are maintained under the widely fluctuating pressures produced in ventilation. These tubules gradually change in structure from thick-walled, rigid tubes to increasingly thinner and softer ones, a change similar to that occurring in blood vessels that accompany them.

UPPER PARTS OF RESPIRATORY TRACT
NASAL PASSAGES

The nose consists of two passageways separated by the cartilage-containing *nasal septum*. Each passageway begins at the *external nares* as an inflection of the keratinized stratified squamous epithelium of the wings (alae) of the nose. The inflected portion forms the *vestibule* of the nose and is covered by numerous hairs (vibrissae). Large sebaceous glands and numerous sweat glands are also found in this region. The connective tissue papillae are deep, and scattered mixed serous and mucous glands may be observed. In the posterior region of the vestibule the epithelium becomes nonkeratinized, or forms only small patches of nonhairy keratinized epithelium. The latter indicates the beginning of the so-called *respiratory* part of the nasal passage, which, in turn, terminates in a small orifice called the *choana* leading into the nasopharynx.

The respiratory portion of each nasal passage includes the sinuses, olfactory organ, the three conchae, including the meati, and the upper surface of the hard palate. In general, the epithelium of this region is ciliated pseudostratified columnar, usually exhibits four to five rows of nuclei, and contains goblet cells. The underlying lamina propria, composed of both

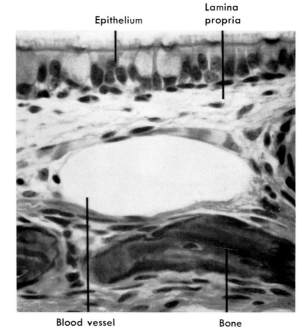

Fig. 16-2. Section through inner surface of nasal cavity showing respiratory epithelium in embryo. In the adult the epithelium is multilayered. (×640.)

elastic and collagenous fibers, is adherent to a nearby periosteum or perichondrium (Fig. 16-2). A basement membrane containing elastic fibers occurs irregularly.

The sinuses indicated are located in certain bones of the head and are usually observed in decalcified sections of the head of an embryo or fetus. They are usually identified by their location rather than by histologic characteristics. The epithelium is ciliated pseudostratified columnar, of approximately half the thickness of other parts of the tract. The sinuses exhibit two or three rows of nuclei and very few goblet cells. The basement membrane is thin and rarely observed. The lamina propria, also thin, is mainly collagenous and is closely adherent to the periosteum. It has few glands but is frequently supplied with lymphoid aggregations and other leukocytic forms.

The superior, middle, and inferior conchae are usually observed in frontal sections through the head of the human fetus as coiled and recurved projections arising from the walls opposite the septa (paraseptally). In animals like the pig, only parts of the conchae are visible because the head is prolonged into a snout. The space inferior to each concha is, in sequence, the superior, middle, and inferior meatus.

The middle and inferior conchae bear the usual thick type of pseudostratified columnar epithelium, containing many goblet cells. The basement membrane is thick and is readily demonstrated. The lamina propria exhibits both serous and mucous alveoli, as well as a large number of prominent venous passages. The latter may be engorged with blood or collapsed, and their walls exhibit both circular and longitudinal bands of smooth muscle. Each meatus bears a thin epithelium containing a few goblet cells, which rests upon a thin basement membrane. The superior concha and parts of the roof of the nasal passage and adjacent septum form part of the olfactory organ. The epithelium of the organ is thick and, since the neural processes are almost impossible to trace in hematoxylin and eosin preparations, its appearance is like that of stratified columnar epithelia. The surface cells contain pigment granules when properly preserved, and the cilia present are covered by a coagulated secretion, which gives the impression that the tissue is covered by a cuticle.

NASOPHARYNX

In the parts of the nasopharynx that do not come into contact with surfaces of other tissues, the epithelium is ciliated pseudostratified columnar and the lamina propria contains mixed or seromucous glands. In certain transitional zones stratified columnar epithelium may occur but it is not easily distinguished from the pseudostratified variety. In the superior and posterior portions of the nasopharynx there are many aggregations of lymphoid cells, which may be extensions of the pharyngeal tonsils or adenoids. Similar aggregations forming the tubal tonsils are found surrounding the entrance of the eustachian tubes into the nasopharynx. At about the lower level of the

tonsils the posterior wall of the nasopharynx is covered by a nonkeratinized stratified squamous epithelium with numerous low papillae. The superior surface of the soft palate and uvula also bear a nonkeratinized stratified squamous epithelium.

LARYNX

The uppermost portion of the larynx is known as the epiglottis. The lingual or anterior surface of the epiglottis is covered by a nonkeratinized stratified squamous epithelium and bears many seromucous glands in the lamina propria, especially near its connection with the base of the tongue. The upper part of the posterior surface of the epiglottis is covered by a nonkeratinized stratified squamous epithelium, which merges into a transition zone and appears as irregularly ciliated stratified columnar epithelium. The lower part of the posterior surface bears ciliated pseudostratified columnar epithelium exhibiting goblet cells, and near the base one may observe scattered taste buds. The lamina propria includes some mucous and serous units. The zone between the two surfaces is occupied by a large area of cartilage containing several thick elastic fibers, the so-called elastic cartilage. In the epiglottis of some animals the cartilage may contain a central zone invaded by fat cells. No perichondrium, however, occurs in the invaded zone (Fig. 16-3).

The epithelium of the true vocal cords is of the nonkeratinized stratified squamous variety and does not contain mucous glands in the lamina propria. Above and below the true vocal cords the epithelium is ciliated pseudostratified columnar with goblet cells, and many mucous glands are present in the lamina propria. Patches of the stratified squamous type are sometimes found in this region.

LOWER PARTS OF RESPIRATORY TRACT

Morphologists have differentiated the lower parts of the respiratory tract on the basis of gross dissection and by the injec-

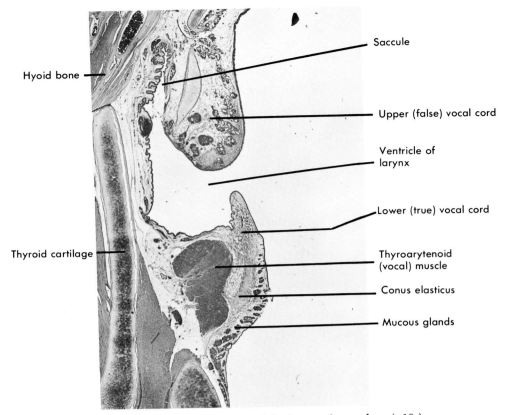

Hyoid bone

Thyroid cartilage

Saccule

Upper (false) vocal cord

Ventricle of larynx

Lower (true) vocal cord

Thyroarytenoid (vocal) muscle

Conus elasticus

Mucous glands

Fig. 16-3. Half of frontal section of the larynx of a monkey. (×10.)

tion of low melting point alloys into the passageways. Thus there are lobes and lobules of the lung (Fig. 16-4), with their attendant blood and lymphatic circulation, containing various air tubules. Ordinarily one does not utilize more than a small portion of a lobule for study. In addition, the former tendency to utilize the diameter of a tubule as a criterion for identification is no more valid here than it is for blood vessels. In routine histology the salient features to observe in the tubules and lungs are (1) the epithelial makeup, (2) the presence or absence of cartilage and its disposition (that is, location, shape, and extent), (3) the glands and their disposition, (4) the disposition of the muscles, and (5) the relation of the parts to each other at the microscopic level. The student should attempt to visualize how each component appears in cross section and longitudinal section.

TRACHEA

The trachea consists of (1) mucosa, (2) submucosa, and (3) a layer of cartilage and muscle that corresponds to the muscularis of the digestive tract (Fig. 16-5). External to the perichondrium of the cartilage is a fibrosa or adventitious layer of connective tissue, which fuses with the tissue of the mediastinum and the similar layer enclosing the esophagus. This layer is usually destroyed during dissection of the trachea.

The mucosa consists of (1) a ciliated pseudostratified columnar epithelium with numerous goblet cells bounded by (2) a prominent basement membrane, which is part of (3) the lamina propria, consisting mainly of reticular or fine areolar tissue containing many elastic fibers (Fig. 16-6). At the outer edge of the lamina propria, coarse elastic fibers are oriented longitudinally to form (4) a relatively compact

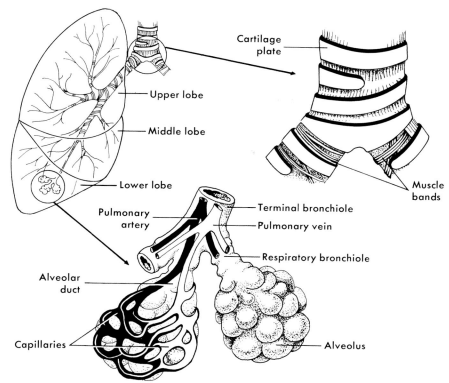

Fig. 16-4. The gross structure of the respiratory passages showing a detail of one respiratory unit. (Drawing by Emily Craig.)

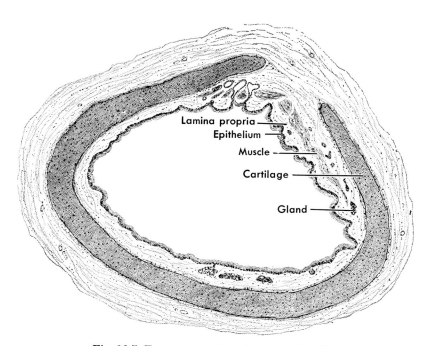

Fig. 16-5. Transverse section of trachea of child.

Adipose tissue   Submucosa   Epithelium

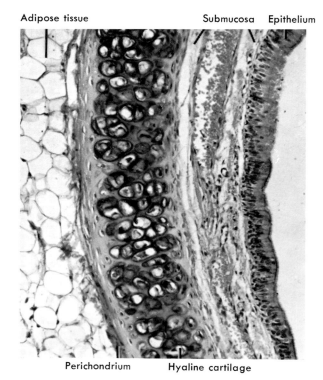

Perichondrium   Hyaline cartilage

Fig. 16-6. Transverse section of trachea of rabbit. (×40.)

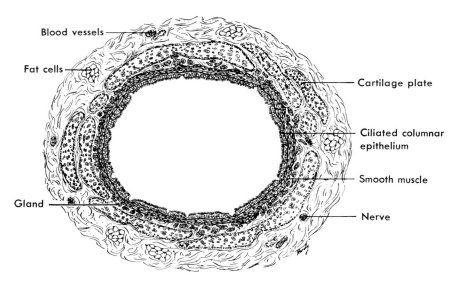

Blood vessels

Fat cells

Cartilage plate

Ciliated columnar epithelium

Smooth muscle

Gland

Nerve

Fig. 16-7. Transverse section of bronchus.

elastic membrane or lamina. The latter is said to be comparable to the muscularis mucosae of the digestive tract and the similar elastic layer in the upper part of the esophagus. In the epithelium, small patches of the stratified squamous variety are encountered, especially in older animals or those with chronic inflammations.

The submucosa is areolar tissue. It contains fat cells, blood vessels, and the secreting portions of mixed glands, with some units exhibiting prominent serous crescents. In longitudinal sections dense clusters of these glands are seen in the triangular regions between the adjacent cartilage rings, to be described below.

In cross sections of the trachea the cartilages appear as a single C-shaped or U-shaped crescent with the open end or prongs directed posteriorly toward the esophagus. The prongs may branch so that more than one piece of cartilage may appear near the open side of the crescent. Bands of smooth muscle fibers transversely arranged appear between the prongs and at times may be observed inserting in the perichondrium, either inside or outside the crescent. External to this muscle band one may observe the cut ends of longitudinally and obliquely arranged muscle fibers and their associated elastic fibers. The tracheal glands frequently penetrate the muscle layers. In longitudinal sections the cartilages appear as two rows of ovoid bodies. Occasionally two adjacent cartilages may fuse or be connected by a small longitudinal bar of cartilage. In the region between cartilages there are longitudinal bands of tough dense connective tissue, which merge with the perichondria of the cartilages. In older animals some cartilages may appear to contain fibers or to be partly calcified.

BRONCHI

The extrapulmonary or primary bronchi are histologically identical with the trachea in practically all details except size. In the lungs the cartilages of the bronchi are arranged in a series of overlapping crescentic plates, which completely encircle these structures. Deeper in the lung these soon give way to irregular masses of car-

tilage with more or less rounded edges (Fig. 16-7) and may or may not overlap when viewed in cross section. The intrapulmonary bronchi differ from the trachea as follows: (1) the elastic membrane of the tracheal lamina propria is replaced by a layer of smooth muscle, which completely encircles both epithelium and the elastic, fiber-containing lamina propria; (2) mucous and seromucous glands are more numerous and more generally distributed in the bronchi than in the trachea and often extend through the muscle and between adjacent cartilage plates; (3) the single crescent-shaped cartilage is replaced by a concentric ring of overlapping crescents. These eventually give way to smaller irregular masses of cartilage, which continue to diminish in size until the tubules are completely devoid of cartilage. In the smallest bronchi only glands may be seen, and the cartilage is completely absent (Figs. 16-8 and 16-9). As the tubules become smaller, the muscle bands that encircle the lumen become more prominent, with the concomitant reduction of the other structures. The muscles are arranged, however, as two opposing spirals, which tend to form looser helices as the tubule branches and narrows. In cross section the looser spirals in smaller tubules appear as gaps between muscle bands at the same level. Upon death, contraction of the spiraling circular muscles throws the pseudostratified columnar epithelium into longitudinal folds, carrying along with it folds of elastic lamina propria. Classification of large, medium-sized, and small bronchi on the basis of definitely overlapping crescentic plates of cartilage, circles of nonoverlapping plates, or no cartilage at all introduces as many problems as it solves and is not a satisfactory criterion to use for identification.

BRONCHIOLES

Bronchioles contain neither glands nor cartilages (Fig. 16-8). The lumen is lined by ciliated simple columnar epithelium, which lacks goblet cells. The lamina propria is elastic and very thin and is surrounded by the same type of loosely spiraling,

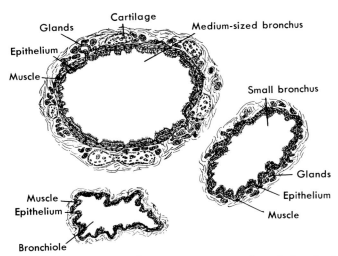

Fig. 16-8. Terminal intrapulmonary passageway of respiratory tract.

smooth muscle bands found in the bronchi. It is interesting to note that ciliated cells are found beyond the point where glands are no longer in evidence. It has been postulated that this is a protection against the accumulation of mucus in the respiratory portion of the lungs. Subdivision of bronchioles into different types according to size is not histologically feasible and accordingly is not elaborated upon in this text.

RESPIRATORY BRONCHIOLES

In the first part of the respiratory bronchiole the epithelium is of the ciliated low columnar or cuboidal type. Distally the epithelium becomes nonciliated cuboidal. The lamina propria is a very thin layer of diffuse reticular, collagenous, and elastic fibers. The spiraling muscle bands are quite prominent, but, between adjacent muscle bands in the region where the lamina propria is not in evidence, one can observe thin walls composed of simple cuboidal epithelium supported on a few helical elastic fibers. Some authors consider this to be respiratory epithelium, and from the appearance of these flattened plates the name respiratory bronchiole has arisen. It should be noted that in some sections the cells are so attenuated that the nuclei in these plates are not visible. In addition, pulmonary alveoli may arise directly from the walls of the respiratory bronchiole so that they appear as pockets in the tubule wall. Near their termini, respiratory bronchioles flare out and give rise to two or more alveolar ducts (Fig. 16-10).

ALVEOLAR DUCTS

The alveolar ducts (Figs. 16-4 and 16-10) are similar to the respiratory bronchioles from which they branch. The walls of the ducts are provided with so many openings into the alveoli that the wall appears discontinuous. Small bits of the branching, spiraling muscle fibers are seen around the openings into the alveoli or the chambers that lead into the alveoli.

Alveoli

In the alveoli of the lung there are respiratory epithelium and elastic tissue. To understand the arrangement of the former one must remember that all the tubules of the fetal lung are lined with cuboidal epithelium and are embedded in embryonic connective tissue. When respiration begins, at birth, some of the epithelium is stretched into the form of thin plates described previously in this discussion. However, at the angles between alveoli, areas remain where the cells are not flattened. The surrounding connective tissue is reduced to a network

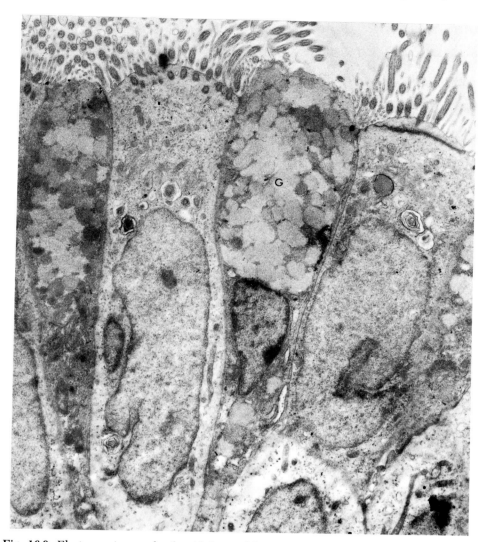

Fig. 16-9. Electron micrograph of epithelium of bronchus of cat. This epithelium is typically ciliated and exhibits numerous goblet cells, G, filled with mucous droplets. (×7,600.)

of elastic fibers and a few fibroblasts between the alveoli. One may see, therefore, in a section of lung, regions where the cells are reduced to a mere line and other regions where they are polygonal and evidently nucleated.

The original shape of each alveolus, or air sac, is round. The mutual pressure of adjacent sacs, however, alters the shape, and they appear as irregular polygonal spaces open on one side. They are grouped so that several of them open into a common central space or atrium, which in turn opens into an alveolar duct.

In humans the atria are rare, and in other animals they are an inconstant feature, so we may well consider this term to be superfluous.

The true relation of the parts described previously is not often clear in a section of the lung. Occasionally one may have the good fortune to see an area in which

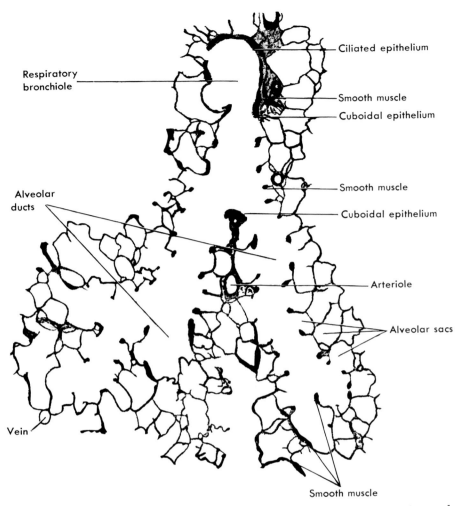

Fig. 16-10. Section through a respiratory bronchiole and two alveolar ducts of a human lung. (After Baltisberger; from Maximow and Bloom: Textbook of histology, Philadelphia, 1952, W. B. Saunders Co.)

the relations of respiratory bronchioles, alveolar ducts, atria, and alveoli appear, as in Fig. 16-10.

With the light microscope one may observe that there are capillaries and some connective tissue between the air spaces of adjacent alveoli (Fig. 16-11). The fine structure of the alveolar wall has now been resolved, and it has been shown that it consists of three basic cell types (Fig. 16-12). (1) The most numerous cells of the alveolar wall are the *endothelial cells*

of the capillaries. The nuclei of these cells are usually smaller and more elongated than those of epithelial cells. (2) Thin attenuated epithelial cells (*squamous alveolar epithelial cells, type I cells*) fit together and form a continuous lining of the alveolar spaces. This lining is so thin that it is not observable at the light level. The cytoplasm is devoid of an endoplasmic reticulum but contains a variety of other organelles. (3) *Great alveolar cells (type II cells)* appear to be epithelium. They are

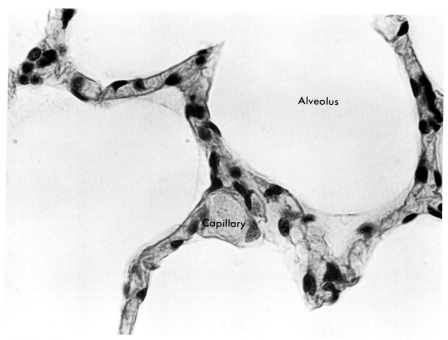

Fig. 16-11. Photomicrograph showing parts of several alveoli of lung. Most of the nuclei shown in the alveolar septa are those of the endothelium. (×640.)

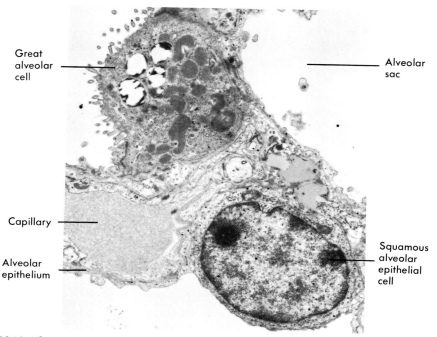

Fig. 16-12. Electron micrograph of part of the alveolar wall of mouse lung. (Original ×14,000.)

cuboidal or rounded and are less numerous than the squamous alveolar cells (only five to eight per alveolus). They usually occur at the junction of the walls of several alveoli but may make up part of the air sac as well. They are much larger than the squamous epithelium cells, averaging 15 to 20 μ in diameter in comparison to 0.5 μ width for type I cells. At the light microscope level the cytoplasm appears vacuolated and the nuclei are large and vesicular. These cells have microvilli on their free borders and the cytoplasm contains osmiophilic inclusions called cytosomes, which consist of peculiar lamellar arrangements of membranes. Since the development of the inclusions coincides with the beginning of surfactant secretion in the fetal lung, the cells may either secrete surfactant or phagocytose it. Surfactant is a surface film that serves to lower the surface tension of the fluid covering the alveolar wall and thus helps hold these small air channels open. It has also been

suggested that the great alveolar cells may give rise to alveolar macrophages, which are different functionally from the usual tissue macrophage in that they do not rely upon glycolysis for energy but require oxygen instead.

Another group of large cells is found in the terminal bronchioles. They are called Clara cells, contain whorls of endoplasmic reticulum, and are packed with mitochondria. They appear to be active secretory cells and it has been suggested that they are the source of surfactant.

The barrier or wall between the alveolar air and the blood is extremely thin (about 1 μ) and consists of the capillary endothelium, a connective tissue space, the basement membrane of the capillary, and the alveolar epithelium (Fig. 16-13). The wall is readily permeable to gases and water, less so to salts, and least of all to proteins. The main barrier to absorption from the alveolar sac into the blood is the alveolar epithelium. This barrier must

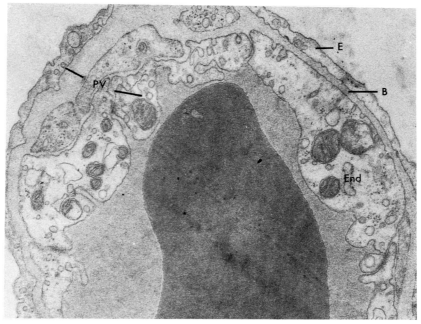

Fig. 16-13. Electron micrograph of alveolar membrane of mouse. The alveolar air is separated from the blood by a thin epithelium, *E;* a basement membrane, *B;* and the capillary endothelium, *End.* Pinocytotic vesicles, *PV,* are present in epithelium and endothelium. (×28,000.)

serve the dual function of preserving a highly permeable membrane for gaseous exchange and maintaining sufficient strength to hold the wall together. It must also include a defense system against foreign particles and invasive organisms that reach the alveolus in the inspired air (see final section of this chapter). The alveolar wall is renewed continuously and is completely replaced every 35 days or so.

In the thicker sections of the alveolus, the basal laminae of the capillary and the epithelial cells are separated by reticular and elastic fibers that tend to increase the resilience of the wall. Fibroblasts and other cells can be found in the thickest parts of the wall. The functional unit of the lung is the respiratory bronchiole with its branching alveolar ducts and terminal alveoli (Fig. 16-4).

The entrance into each of these units at the mouth of a respiratory bronchiole is quite narrow and is a vulnerable area because of the possibility of becoming clogged with mucus during inflammatory reactions. It is also a transitional point in the lung defense system, having neither a mucousciliary escalator to remove debris nor a good local macrophage population capable of phagocytosis of debris. It is accordingly a frequent site of invasion by infectious agents such as viruses.

BLOOD SUPPLY OF LUNGS

The lungs have a dual blood supply: (1) the *pulmonary arteries* and (2) the *bronchial arteries*. The pulmonary arteries carry deoxygenated blood from the right ventricle to the lungs to be purified. The pulmonary artery gains access to the lung with the corresponding chief bronchus. It follows the branching of the bronchus, and, on reaching the alveolar duct, the artery divides into a capillary plexus located in the alveolar walls. Veins arise from these capillaries, which pass first through the septa, then along the bronchioles to the root of the lung.

The *bronchial arteries* arise from the aorta. They accompany the bronchi and supply them, as well as the connective tissue of the lung, with oxygenated blood.

These vessels terminate in capillaries, which anastomose with capillaries of the pulmonary plexus. Part of the blood carried by the bronchial arteries reaches the pulmonary veins through this anastomosis, the remainder via the bronchial veins.

Lymph supply of lungs

Two groups of interconnected lymphatic vessels are present in the lung. One, a superficial or pleural group, occurs in and drains the pleura; the other deep group follows the bronchi, pulmonary artery, and vein. All drain centrally to the hilum, where they communicate with the efferent vessels of the superficial group.

NERVE SUPPLY OF THE LUNGS

The lungs are supplied by branches of the vagus nerve and also fibers of the thoracic ganglia. The fibers that supply the constrictor elements are derived chiefly from the vagus. Those that innervate the dilators of the bronchi are, in the main, sympathetic in character; they are said to arise from the inferior cervical and upper thoracic ganglia.

DEFENSE SYSTEMS IN THE RESPIRATORY TRACT

Small dust particles are dangerous only if they reach the alveoli. To prevent this, there are two basic adaptations of the airconducting passageways: the mucociliary escalator and the tortuosity of the channels themselves. Particles 5 to 10 μ or larger are filtered out in the nasal cavities as air swirls past the turbinate bones, which project from the walls of the nasal cavity. They are swept into the oral pharynx by the ciliary movement of a mucous sheet. Many of the smaller particles are deposited on the mucosa of the larger tubes such as the trachea and large bronchi and are cleared from the tract by moving along with the mucus as it is swept up toward the pharynx by the cilia on the lining cells. These cilia move mucus up toward the pharynx (a mucociliary escalator) at the rate of 1 to 3 cm. per minute in the larger bronchi and more slowly in the bronchioles (0.1 cm. per minute). The surface coat that is moved along is about 5 μ thick and is made up of a watery film covered by a thick viscous layer of mucus. This mucus is produced by the goblet cells located in the mucosal lining of the wall and by mixed serous-mucous glands located beneath the epithelium (about one per square millimeter).

Small particles 0.1 to 2 μ in size probably reach the alveoli. Some of these are innocuous but some, particularly industrial dusts such as coal dust, silica, and asbestos, may result in considerable damage to lung tissue. Insoluble particles such as silica or carbon are retained permanently and accumulate in local macrophages (appropriately called dust cells), where they may elicit a slow inflammatory reaction leading to the accumulation of fibrous tissue in the walls of the respiratory passage-

ways. There are around seven dust cells in each alveolus, lodged in small niches near the capillaries. Dust does not usually accumulate in the cells lining the alveolar wall. The macrophages in the lung may come from the bloodstream, but there is also a small area between the blood and the air sacs that seems to serve as a compartment for cell division and maturation of new macrophages from alveolar type II cells. There are no lymphatics in this space. The lymphatics penetrate only as far as the alveolar ducts, yet dust particles entering an alveolus may reach the lymphatic circulation quickly. It is not certain how this occurs. The efficiency of the alveolar macrophages in defending against local accumulation of dust particles and infectious agents is much diminished by hypoxia.

17

Urinary system

In mammals the main excretory pathways are the respiratory, integumentary, and urinary systems. The urine formed in the kidneys is transported with the aid of peristalsis through the ureters to a urinary bladder. As the sphincters leading out of the bladder relax, the whole bladder contracts and urine is forced out through the urethra.

KIDNEY

Study of the kidney offers two unusual opportunities to the student. (1) The gross structure of the dissected kidney correlates well with the pattern observed microscopically. (2) Rather than a vague mass of unnamed blood vessels, each one is named and exhibits definite microanatomic relations easily recognizable by beginning students. Because of its simplicity, we will describe the rabbit kidney first, then the human kidney.

Gross structure of the unilobar kidney

The kidney of the rabbit is a bean-shaped gland covered by a fibrous tunic or *renal capsule,* which involutes into the kidney parenchyma along the medial aspect to form the *kidney sinus.* The external orifice of the sinus is called the *hilum,* or hilus. The ureter expands into an *extrarenal pelvis,* which enters the kidney sinus and gives rise to an *intrarenal pelvis* (Fig. 17-1). The distal portion of the latter is expanded into a trumpet-shaped cup, or *calyx.* The lateral walls of the calyx fuse with the tissue lining the sinus. In addition to the ureter, the renal sinus contains a prominent fat pad, nerves, lymphatics, and branches of the renal artery and vein. (The highly vascularized perirenal fat body in the abdominal cavity functions to cushion and support the kidney.)

A rabbit kidney sliced lengthwise is seen to be composed of a single, large, mushroom-shaped lobe (unilobar kidney). The cap of the structure appears granular and is known as the kidney *cortex.* The stemlike portion appears triangular, striated, and in three dimensions resembles a *pyramid* (from which is derives its name). The tip of the pyramid is called the *papilla,* and it is this part that projects into and is received by the calyx. In the unilobar, unipyramidal kidney the term *medulla* applies to the pyramid itself, whereas the region near the base of the pyramid in the cortex is called the *juxtamedullary region.* Examination of the juxtamedullary region reveals fine strands of medullary substance penetrating and subdividing the cortical parenchyma. The former are called *medullary rays* (rays of Ferrein) and the latter are the *cortical labyrinths.* Also found in the juxtamedullary region are arched blood vessels running parallel to the base of the pyramid, which give rise to radial branches supplying and draining the cortical labyrinths.

Each lobe is subdivided into *lobules.* Most authors describe a lobule centered about a medullary ray and bounded by *interlobular arteries* running parallel to the ray in all the adjacent cortical labyrinths (Plate 3, medullary ray lobule). Valid reasons have been given for supporting the idea that the artery located in the cortical labyrinth should be considered the center

237

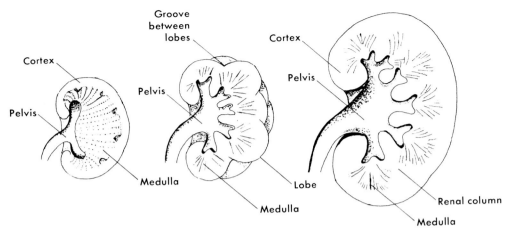

Fig. 17-1. Diagram showing topography of a unipyramidal rabbit kidney (left), a newborn human kidney (middle), and an adult multipyramidal human kidney (right). (Drawing by Emily Craig.)

of the lobule (Plate 3, vascular lobule), which is then bounded by the centers of adjacent medullary rays. In the vascular lobule the artery becomes a *lobular artery*, which is synonymous with the interlobular artery of the previous system.

Gross structure of the multilobar kidney

Examination of the external aspect of the kidney of a 6-month-old infant reveals remnants of many lobes (twelve to eighteen). With maturation the external evidence of lobation in man is obliterated. In the larger mammals, for example, ox, elephant, or seal, the lobes are externally visible, and each one appears to act like a separate kidney. Man has a multilobed, multipyramidal kidney (Fig. 17-1).

In man the intrarenal pelvis branches into three anterior and posterior tubes called the *major calyces,* which in turn branch to form a total of eight *minor calyces* (Plate 4). Each minor calyx receives a papilla from a single pyramid or a papilla formed by the fusion of two or more pyramids. As a result of fusion there are fewer papillae (four to thirteen) than pyramids (eight to eighteen). In multipyramidal kidneys, trabeculae of the cortical parenchyma fill in the spaces between adjacent pyramids and are called

the *renal columns,* or columns of Bertini or Bertin. The physiologist considers only the renal pyramids and medullary rays as medulla and the cortical labyrinths and renal columns to constitute the cortex of the kidney.

Circulation

Each kidney (Plate 4) is supplied by a single *renal artery,* which divides in the renal sinus into two sets of *secondary renal arteries.* One set supplies the anterior two thirds of the kidney, whereas the other supplies the posterior one third. As they pass through the fat body of the sinus, they divide again prior to penetrating between adjacent pyramids or between a pyramid and an adjacent renal column. The latter are called *interlobar arteries* (a term obviously not suited to unilobar kidneys). Each lobe is supplied by numerous interlobar arteries (six to fourteen), which curve abruptly in the juxtamedullary region to form incomplete arterial arches known as *arciform arteries* (arcuate arteries). Along their entire path over the base of the pyramid the arciform arteries give rise to radial or perpendicular *lobular arteries* (interlobular arteries), which supply the cortical labyrinths. In the cortical labyrinths the lobular arteries give rise to

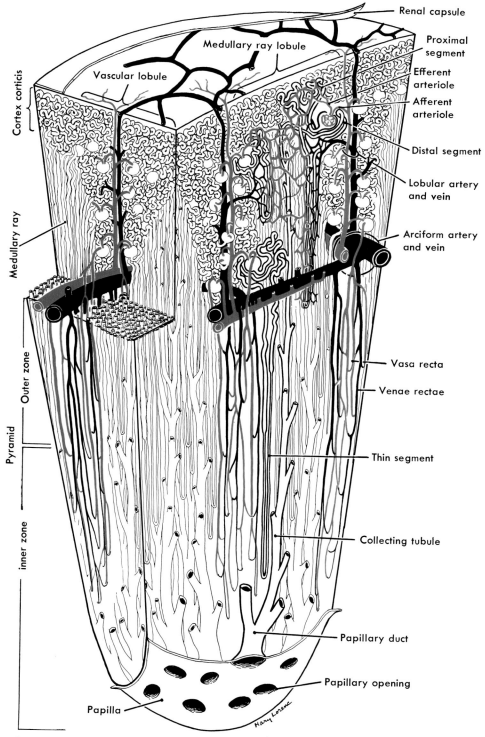

Labels on figure:

Cortex corticis

Medullary ray

Pyramid

Outer zone

inner zone

Vascular lobule

Medullary ray lobule

Renal capsule

Proximal segment

Efferent arteriole

Afferent arteriole

Distal segment

Lobular artery and vein

Arciform artery and vein

Vasa recta

Venae rectae

Thin segment

Collecting tubule

Papillary duct

Papillary opening

Papilla

Mary Lorenc

Plate 3. Details of a renal pyramid and cortex. (From Smith: Principles of renal physiology, New York, 1956, Oxford University Press, Inc.)

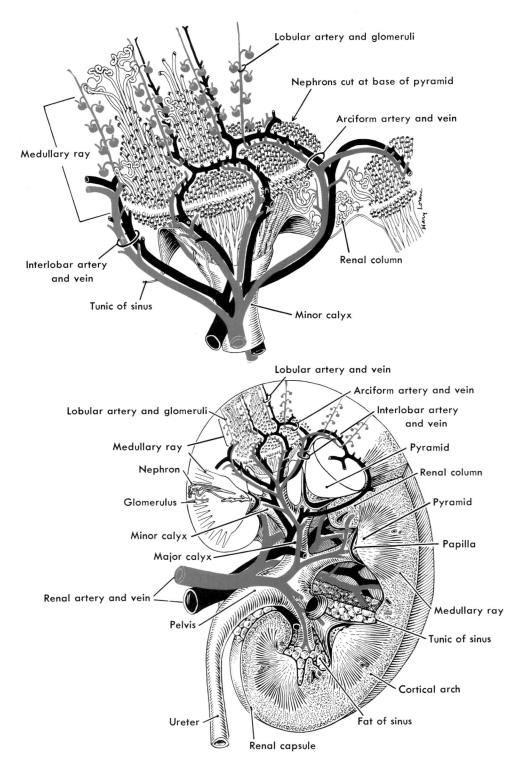

Plate 4. Circulatory plan of kidney. (From Smith: Principles of renal physiology, New York, 1956, Oxford University Press, Inc.)

numerous short straight *afferent arterioles,* which supply small tufts of blood vessels called *glomeruli.* The lobular arteries become progressively smaller and terminate in the subcapsular region in a plexus of arterioles and capillaries, which supply part of the capsule.

The blood flow leaving the glomeruli differs according to the location of the latter. Each of the *cortical glomeruli* (outer two thirds of the cortex) gives rise to an *efferent arteriole* of a diameter smaller than that of the afferent vessel. The efferent arterioles divide shortly to form a *peritubular capillary network* within the cortical labyrinths and medullary rays found in the cortical region. An efferent arteriole apparently supplies all or nearly all of the tubule derived from that same nephron. Each *juxtamedullary glomerulus* (located in the inner third of the cortex) gives rise to an efferent arteriole whose diameter is equal to or larger than the afferent vessel. The efferent arterioles of these glomeruli penetrate the pyramid and divide there into a series of long, straight parallel blood vessels passing into the papilla. They are collectively referred to as the *vasa rectae.* Their diameter is roughly equal to that of the efferent vessels, and the presence of intermittent, circularly arranged, smooth muscle elements indicates the source of the name *arteriolae rectae.* Careful observation is necessary to differentiate these from ordinary capillaries. An incomplete inner elastic membrane may occur in afferent arterioles but not in the efferent or glomerular vessels. The smooth muscle elements of the efferent arterioles may be lacking or replaced at intervals by groups of contractile pericytes or Rouget cells.

If the renal capsule is stripped away carefully, one may observe that a series of subcapsular blood vessels merge at certain points. These give the impression that the kidney surface is covered by several star-shaped blood vessels. These are the so-called *stellate veins,* and the central point of fusion marks the beginning of the *lobular vein* (interlobular vein). The lobular veins pass through the cortical labyrinths together with the lobular arteries. The freely anastomosing peritubular capillaries drain into short cortical veins (intralobular veins), which in turn join the lobular veins. In the juxtamedullary region the lobular veins join the *arcuate veins* (arciform veins). In contrast with the arcuate arteries the arcuate veins form complete arches over the surface of the pyramidal base (see Plates 3 and 4). The papilla is drained by a series of straight blood vessels, *venae rectae* (vasa rectae). The walls of these veins contain smooth muscle spirally arranged and have a thinner endothelial lining than do the descending vessels. The vasa rectae and venae rectae are extensions of the peritubular capillary network that penetrate deeply into the medulla in association with the long loops of Henle of the juxtamedullary nephrons and return toward the cortex in a hairpin loop. They are closely associated with exchanges of water and salt between the loop of Henle and the blood. The venae rectae drain directly into the arcuate veins in the juxtamedullary region. The renal artery sends a branch to the adrenal gland, as well as much smaller branches to the ureter, renal pelvis, adipose tissue, and nerves of the sinus, calyces, and the vasa vasorum of the larger blood vessels entering the kidney parenchyma.

Finer structure of the kidney

The urinary functions of the kidney are carried out by three groups of structures: (1) the glomeruli, (2) the nephrons, and (3) the collecting tubules and papillary ducts. Urine is formed by the activity of the nephrons, and they are described as the functional units of the kidney. There are about 1 million nephrons in each human kidney.

Glomeruli. In tissue sections each glomerulus is observed as an oval or rounded body consisting of a mass of capillaries containing many red blood cells and bounded by a small space (Figs. 17-2 and 17-4). The space is the cavity of Bowman's capsule and is formed by invagination of the capillary into an enlargement of the end of the nephron. Thus Bowman's capsule is a double-layered structure com-

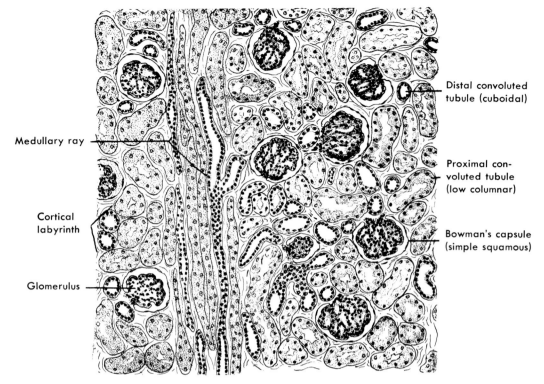

Medullary ray

Cortical labyrinth

Glomerulus

Distal convoluted tubule (cuboidal)

Proximal con- voluted tubule (low columnar)

Bowman's capsule (simple squamous)

Fig. 17-2. Section of part of cortex of human kidney.

posed of simple squamous epithelium, with nuclei bulging into the capsular space. The inner layer of Bowman's capsule is known as the *visceral layer* and is in intimate contact with all the exposed surfaces of the glomerular tuft. The *parietal layer* forms the outer boundary of the capsule. A prominent basement membrane is visualized by the PAS technique and is located around the parietal layer of the capsule and between the visceral layer and the glomerular capillaries.

The side of the glomerulus where the afferent and efferent arterioles enter and leave and approximate each other forms the vascular pole of the glomerulus. The end directed toward the tubular portion of the nephron is known as the urinary pole of the glomerulus (Fig. 17-4).

As the afferent arteriole approaches the vascular pole it gives rise to the juxta-glomerular apparatus (Fig. 17-4). As it

enters Bowman's capsule the afferent arteriole loses its inner elastic membrane and gives rise to four to eight primary capillaries, which branch and form several anastomosing secondary capillaries. They, in turn, merge to form primary capillaries draining into the efferent arterioles. As a result of this arrangement of capillaries, the glomerulus is described as *lobulated*. In section, however, the mass of capillaries observed in glomeruli rarely appears lobulated.

The glomerulus and its enveloping Bowman's capsule form the *malpighian corpuscle*, or renal corpuscle. Although they vary considerably in size, the juxtamedullary glomeruli appear to be larger and in man may average approximately 0.2 mm. in diameter. Glomeruli are limited to the cortical labyrinths and renal columns and are not ordinarily found in the medullary rays or pyramidal tissue of the kidney

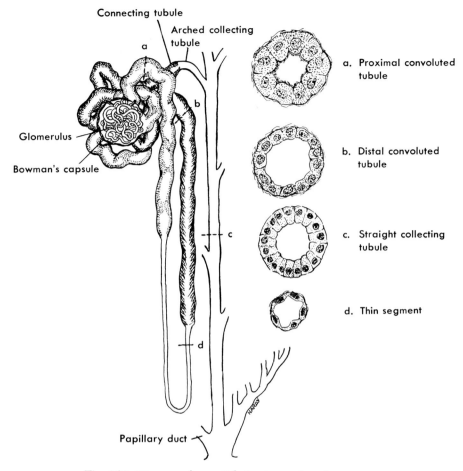

Connecting tubule

Arched collecting tubule

a

a. Proximal convoluted tubule

Glomerulus

b

b. Distal convoluted tubule

Bowman's capsule

c

c. Straight collecting tubule

d

d. Thin segment

Papillary duct

Fig. 17-3. Diagram of essential structures of nephron.

(Plates 3 and 4). *Note:* Many lower chordates, for example, certain fishes, possess aglomerular kidneys.

Nephron. On an anatomic basis the nephron consists of four parts: Bowman's capsule, proximal convoluted tubule, loop of Henle, and the distal convoluted tubule (Fig. 17-3). Bowman's capsule has been described previously as an invaginated dilation of the nephric tubule. The parietal layer leads into a small necklike constriction, which contains ciliated cells in submammalian forms but not in human beings. The tubule leading from the capsule almost immediately begins a twisted and tortuous path through the cortical labyrinth and is

accordingly named the proximal convoluted tubule. In sections, this is indicated by tubules cut in several planes (Fig. 17-2); most, however, appear in transverse or tangential section.

The proximal tubule enters a medullary ray at the site where it bends toward the papilla and forms a relatively straight tube, the *descending arm* of Henle's loop. This extends for a variable distance and then reverses its direction to form the so-called *ascending arm* of Henle's loop, which is approximately parallel to the descending arm. In the region of the actual curvature the tubule becomes extremely thin, giving rise to the *thin segment* of Henle's loop. The

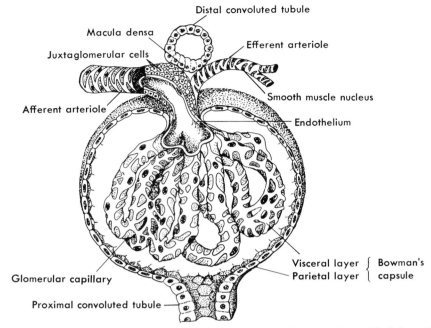

Distal convoluted tubule
Macula densa
Juxtaglomerular cells
Efferent arteriole
Afferent arteriole
Smooth muscle nucleus
Endothelium
Glomerular capillary
Visceral layer ⎰ Bowman's
Parietal layer ⎱ capsule
Proximal convoluted tubule

Fig. 17-4. Representative drawing of renal corpuscle. (Redrawn and modified from Bailey.)

thin segment is a variable structure, since it may be located on the ascending side, the descending side, or both. Thin segments of nephrons arising from cortical glomeruli are abbreviated or lacking entirely, whereas nephrons originating in the juxtamedullary region bear long thin segments penetrating deeply into the pyramids (Plate 4). In summary, the loops of Henle are located entirely within the medullary rays and pyramids. They consist of a thick descending limb, a thin segment, which varies in location and length, and a thick ascending limb.

The ascending limb enters the cortical labyrinth slightly below the level of the glomerulus of origin and passes between the afferent and efferent vessels and makes tangential contact with the vascular pole of the glomerulus. The region of tangential contact is specialized to form the *macula densa* (Fig. 17-4). The portion of the tubule extending beyond the vascular pole is known as the *distal convoluted tubule*. It is less convoluted than the proximal tubule. The distal tubule leads to an arched tubule,

which enters the medullary ray to join the system of collecting tubules.

On a cytologic-physiologic basis only four subdivisions of the nephron are designated: Bowman's capsule, a proximal segment, a thin segment, and a distal segment.

Bowman's capsule. The *parietal* layer of Bowman's capsule consists of squamous epithelium with prominent nuclei that protrude into the capillary space (Fig. 17-5). The inner or *visceral* epithelium forms a thin sheet over the loops of the glomerular capillaries. This fact was not clearly demonstrated until observed by electron microscopy. Studies utilizing the electron microscope have shown that the cells comprising the visceral epithelium are branching cells called *podocytes* (Fig. 17-6). Each cell consists of a central mass containing a nucleus and several radiating processes, which, in turn, give rise to smaller processes known as *pedicles*. The pedicles make contact with the basal lamina of the capillary. Pedicles from adjacent cells interdigitate and leave slits (filtration slits) that communicate with the larger spaces

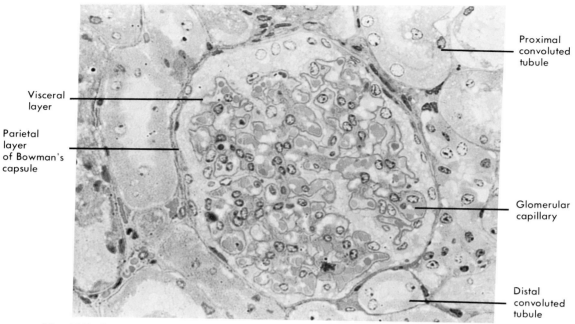

Visceral layer

Parietal layer of Bowman's capsule

Proximal convoluted tubule

Glomerular capillary

Distal convoluted tubule

Fig. 17-5. Photomicrograph of section of glomerulus of monkey's kidney. (Plastic section; ×400.)

between major extensions. They all empty into the capsular (urinary) space.

The endothelium of the capillaries is composed of thin flattened cells with a mass of cytoplasm in the area of the nucleus. In the thinner portions, they exhibit a specialization that consists of numerous round openings (fenestrations), which are regularly arranged and lie near one another.

Another component of the glomerulus consists of cells and intercellular matrices occupying a position between the capillary loops known as the *mesangium*. The mesangial cells have been described as having a dense cytoplasm and radiating cytoplasmic processes and tonofilaments. Since they have been shown to contain a myosin-like protein by immunofluorescent techniques, these cells are probably contractile. They maintain close contact with the macula densa of the distal tubule via cellular interdigitations.

Proximal segment. The proximal segment consists of tubules with low columnar epithelium (Fig. 17-3) bearing a brush bor-

der at the free surface and basal striations in the subnuclear position. The latter represent infoldings of the cell membrane along which mitochondria may be visualized by special methods. Inasmuch as adjacent cells interdigitate freely, the cell outlines are rarely seen in cross sections of the tubule. The coarsely granular eosinophilic cytoplasm bulges into the lumen, and the nuclei are basally located. The brush border is not ordinarily well preserved; accordingly, the free edge of the cell appears rounded and slightly ragged. Similarly mitochondria and basal striations are not well preserved in routine preparations and are not usually apparent to the novice. The basal striations become less distinct as the thin segment is approached. Despite considerable postmortem degeneration, these cells are considerably more eosinophilic than are those found in adjacent tubules.

The proximal segment consists of a convoluted portion in the cortical labyrinth and a straight descending limb in the medullary ray and pyramid.

At the electron microscope level, the

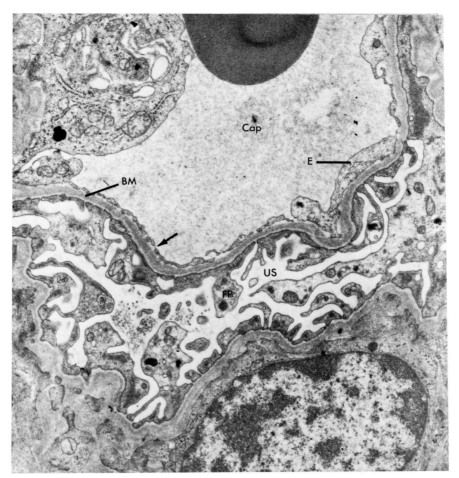

Fig. 17-6. Electron micrograph of part of the glomerulus of a monkey's kidney. The capillary, *Cap*, is lined with endothelium, *E*, which at intervals contains pores (arrow). The outer walls of the capillaries are invested by the cytoplasm of podocytes, whose fingerlike processes, called pedicles, *FP*, extend from the capillary into the lumen of the urinary space, *US*. The cytoplasm of the basal portions of the endothelial cells and the podocytes are separated by a prominent basement membrane, *BM*. (×10,000.)

brush border is shown to consist of numerous thin microvilli. Frequently small vesicles appear between the bases of the microvilli, and it has been suggested that tubular reabsorption may be accomplished in part by pinocytotic activity. A Golgi complex located in the supranuclear position is a constant feature of these cells (Fig. 17-7).

A prominent feature of the cells of the proximal tubule is the basal portion that is divided into compartments by prominent infoldings (Fig. 17-8). These compartments contain numerous elongated mitochondria and polyribosomes. They rest upon a continuous basal lamina, which separates them from the walls of the surrounding (peritubular) capillaries.

Thin segments. The thin segments are tubular structures consisting of squamous cells. The cytoplasm appears agranular, and the nucleus is slightly compressed. In cross section they may be confused with capil-

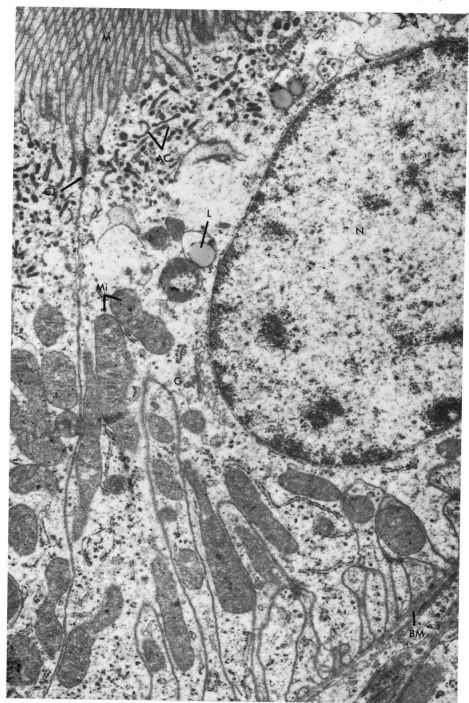

Fig. 17-7. Electron micrograph of part of epithelial cell of proximal convoluted tubule of mouse kidney. *AC,* Apical canaliculi; *BM,* basement membrane; *CJ,* cell junction; *G,* Golgi apparatus; *L,* lipid granule; *M,* microvilli; *Mi,* mitochondrion; *N,* nucleus. (×17,000.)

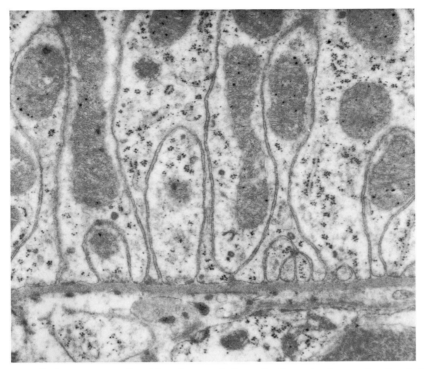

Fig. 17-8. Electron micrograph of basal part of the cell of proximal convoluted tubule of a mouse kidney. Note extensive infolding of cell membranes enclosing densely packed mitochondria and scattered ribosomes. (×25,000.)

laries and arteriolae rectae, especially since red blood cells are sometimes forced into the thin segments during preparation of the tissue. They are distinguished from capillaries by the more extensive protrusion of nuclei into the lumen and the greater number of cells visible in cross section through a tubule.

Thin segments are demonstrable in profusion in the deeper portions of the pyramids since they extend almost to the papillae. Thin segments of the kind described are lacking in reptiles, most birds, amphibians, and fishes.

Distal segment. The thin segment joins the distal segment, which is composed initially of low cuboidal cells with indistinct boundaries. As the ascending limb approaches the cortex the cells are taller but are still cuboidal and bear irregular projections into the lumen. Upon entering the cortical labyrinths the tubule passes the vascular pole of the glomerulus of origin and makes tangential contact wtih the afferent arteriole. At the point of contact the cuboidal cells become more closely packed so that the cells appear taller (sometimes columnar), and many nuclei are visible and crowded together to form the *macula densa* (Fig. 17-4). Beyond this structure the tubule becomes convoluted, consisting of smaller cuboidal cells, the free surfaces of which are smooth. These cells are less eosinophilic (or more basophilic) than are those found in the proximal tubule. The cells do not bear a striated border or brush border or basal striations, neither do they exhibit definite cell boundaries in sectioned material. The basement membrane is prominent along all parts of the tubule except in the region of the macula densa. Since the convoluted portion is short, fewer sections

Cuboidal cells   Basement membrane

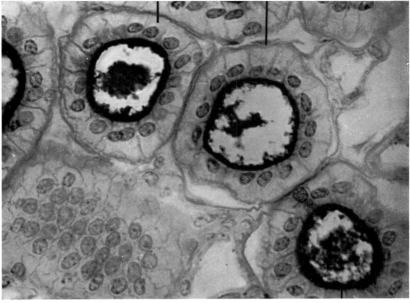

Alkaline phosphatase

Fig. 17-9. Section of kidney of a skate showing collecting tubules treated to show localization of the enzyme alkaline phosphatase. (×640.)

through this segment are seen in the cortical labyrinths.

Collecting tubules and papillary ducts. At the termination of the distal convoluted tubule, a short connecting tubule can be observed sometimes. It contains a mixture of the cuboidal cells characteristic of the distal segment and occasional isolated large granular cells (intercalated cells). This is supposedly the region of embryonic fusion between the nephron and the collecting tubule.

The connecting tubule is continuous with the *arched collecting tubule* that passes into the medullary ray, where it joins the *straight collecting tubule* (Fig. 17-3). The straight tubules, along with Henle's loops, lie in parallel bundles and occupy most of the medulla, with the exception of the papilla. The cells of the collecting tubules are noted for their distinct boundaries, spherical nuclei at approximately the same level in the cell, and relatively agranular cytoplasm (Fig. 17-9). Eventually the

straight tubules (Plate 3) reach the papillary region and fuse to form relatively large ducts, the *papillary ducts* (ducts of Bellini). The latter consist of tall columnar cells. In each papilla are formed sixteen to twenty papillary ducts, which penetrate the apex of the papilla to form a sievelike region or *area cribosa* (Plate 3). From this site the urine formed in the nephrons is drained into a minor calyx (Fig. 17-1).

Juxtaglomerular apparatus. At the vascular pole of the glomerulus (Fig. 17-4) the media and adventitial reticulum of the afferent arteriole are replaced by cells that vary from cuboidal to columnar. These form a thickening or cuff around the arteriole (periarteriolar pad). Numerous cells may spill into the cleft between the afferent and efferent vessels to form an asymmetric cap (polkissen or polar cushion). This complex of cells is referred to as the *juxtaglomerular apparatus*. The polkissen and periarteriolar pad both may be in contact with the macula densa, and their region of contact is marked by the absence of a PAS-positive basement membrane. The polkissen cells of certain rodents exhibit some large epithelioid cells containing brilliant fuchsinophil granules. In canines and man the cells are small and agranular. In addition, the juxtaglomerular apparatus is not demonstrable in man for the first two years of postnatal life. The presence of epithelioid cells similar to those found in certain endocrine organs suggests an endocrine function. Physiologic experiments indicate that these cells produce renin. Renin is a proteolytic enzyme secreted by the juxtaglomerular apparatus that reacts with a precursor in the blood to form an active vasopressor substance, angiotensin II. Present techniques have not adequately demonstrated whether renin is made in the macula densa of the distal convoluted tubule, the juxtaglomerular (JG) cells of the afferent arteriole or cells between them. Current evidence favors the juxtaglomerular cells as the source of renin, but the cellular membranes of the juxtaglomerular cells and the macula densa cells interdigitate and some exchange of materials between them is likely.

Lymphatic circulation. The lymphatic plexuses are found in three main regions as follows. (1) A network of lymphatic capillaries permeates the cortex and renal columns; these capillaries form an anastomosing network around blood vessels, especially the larger arteries. The plexus drains into the lymphatic vessels leaving the hilum of the kidney; then it goes into the lateral aortic nodes (2) beneath the renal capsule in intimate association with the stellate veins and subcapsular plexus of blood capillaries. This group communicates with (3) the lymphatics draining the perirenal fat body. The perirenal lymphatic plexus drains into the lateral aortic nodes.

Lymphatics are lacking in the renal pyramids and glomeruli and do not enter the tubules. No specific function has been demonstrated for the kidney lymphatics.

Connective tissue. The renal capsule is formed of a dense fibrous connective tissue that is primarily collagenous, with some elastic fibers and a few scattered smooth muscle cells. A thin inflexion of this capsule lines the renal sinus and fuses with the adventitia of the blood vessels and epineurium of the larger nerves. It also disperses into fine strands in the fat body of the renal sinus. The renal capsule is easily stripped from normal kidneys because of a lack of trabeculi from the capsule.

The basement membrane entirely envelops all parts of the nephron and collecting tubules except as noted previously. The ground substance of the basement membrane is PAS positive, and the reticular fibers are typically argyrophile and quite fine. In the pyramids the reticular fibers form an extensive network binding ducts and blood vessels together.

Excretory passages. The excretory passages consist of the calyces, renal pelvis, ureter, bladder, and urethra. All of these structures, with the exception of the urethra, have a similar basic structure. The wall consists of an inner mucosa lined with transitional epithelium, a middle muscular layer that becomes thicker as the ureter reaches the bladder, and an outer adventitia that blends into the surrounding connective tissue. There is no distinct submucosa (Fig. 17-10).

URETER

Urine collects in the pelvis of the kidney and passes into the ureter, a thin duct leading to the bladder.

Mucosa. The mucosa includes an epithelium of the transitional type resting on a lamina propria of reticular and fine areolar tissue. The basement membrane separating the epithelium from the lamina propria is not distinct, although one can be detected at higher magnification. The epithelium is two or three cell layers thick in the renal pelvis; it gradually increases to six or more layers in the undistended bladder. When the organ is stretched, the cells flatten and interdigitation between the cells is reduced. The epithelium lining the ureter and bladder is reduced to a layer approximately three cells thick in the distended state. The muscularis mucosa is lacking.

Adipose tissue   Muscularis

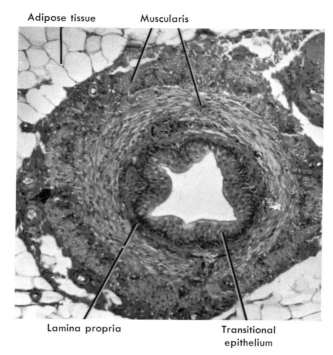

Lamina propria   Transitional
                              epithelium

Fig. 17-10. Ureter of cat. (×160.)

Muscularis. In the muscularis the usual arrangement of coats is reversed, there being an inner longitudinal and an outer circular layer. The lower portion of the ureter contains a third layer of muscle, longitudinally disposed, outside the circular layer. All three layers are somewhat loosely arranged, with a great deal of areolar tissue among the muscle fibers.

Adventitia. The adventitia is formed of loose connective tissue.

URINARY BLADDER

The wall of the urinary bladder is composed of the same elements as those of the lower part of the ureter, that is, transitional epithelium, lamina propria, three layers of muscle, and adventitia (Fig. 17-11). In the bladder the epithelium varies in thickness according to the degree of distention of the organ. (See discussion on transitional epithelium, Chapter 2.) The muscular layers of the bladder are not so regular in their arrange-

ments as those of the ureter, but they form a thicker layer (Fig. 17-12). Where present, the adventitia is composed of fibroelastic tissue.

URETHRA

The urethra of the female serves as an outlet for urine from the bladder, whereas that of the male functions also as the terminal portion of the ducts of the reproductive system. The organ is, therefore, somewhat different in the two sexes.

Female urethra

In the female the tube is composed of an epithelial lining, a connective tissue layer, and a muscular coat. The epithelium of the proximal part is like that of the bladder. This type is replaced further down the tube first by stratified columnar or pseudostratified columnar epithelium and later, toward the distal end, by stratified squamous epithelium.

The connective tissue layer contains elastic fibers and a rich plexus of veins, which

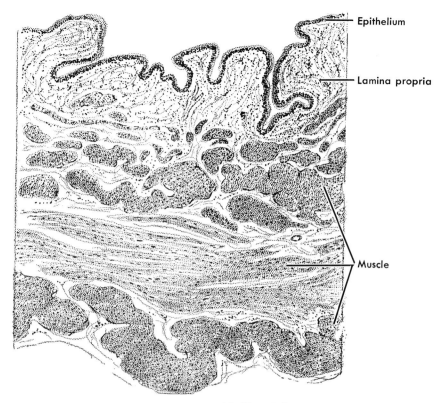

Epithelium

Lamina propria

Muscle

Fig. 17-11. Urinary bladder of dog.

may be compared with the corpus cavernosum of the male urethra (see next section)
though it is much less extensive. The lumen
of the organ is irregular, since the connective tissue and epithelium are thrown into
longitudinal rugae. There are also small
diverticula from the lumen (lacunae) into
which open the mucus-secreting glands of
Littré.

The muscularis consists of two sets of
smooth muscle fibers intermingled with
connective tissue. The fibers of the inner
set are longitudinally placed, the outer
have a circular direction. Note that this is
different from the arrangement of muscle
in the gut wall, where the inner muscle
coat is circular and the outer is longitudinal. At the distal end of the urethra
there is, in addition, a sphincter of striated
muscle.

Male urethra

The male urethra shows modifications
of the structure just described. It is divided
into three portions: prostatic, membranous,
and cavernous (Fig. 18-1).

Prostatic portion. The proximal end of
the prostatic urethra is homologous to the
female urethra and resembles it in structure as well as in function. As the tube
passes through the prostate gland it receives the openings of the ducts from the
testes and numerous small ducts from the
prostate.

Membranous portion. The membranous
portion of the urethra, which passes
through the urogenital diaphragm, is also
somewhat like the female urethra. The epithelium changes in or about this region
from transitional to stratified columnar or
pseudostratified, but the location of the

Lamina propria   Transitional epithelium

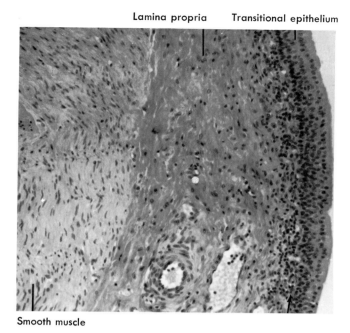

Smooth muscle

Fig. 17-12. Section of human urinary bladder showing mucosa and part of muscularis. (×40.)

change varies considerably in different individuals. Glands are more common than in the female urethra. The bulbourethral (mucous) glands of Cowper are situated in the muscle near the distal part of the membranous urethra, but their ducts enter the cavernous urethra.

Cavernous portion. The cavernous portion is the longest segment of the urethra, lying in the penis. The tissues surrounding it will be discussed more fully in Chapter 18. The epithelial lining of the urethra changes at the distal end to stratified squamous with well-developed connective tissue papillae. The lamina propria contains an extensive plexus of blood vessels, which forms the corpus cavernosum urethrae, and the glands of Littré are most numerous in this portion of the tube. The muscular coat is broken up into scattered groups of fibers.

Blood and nerve supply of the excretory passages

The blood supply of the ureter, bladder, and urethra comes from arteries that penetrate the muscular coats of the organs and form plexuses in the deeper layers of the lamina propria. From here, vessels continue inward, forming other plexuses just below the epithelium. The deeper layers of the connective tissue and probably the muscular layers have a rich lymphatic supply.

Plexuses of medullated and nonmedullated nerves occur in the walls of the ureter and the bladder. The nonmedullated nerves supply the muscles; the medullated, the mucosa. Numerous ganglia are present in the connective tissue.

18
Male reproductive system

The male reproductive system consists of (1) the testes, which produce sperm and male hormones, (2) the system of ducts that carry the sperm from the testes to the urethra and in which sperm continue their maturation, (3) several accessory glands associated with the duct system that secrete components of the seminal fluid, and (4) the penis (Fig. 18-1).

TESTIS

The testis is covered by a two-layered connective tissue capsule. The outer layer of tunica albuginea is composed of dense collagenous fibrous tissue; the inner or vasculosa layer is of looser areolar tissue richly supplied with blood vessels. From the capsule, trabeculae extend inward to a central mass of connective tissue, the mediastinum, which contains the proximal portions of the duct system. The parenchyma of the testis is thus divided into many pyramidal lobules, which contain the closely packed coils of the seminiferous tubules and a stroma of interstitial connective tissue (Figs. 18-2 and 18-3). In the connective tissue are blood vessels and groups of endocrine cells called the interstitial cells of the testes *(Leydig cells)*, which produce steroid hormones.

The convoluted seminiferous tubules are lined with germinal epithelium that may contain as many as five layers of cells (Fig. 18-3). This epithelium is composed of spermatogenic or sperm-forming cells (Fig. 18-4) and Sertoli or "supportive" cells. These two cell groups are generally believed to be derived from two independent cell lines. At birth, the testes contain recognizable spermatogonia, but within a few

months they disappear, reappearing again at the onset of puberty. With the beginning of sexual maturity, the Leydig cells become more prominent and spermatogenic cells in diverse stages of development appear within the tubules (Figs. 18-4 and 18-5). The epithelium rests upon a thin basement membrane that, in turn, is surrounded by a capsule consisting of fibroelastic connective tissue. Most closely applied to the outside of the wall of the tubules are the spermatogonia or primordial germ cells separated from the wall by fine Sertoli cell processes. These cells are small, cuboidal, or rounded with vesicular nuclei. Proceeding toward the lumen one observes the primary spermatocytes. They are larger cells and exhibit dense clumps of chromatin in the nuclei. Next in order are the secondary spermatocytes, which are rarely seen but which are similar in appearance to the primary spermatocytes but somewhat smaller. Superimposed on these are the spermatids, which are much smaller cells with vesicular nuclei. Bordering on the lumen one may observe the fully formed spermatozoa, possessing dark, elongated nuclei and flagellae (Fig. 18-6).

The process involved in the development of the spermatozoa consists of (1) a reduction of the chromosomal number from the diploid or somatic number (forty-six) to the haploid or germ cell number (twenty-three) and (2) the formation of elongate, tail-bearing motile cells from the primitive oval spermatogonia. In males, chromosomal redistribution (meiosis, spermatogenesis) occurs before the cell becomes differentiated (spermiogenesis). In females, the egg is formed while the cell

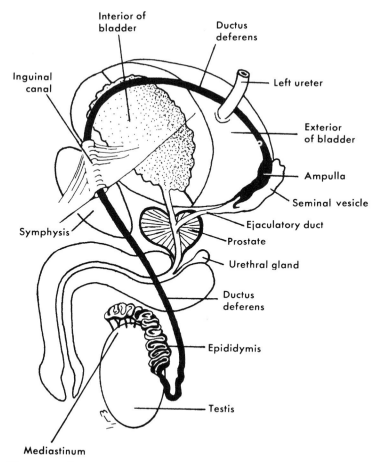

Fig. 18-1. Diagrammatic representation of the male reproductive organs. (Drawing by Emily Craig.)

is in the first stage of meiosis. In ordinary cell division (mitosis), the chromosomal material is replicated before the onset of nuclear division. Following this, each daughter cell then receives one full set of chromosomes. The number of chromosomes in each mitotic cell is constant and characteristic for each species of animal. In man there are forty-four autosomes and two sex chromosomes (X and Y), making a total of forty-six. This number is also found in the nucleus of spermatogonia and is replicated during division of the spermatogonia. Mature sperm have the haploid number of chromosomes. To achieve the duplication and distribution of chromosomes in meiosis, two divisions

(maturational divisions) are required. In the first maturational division, which occurs in primary spermatocytes (Fig. 18-4), the forty-six chromosomes become arranged as twenty-three homologous pairs, each chromosome being joined by its replicate. One member of each pair, accompanied by its duplicate, is distributed to each daughter cell. The resulting cells are the *secondary spermatocytes,* which almost immediately enter the second maturational division. In this stage, each daughter cell receives one copy of the twenty-three chromosomes contained in the primary spermatocyte. The resulting daughter cells, called *spermatids,* contain the haploid number of chromosomes and have completed the first step in

Secondary spermatocyte   Lumen   Spermatids

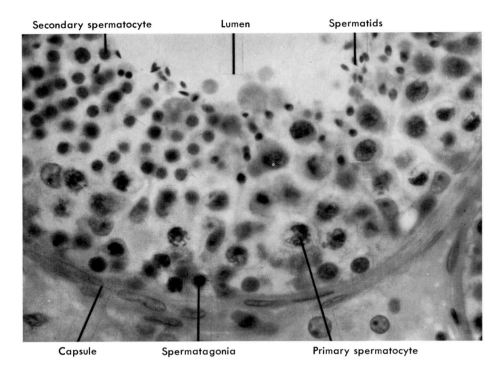

Capsule   Spermatagonia   Primary spermatocyte

Fig. 18-2. Section of portion of human seminiferous tubule. (×640.)

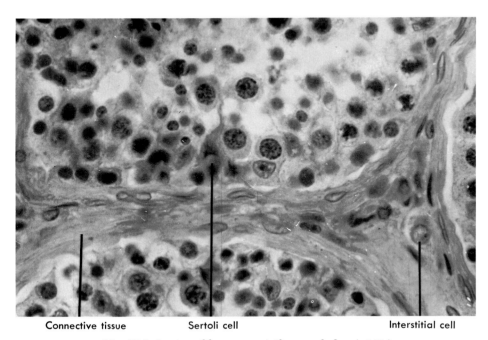

Connective tissue   Sertoli cell   Interstitial cell

Fig. 18-3. Section of human seminiferous tubules. (×640.)

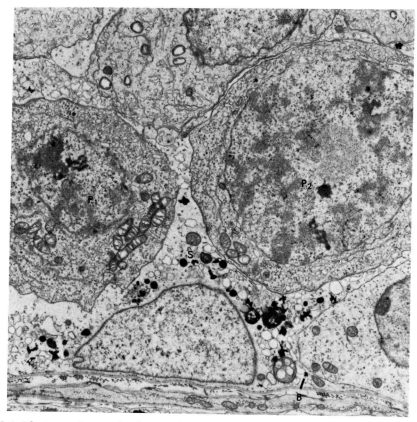

Fig. 18-4. Electron micrograph of part of a seminiferous tubule of mouse. *B*, Basement membrane; *P₁, P₂,* primary spermatocytes in prophase; *S*, Sertoli cell. (×7,000.)

formation of a mature sperm. Each spermatid will now be remodeled to form a mature sperm cell. A similar set of events must take place in the ovum, the female germ cell, but the timing of the events is different (see Chapter 19). The result of meiosis is to produce a spermatozoan containing twenty-three chromosomes and an ovum, also containing twenty-three chromosomes. When these two unite, the resulting zygote is provided with the original forty-six chromosomes contained in all body cells other than germ cells. Since the chromosomes are the bearers of hereditary characteristics, their distribution is of great interest to geneticists.

Spermiogenesis is the maturation of the spermatids to form spermatozoa. This oc-

curs by means of a series of orderly changes that transform the small, round spermatid into the elongated, tail-bearing spermatozoan (Fig. 18-7). This process occurs after meiosis is complete. The stages in this process are shown diagrammatically in Fig. 18-7. The main stages are (1) the formation of an acrosome (a large lysosomal derivative from the Golgi apparatus), (2) a change in the shape and degree of condensation of the nucleus, (3) the formation of a flagellum that will later become motile, and (4) an extensive remodeling of the cytoplasm including the formation of an elaborate mitochondrial sheath surrounding the flagellum beneath the sperm head.

The spermatid exhibits a large centrally

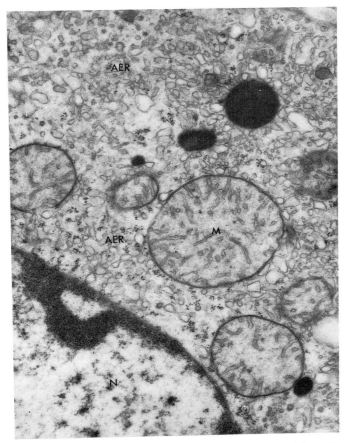

Fig. 18-5. Electron micrograph of part of an interstitial cell of mouse. Note abundant, tubular, agranular endoplasmic reticulum, *AER*. *N*, Nucleus; *M*, mitochondrion. (×23,000.)

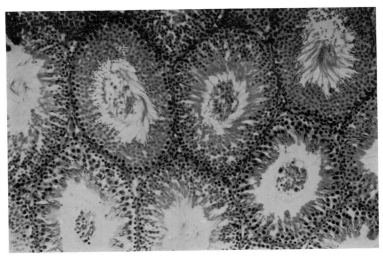

Fig. 18-6. Section of seminiferous tubules of rat showing mature sperm.

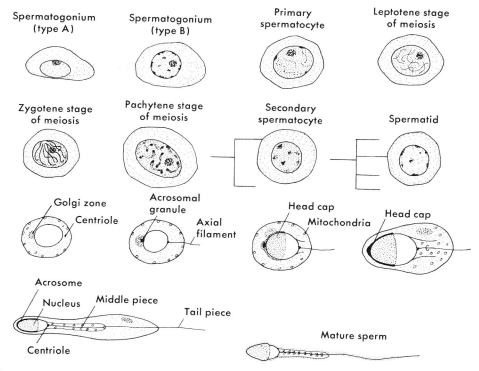

Fig. 18-7. Stages in sperm formation. It takes about 74 days for a group of spermatogonial cells to progress through the stages of sperm formation to the mature sperm with head and tail. Large numbers of spermatogonia tend to enter the maturational process together and to divide synchronously. New groups of spermatogonia enter the cycle before the older "generations" have completed their sequence, resulting in a patchwork arrangement of cell communities with the youngest generations next to the wall of the seminiferous tubule and the more mature cell clusters near the lumen. (Drawing by Emily Craig.)

located nucleus, numerous mitochondria, and a pair of centrioles. The prominent supranuclear Golgi apparatus consists of numerous lamellae and vesicles. Granules that appear in these vesicles coalesce to form the *acrosome* within the acrosome vesicle (Fig. 18-8). It is believed that the acrosome contains enzymes necessary for sperm penetration of the egg. The acrosome and its vesicle lie between the Golgi apparatus and nuclear membrane. The vesicle enlarges and eventually envelopes approximately half of the surface of the nucleus; finally it collapses and forms a closely applied membrane covering the acrosome, known as the *head cap*. During the formation of the acrosome at one pole of the nucleus, one of the centrioles becomes modified into a slender flagellum at

the opposite pole. Further differentiation consists in the application of a filamentous sheath around the axial filaments of the flagellum. Meanwhile, the other centriole migrates toward the surface of the cell and gives rise to the annulus encircling the longitudinal axial filaments. The nucleus decreases in size, becomes flattened and elongated, and is then known as the sperm head. Development of the tail consists in a shift of the cytoplasm and a rearrangement of the mitochondria to the region between the basal centriole and the annulus. In this region, the mitochondria become aligned in helical fashion and make up the mitochondrial sheath of the middle piece of the developing sperm. As differentiation continues, the excess cytoplasm is shed as the residual body; thus, eventually

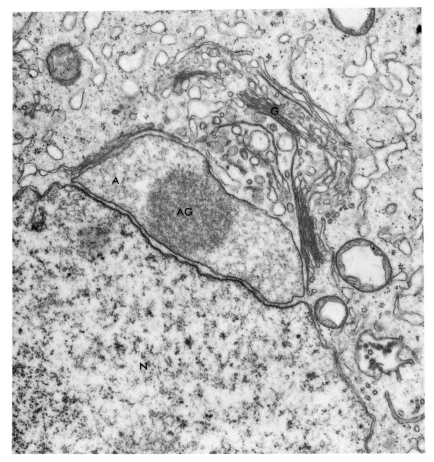

Fig. 18-8. Electron micrograph of developing spermatid of mouse showing relation of Golgi apparatus, *G*, to acrosome. *A*, Acrosomal vesicle; *AG*, acrosomal granule; *N*, nucleus. (×28,000.)

the spermatozoon is covered by a very thin layer of cytoplasm (Fig. 18-9).

The mammalian sperm is comprised of three main components: the head, neck, and tail (Fig. 18-10). The head mainly consists of a dense nucleus that is surmounted by a small crescentic acrosome. The neck, or connecting piece between the head and the tail, contains linear fibrils surrounded by a mitochondrial sheath. The middle piece of the tail consists of two central filaments and nine doubled peripheral ones (Fig. 18-11, *B*). External to the latter are nine, outer, coarse fibers of uneven size that extend varying distances down the tail enclosed by a helical mitochondrial sheath. The main segment of the tail has two central and nine peripheral filaments and except in the terminal portion is enclosed by a thin layer of cytoplasm (Fig. 18-11, *A*).

The process of spermatogenesis in man takes place in six basic stages (Fig. 18-12). These stages are characterized by the cells found in association with each other. The various generations of germ cells are not associated at random but are always found in certain configurations. These stages can be ascertained in Fig. 18-12 by examination of the vertical columns. The resulting orderly sequence of associations is called the "cycle of the seminiferous epithelium."

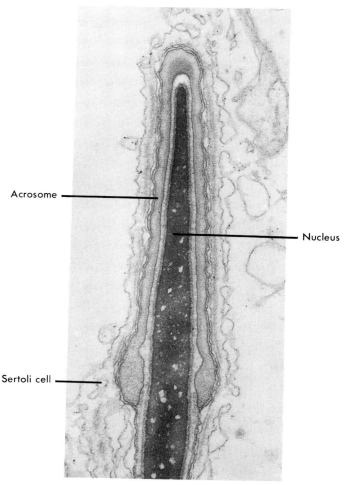

Acrosome

Nucleus

Sertoli cell

Fig. 18-9. Electron micrograph of nearly mature sperm head of dog. (×18,000.)

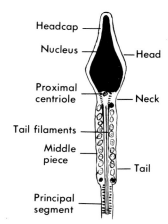

Headcap

Nucleus

Head

Proximal
centriole

Neck

Tail filaments

Middle
piece

Tail

Principal
segment

Fig. 18-10. Diagrammatic longitudinal section of human sperm. (Redrawn and somewhat modified after Fawcett.)

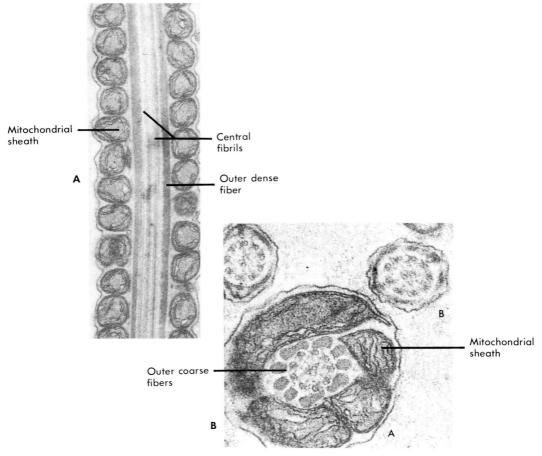

Fig. 18-11. A, Electron micrograph of part of middle piece of sperm tail of a mouse. **B,** Electron micrograph of transverse section of tail of mouse sperm. *A,* Middle piece; *B,* principal piece. The middle piece shows an internal core of one central pair and nine peripheral pairs of fibers surrounded by nine outer coarse fibers enclosed by a mitochondrial sheath. (**A,** ×38,000; **B,** ×60,000.)

In man, the stages of this cycle are more difficult to see than in other mammals. The length of time that it takes for a complete cell cycle of sperm formation to be completed is estimated to be 16 days based on the time observed for the incorporation of ³H-thymidine by germ cells. The maturation of spermatozoa occurs in a series of irregularly shaped zones in which all the cells are in the same stage. For this reason, a transverse section through the testis will show some profiles of seminiferous tubules in which all six stages are visible and others in which only three or four stages are observed.

It will be noticed that the germinal epithelium of the testis, although stratified, is not to be classed with any other type of epithelium. In those already studied, the stratification has as its purpose the formation of a protective layer. In the germinal epithelium it is simply the accidental result of the piling of one stage of development on another. The tissue differs from

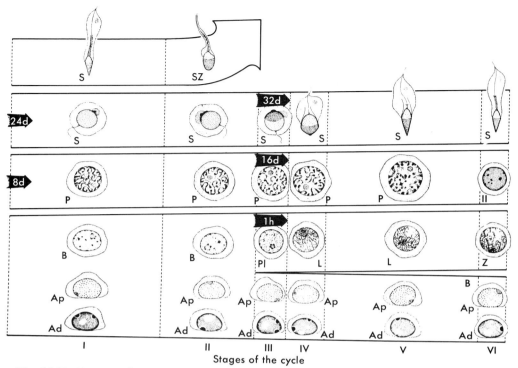

Stages of the cycle

Fig. 18-12. Diagram showing the cells found associated together in the six stages of the cycle of the seminiferous epithelium in man. Stages are indicated by Roman numerals (*I* to *VI*). After stage VI, the cycle starts again at I. *Ad,* Dark spermatogonium; *Ap,* pale type A spermatogonium; *B,* type B spermatogonium; *PL, L, Z, P,* preleptotene, leptotene, zygotene, and pachytene primary spermatocytes; *II,* secondary spermatocyte; *S,* spermatid; *SZ,* spermatozoan. Arrows refer to most advanced cell types labeled at various times after an intratesticular injection of 3H-thymidine. (From Clermont; in Rosenberg and Paulsen, editors: The human testis, New York, 1971, Plenum Publishing Corp.)

other epithelia also in the relation of the cells to each other. In stratified squamous epithelium, for instance, the cells are closely applied to each other and are held together by cement substance. In germinal epithelium the cells are so loosely piled that many of them retain their spherical shape.

Besides the cells that represent stages of spermatogenesis, the seminiferous tubule has in its wall several supporting cells, the sustentacular or Sertoli cells. These are irregular elongated elements, the bases of which lie against the basement membrane and the apices of which border on the lumen (Figs. 18-3 and 18-4). The nucleus, located either basally or somewhat re-

moved from the base of the cell, is ovoid in shape, appears pale, and contains finely dispersed chromatin and usually one or more prominent nucleoli that stain unevenly with a central acidophilic core and a basophilic rim. The nuclear membrane may exhibit a longitudinal spiral groove. Above the nucleus, in addition to mitochondria and other cytoplasmic inclusions, an unusual spindle-shaped crystalloid structure is often present in the Sertoli cell of man only. Although the Sertoli cells do not contribute to or take an active part in the production of sperm, they do undergo a cyclic activity that is correlated with spermatogenesis. When mature spermatozoa are present, they tend to gather in groups with their heads (nuclei) embedded in the free end of the Sertoli cell, and this fact will aid the student in viewing the groups of spermatozoa. The sustentacular cells furnish nourishment to the spermatozoa and also form a supporting framework for the other germinal cells.

In the mature testis, there are fewer Sertoli cells than germinal cells, and the former tend to be evenly spaced around the seminiferous tubule. The Sertoli cells (Fig. 18-3) are fairly resistant to many noxious agents and to the effects of aging. Two types of Sertoli cells may be seen, one that stains darkly, the other that stains lightly. The functional significance of these staining differences is unknown. It has been suggested that the Sertoli cells produce a substance that can inhibit gonadotrophin secretion by the anterior pituitary and further that these cells can metabolize steroid hormones. The relative importance of the endocrine function of Sertoli cells in addition to their supposed nutritive and supportive roles in unknown.

The spermatogenic tubules lie coiled in a stroma of loose connective tissue. In the latter and separated from the tubules are groups of cells either aggregated in clusters or arranged in thin layers along blood vessels. These are the *Leydig* cells. They are the source of testicular androgens (the male hormones) and may also produce trace amounts of female hormones such as estrone. The cells are fairly large and are ovoid or polygonal in shape. The nuclei are large and eccentrically placed. The cytoplasm near the nucleus is dark and granular while peripherally it is vacuolated and stains lightly. Pigment granules (lipochromes) and crystalloids (of Reinke) may be present (Figs. 18-3 and 18-4).

The most striking feature of the cytoplasm of the Leydig cells, like that of most steroid-secreting cells, is the presence of an extensive smooth endoplasmic reticulum composed of interconnecting tubules that extend throughout much of the cytoplasm (Fig. 18-5). The mitochondria are rod shaped and of variable diameter; the cristae appear to consist of fenestrated lamellae. The Leydig cells of the human secrete a moderate amount of steroid when compared with some other mammals.

The action of male hormones has been ascertained by direct observation and by many experimental procedures involving castration at various stages of sexual maturity. Briefly, it has been shown that male hormone is necessary for the appearance of the so-called secondary sex characters in the developing mammal. If castration is performed after sexual maturity has occurred, the effect on already established secondary sex characteristics is less pronounced than in the developing individual. In the latter situation, involution of the epithelium of the genital ducts and accessory glands is the most constant feature observed.

From the convoluted seminiferous tubules the spermatozoa pass into the proximal part of the duct system of the testis, which lies in the mediastinum of the organ (see Fig. 18-1). They traverse the straightened necks of the seminiferous tubules (called tubuli recti or straight tubules) into the rete testis, consisting of a network of fine spaces occupying part of the mediastinum. The walls of the straight tubules and rete testis are lined with a low cuboidal epithelium. The surrounding connective tissue is tightly woven and extremely vascular. Scattered strands of smooth muscle can be found next to the tubules but do not form a definite coat. The rete drain into eleven to twenty efferent ductules that penetrate the tunica to form the head of the epididymis. Each tubule is arranged as a tightly woven cone held together by loose connective tissue. The separate efferent ductules are lined with alternating groups of high columnar cells with motile cilia and shorter columnar cells without cilia. The nonciliated cells can be classified into functional groups on the basis of their ultrastructural appearance as either secretory or absorptive. It has been suggested that these cells, which are derived from the primitive kidney (mesonephros) may absorb fluids secreted by the seminiferous tubules and also to aid in sperm transport. The tubules are surrounded by smooth muscle responsible

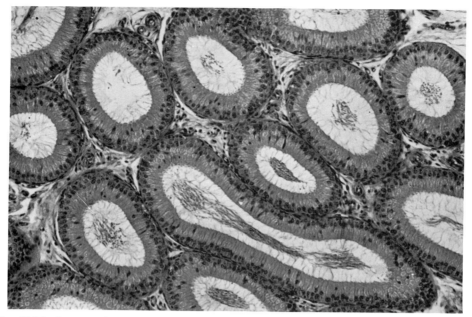

Fig. 18-13. Section of epididymis of dog showing several sections through the ductus. The stereocilia are prominent and the lumen contains spermatozoa. (×160.)

for the production of peristaltic waves that pass along the tubules at the rate of about one every 15 seconds. It has been estimated that the time necessary for the sperm to traverse the epididymis is approximately 1 to 3 weeks. The sperm traversing the efferent ductules empty into a single duct, the ductus epididymis.

EPIDIDYMIS

The epididymis lies near the testis and is surrounded in part by a fold of the tunica vaginalis, which is enclosed within a connective tissue capsule (Figs. 18-13 to 18-15). It consists of one long extensively coiled tubule, the ductus epididymis, which if stretched out would measure over 20 feet in length. A slide prepared from this region of the tract will show a great number of tubule profiles cut tangentially, transversely, or longitudinally (Fig. 18-13). The epithelium is pseudostratified columnar and contains small rounded basal cells as well as tall columnar cells that together form a smooth luminal surface. The surface cells contain secretory gran-

ules. Their free surfaces exhibit projections that resemble cilia but lack axial filaments. The function of these stereocilia ("solid cilia") is not known. The sperm spend from 1 to 3 weeks in the epididymis and during this time changes occur in appearance, motility, size, membrane permeability, temperature sensitivity, and metabolic function. The composition of the secretions of the epididymis change from the head to the tail and the epithelium gradually gets taller in the region of the vas deferens. A corresponding change occurs in the thickness of the muscle coat, which is maximum as the epididymis leads into the vas deferens (Fig. 18-1). The blood supply of the head and tail of the epididymis is more abundant than in more proximal parts of the male reproductive tract.

DUCTUS (VAS) DEFERENS

The vas deferens is a continuation of the ductus epididymis. It is lined by a somewhat lower epithelium. The epithelial cells lack cilia and rest upon a well-developed

Sperm in lumen   Smooth muscle fibers

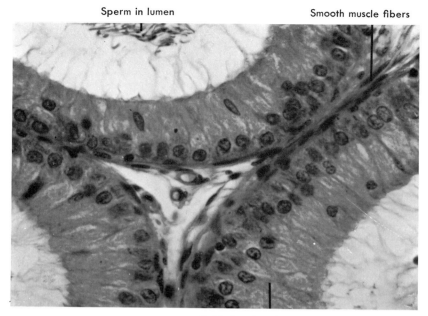

Epithelium bearing stereocilia

Fig. 18-14. Section of epididymis of dog.(×640.)

lamina propria. The muscularis has three layers: a thick intermediate circular layer and two thin longitudinal layers, one on the inner and the outer surfaces, respectively (Fig. 18-16). On reaching the prostate gland, the ductus deferens dilates to form the ampulla, a thin-walled structure with a complexly folded mucosa. As it passes into the substance of the prostate, the ampulla narrows again to form the ejaculatory duct that opens into the prostatic part of the urethra.

ACCESSORY GLANDS

Many cells in the epithelial lining of the male reproductive tract are secretory. In addition, all male mammals have several specialized glands associated with specific regions of the reproductive tract. These glands elaborate the major portion of the seminal fluid. Usually the secretory epithelium of these glands is characterized by infoldings of the mucosa and loosely arranged subjacent connective tissue. These structural features facilitate expansion of the gland and an increase in the surface epithelium. There is also a mass of smooth muscle within the connective tissue that helps to empty the glands quickly during entrance of the seminal fluid into the urethra (emission). The secretory activity of these glands depends upon testicular hormones, and the appearance and function of the cells varies greatly with hormonal status.

The two major accessory glands in man are the seminal vesicles, which are derived from the mesonephric or wolffian duct as are the ductus deferens and the prostate. In addition, a pair of small compound tubuloalveolar glands called the bulbourethral or Cowper's glands empties into the proximal urethra. These glands, similar to mucous glands, elaborate a fluid believed to function as a lubricant during intercourse. Opening into the urethra along its entire length are also small mucous glands (glands of Littré).

SEMINAL VESICLE

The seminal vesicle is an elongated saccular organ lying near the ampulla of the

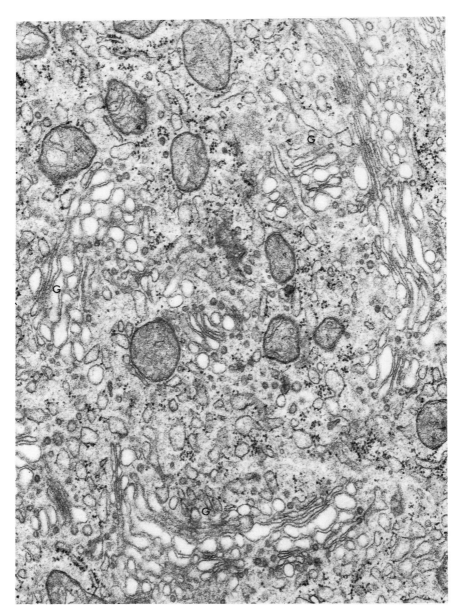

Fig. 18-15. Electron micrograph of part of epithelial cell of mouse epididymis showing very prominent Golgi complex, G. (×38,000.)

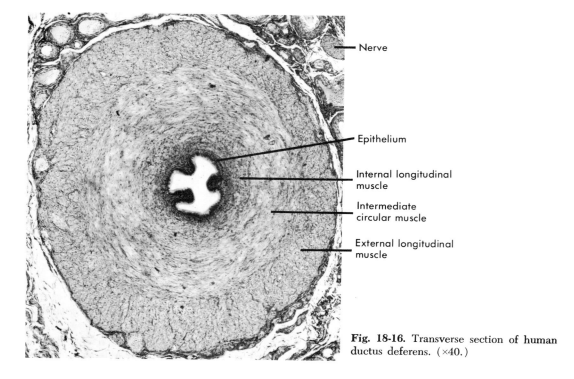

Nerve

Epithelium

Internal longitudinal muscle

Intermediate circular muscle

External longitudinal muscle

Fig. 18-16. Transverse section of human ductus deferens. (×40.)

Crypts

Epithelium

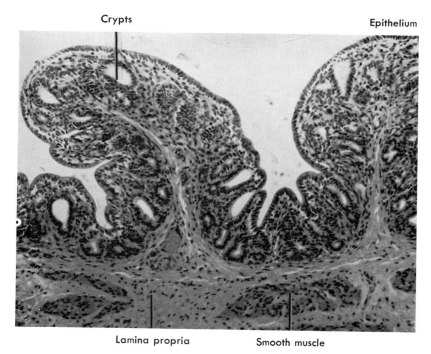

Lamina propria

Smooth muscle

Fig. 18-17. Mucosa of seminal vesicle of cat. (×160.)

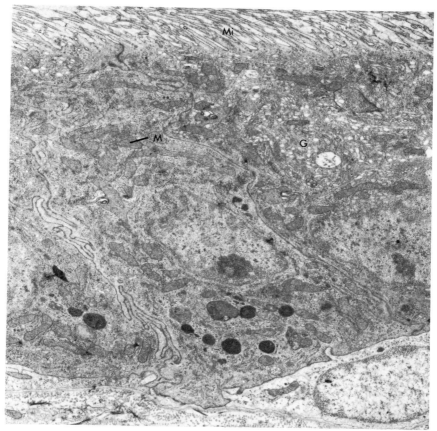

Fig. 18-18. Electron micrograph of the epithelium of mouse seminal vesicle. *Mi,* Microvilli bordering lumen; *M,* mitochondrion; *G,* Golgi complex. (×10,000.)

ductus deferens and opening into the latter at the point where it narrows to form the ejaculatory duct. When uncoiled it extends over 15 cm. The most striking histologic characteristic of the seminal vesicle is the folding of its mucosa (Fig. 18-17). In sections, this produces a great number of projections and pockets, and, since the latter are often tangentially cut, there appear to be follicles in the mucosa much like those occurring in the gallbladder.

The epithelial cells of the seminal vesicle are columnar. They have a prominent, centrally located nucleus and at times exhibit several vacuoles and granules. At the electron microscope level additional cytologic details observed consist of microvilli lining the lumen, numerous scattered mitochondria, rough endoplasmic reticulum, and a large prominent supranuclear Golgi complex. Scattered secretory granules and vacuoles are transitory structures (Fig. 18-18).

PROSTATE

The prostate is a bean-shaped structure made up of clusters of glandular tissue surrounding the urethra at the site where it emerges from the bladder. The firm glandular tissue is surrounded by a thin connective tissue capsule containing some smooth muscle. The gland as a whole is composed of secretory channels (50%), smooth muscle (25%), and fibrous tissue (25%). The bulk of the glandular tissue

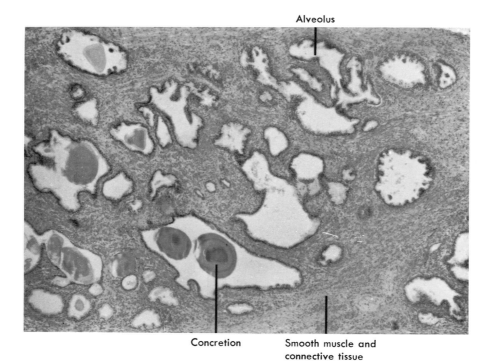

Alveolus

Concretion

Smooth muscle and
connective tissue

Fig. 18-19. Section of human prostate gland. (×40.)

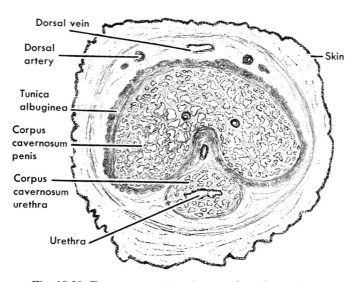

Dorsal vein

Dorsal
artery

Skin

Tunica
albuginea

Corpus
cavernosum
penis

Corpus
cavernosum
urethra

Urethra

Fig. 18-20. Transverse section of penis of newborn infant.

consists of thirty to fifty large glands that open into the urethra on the seminal colliculus along with the ejaculatory ducts. In addition there are some smaller mucosal and submucosal glands that contribute to the prostatic secretion. The gland can be divided rather imperfectly into lobes produced by the passage of the ejaculatory ducts through the glandular mass. The lobes are further subdivided into lobules, each drained by a duct that empties into the urethra. The lobes are of interest since some of them tend to be the site of prostatic tumors (posterior and dorsal lobes) while others may give rise to benign hypertrophy (anterior and ventral lobes). The glands are of the tubuloalveolar type and show considerable infolding of their epithelium to accommodate the distention required during storage of prostatic fluid. The secretory portions of the gland are lined with columnar epithelium superimposed on a few flattened cells. Within the contorted, large irregular lumina of these glands one can sometimes observe lamellar bodies that stain red with eosin. These are called *prostatic concretions*. The epithelium of a lumen containing a prostatic concretion is often flattened. These concretions are often calcified, especially in older men. A characteristic feature of the prostate is the presence of scattered fibers of smooth muscle in the connective tissue surrounding the glands. The muscle does not form organized layers around the glandular portions but is distributed in groups or strands of fibers running in various directions.

SEMINAL PLASMA

The fluid in which the sperm are suspended originates from several accessory glands as well as from the isolated secretory cells lining the male reproductive tract, including the epididymis, ductus deferens, seminal vesicle, prostate, and bulbourethral glands. It is different in composition from blood plasma and other body fluids. It has, for example, a high concentration of fructose and certain amino acids, as well as several unique substances

such as spermidine, an amine with a characteristic odor. At emission, prostatic secretion enters the urethra first, followed by the ampullar sperm and then the secretions of the seminal vesicle. Attempts to determine probable fertility using analysis of seminal plasma have relied on the number of sperm (over 20 million per milliliter represents a probably fertile specimen), the appearance of the sperm heads (over 70% normal), and the motility of the sperm (over 50% motile). A low score on any of these traits may mean reduced fertility. Variations in the chemical composition of seminal fluid may also affect fertility, for example, fructose and glucose concentrations (necessary energy substrates for sperm) or prostaglandin content (affects motility of smooth muscle in reproductive tract and elsewhere).

PENIS

A section of the penis shows, under low microscopic power, three large masses of erectile tissue, each of which contains a great number of anastomosing blood vessels (Fig. 18-20). The two dorsal masses of erectile tissue, connected by a bridge of the same kind of tissue, are the *corpora cavernosa penis*. The smaller ventral mass surrounding the urethra is the *corpus cavernosum urethrae*, called also the *corpus spongiosum*.

The cavernous bodies are surrounded by a sheath of dense connective tissue, the tunica albuginea. Outside this is a stroma of loose connective tissue containing blood vessels, nerves, and pacinian corpuscles. There is no well-defined corium of the skin covering the penis, and it has a thin epidermis.

Blood is brought to the penis by the arteria penis, which branches to form the dorsal artery and the paired deep arteries. The dorsal artery sends branches to the tunica albuginea and to the large trabeculae of the carvernous bodies. Such branches break up into capillaries from which blood passes into the lacunae of the erectile tissue and then to a plexus of veins in the albuginea. The deep arteries run lengthwise, giving off branches that open into the cavernous spaces. During times of sexual excitement the flow of blood into the cavernous spaces is greatly increased, especially that coming from the deep arteries. The veins that drain the blood spaces leave at an oblique angle. The central spaces are filled first, and their distention compresses the peripheral spaces and obstructs the flow of blood through the angular openings into the veins, thus producing rigidity of the penis. In the flaccid condition of the organ, the incoming flow of blood is less and the passage into the veins remains open.

The penis has an abundant supply of spinal, sympathetic, and parasympathetic nerve fibers and many sensory end organs.

19

Female reproductive system

The female reproductive system consists of the ovaries, the fallopian tubes (oviducts), the uterus, and the vagina. Because of its functional relation to the reproductive tract, the mammary gland is discussed with the group of genital organs.

OVARY

The ovary, like the testis, is concerned with the formation of gametes and with the development and maintenance of the secondary sexual characteristics. In this latter function the ovary serves as an endocrine gland.

The paired ovaries are slightly flattened, ovoid structures lying within the pelvis near the fringed open ends of the oviducts. They are attached to a strand of connective tissue, the *broad ligament,* by a fold of mesentery called the mesovarium, which in turn inserts into the ovary at its stalk or hilus. The hilus is the margin of the ovary that serves as an entrance point for nerves, blood vessels, and lymphatics. A section through the whole ovary shows that it is divided into a wide outer cortex and a smaller inner medulla (Fig. 19-1). The central deep zone or medulla consists of a loose connective tissue stroma rich in elastic fibers in which are embedded many large, coiled blood vessels, a rich lymphatic bed, and a nerve supply. Occasionally vestiges of fetal tissue, the rete ovarii, may be observed. Closely associated with the nonmyelinated nerves and vascular spaces along the length of the hilum and occasionally trailing onto the adjacent mesovarium are the hilus cells.

These cells resemble the Leydig cells of the testis in the appearance of the nucleus and cytoplasm and also in the presence of lipids, lipochromes, and crystalloids. They are believed to secrete androgens, and overgrowth of the hilus cells can cause masculinization in women.

The cortex is a broad peripheral zone consisting of a compact cellular stroma punctuated by fluid-filled follicles containing maturing ova. The connective tissue cells of this zone are long and spindle shaped with elongate nuclei resembling those of smooth muscle. These cells are embedded in a matrix of delicate collagenous fibers. The matrix also contains clusters of interstitial cells, especially prominent during pregnancy and lactation. These cells may produce progesterone. The ovary is covered by a simple columnar epithelium called the germinal epithelium, so called because formerly it was held that the oogonia or germinal cells were derived from this epithelium. Immediately underneath the germinal epithelium is a denser stroma, the tunica albuginea, which contains a few scattered cells amidst tightly packed collagenous fibers (Fig. 19-2).

Origin of ova and follicles

The germ cells of the female are derived from cells that migrate into the developing ovary from the endoderm of the primitive yolk sac. The oogonia thus formed continue to divide during early fetal life and in some species such as the pig continue to divide for as long as sev-

273

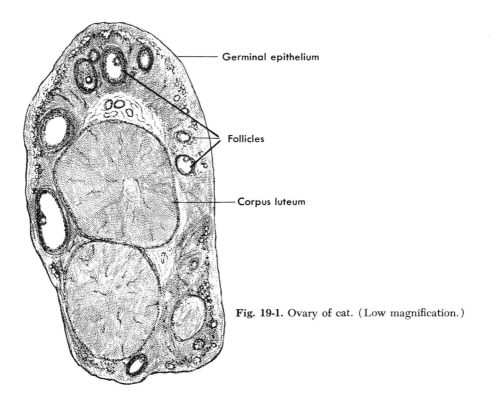

Fig. 19-1. Ovary of cat. (Low magnification.)

Germinal epithelium

Follicles

Corpus luteum

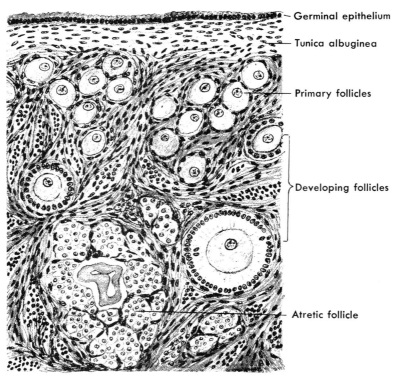

Germinal epithelium

Tunica albuginea

Primary follicles

Developing follicles

Atretic follicle

Fig. 19-2. Cortex of ovary.

Primary follicles

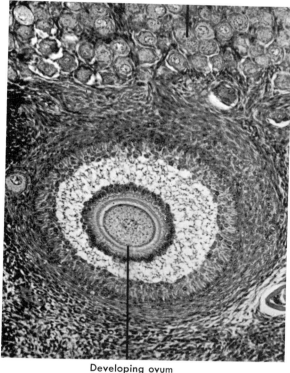

Developing ovum

Fig. 19-3. Section of cortex of rat ovary showing ovum within a follicle. (×640.)

eral weeks postnatally. In humans, the process of oogenesis (the formation of new germ cells by mitosis, in a manner comparable to the continuing process of spermatogenesis in males) is thought to be completed by approximately the fourth prenatal month. At this time the ovary may contain as many as 5 million oocytes. Each oocyte is surrounded by a single layer of smaller cells called the follicular or granulosa cells; each egg and its associated granulosa cells is called a primordial follicle (Fig. 19-2).

Growth of the follicles

Before an oocyte is released from the ovary (the process called *ovulation*) it will undergo marked changes in organization and size. The oocyte will grow from about 30 μ in diameter to about 120 to 150 μ. It will complete the first stage of

meiosis and will enter the oviduct in the second stage of meiosis. Of the oocytes remaining in the ovary at birth, approximately 400 will eventually be released, leaving the remainder to degenerate (atresia).

The primordial follicle contains a small oocyte measuring about 20 μ in diameter (Fig. 19-2), with a large eccentric nucleus and relatively few organelles located near one pole of the nucleus. Surrounding the egg is a single layer of flat cells *(follicle cells)* attached to the cell membrane by desmosomes. Occasional outpocketings of ova cytoplasm indent the follicle cells (Fig. 19-5). Outside the follicle wall a thin basement membrane is present. As the oocyte begins to grow, the single layer of flat follicular cells becomes cuboidal or columnar, forming the *granulosa layer*. Continued development results in the for-

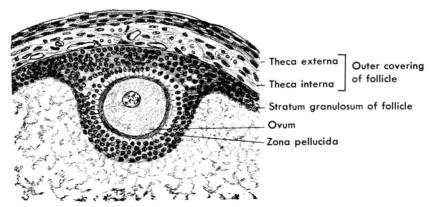

Theca externa ⎤ **Outer covering**

Theca interna ⎦ **of follicle**

Stratum granulosum of follicle

Ovum

Zona pellucida

Fig. 19-4. Part of graafian follicle showing ovum and surrounding structures.

mation of a nucleolus and a Golgi apparatus within the egg. The mitochondria form clusters called rosettes. The cell surface becomes coated with protein polysaccharides apparently secreted by the follicular cells. This coat, the *zona pellucida,* remains as a covering for the oocyte even after fertilization. It is finally shed shortly before blastocyst formation. As the follicle cells divide, the oocyte becomes surrounded by a multilayered wall of cells and is now called a *secondary follicle.* The stroma around the follicle subsequently undergoes a change, in which the inner zone nearest the basement membrane separating the follicle wall from the surrounding connective tissue develops into a highly vascular region *(theca interna).* The outer, more densely organized connective tissue remains as the *theca externa.* Throughout the development of the follicle, the granulosa remains avascular.

In the secondary follicle, the cells of the granulosa are cuboidal and rather loosely attached to one another. The follicle gradually assumes an oval shape and the egg shifts to an eccentric position on the far side of the follicle from where the eventual rupture of the wall occurs at ovulation. Fluid gradually accumulates between the follicle cells and finally coalesces to form a vesicle of fluid called the *antrum.* In the human, a follicle destined for ovulation takes about 12 to 14 days to

reach maturity (the vesicular or graafian follicle). At maximum size, the mature follicle is a large fluid-filled vesicle about 10 to 20 mm. in diameter that may span the entire thickness of the ovarian cortex and produce a bulge visible on the ovarian surface. As ovulation approaches, the cluster of cells surrounding the ovum (Fig. 19-4), called the *cumulus oophorus,* gradually is undercut as the cells swell and the matrix between them depolymerizes. Finally the egg with a surrounding halo of cells (the *corona radiata*) floats free in the antrum. About 36 hours before ovulation, the ovum completes its first maturational division and enters the second division of meiosis. During the last few hours before ovulation, the wall of the follicle facing the surface of the ovary undergoes a reduction in thickness and the cells separate from each other under the influence of luteinizing hormone (LH) secreted by the anterior pituitary gland. It is currently believed that LH stimulates the synthesis of local steroids that are involved in the breakdown of the follicle wall shortly before ovulation. At ovulation, the ovum with its surrounding corona radiata passes slowly through the weakened and ruptured follicle wall and the ovarian surface and is swept into the oviduct. The number of ova discharged at one time and the intervals between ovulations vary in different animals. In the

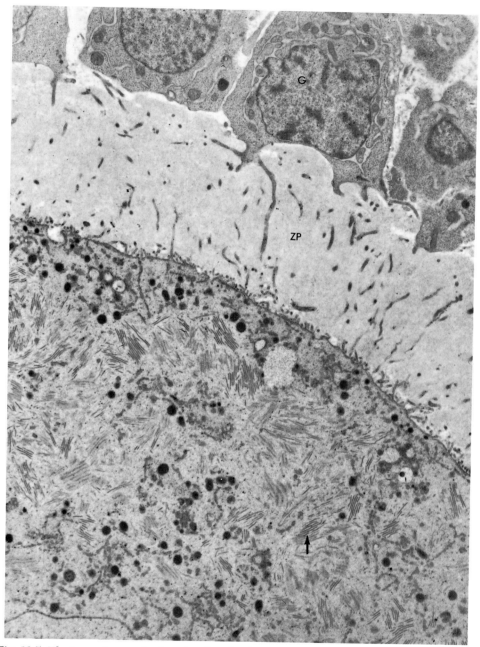

Fig. 19-5. Electron micrograph of ovulated, unfertilized rat ovum surrounded by granulosa cells, G, whose processes extend through the zona pellucida, ZP. Note the abundance of protein plaques (linear structures) in the ovum (arrow). (×6,100.) (Courtesy Dr. Enders, St. Louis, Mo.)

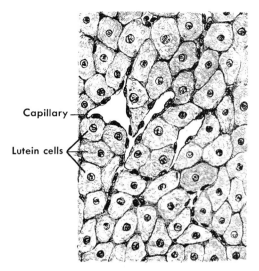

Capillary

Lutein cells

Fig. 19-6. Part of corpus luteum.

human, one ovum is usually discharged from the ovary every 4 weeks. In about 1% of cycles, multiple ovulations occur. In every cycle, three to thirty primary follicles will begin to mature. Those that do not undergo ovulation will become atretic.

The local ovarian mechanisms responsible for rupture of the follicle wall and the extrusion of the ovum are not known. Various explanations that have been proposed to account for this process are: increased intrafollicular pressure (evidence fails to support this idea), enzymatic breakdown of the connective tissue matrix, local vascular changes, and smooth muscle contractility within the ovary.

CORPUS LUTEUM

At ovulation the majority of the follicular cells remain in the ovary and the follicle undergoes changes leading to the formation of the corpus luteum. The first of these is the formation of blood clot, derived from the vessels of the theca interna, which ruptures at ovulation. The following change involves the alteration of the character of the follicular cells and the cells of the theca interna. In the mature graafian follicle the former are rather small elements with relatively little cytoplasm.

They now enlarge and begin to invade and resorb the blood clot. Ultimately the follicular cells fill the center of the follicle with large, pale cells (Figs. 19-6 and 19-7).

The nuclei become vesicular, and the abundant cytoplasm, which at first appears granular, gradually accumulates lipid and yellow pigment granules, which are the basis for the appearance of these cells, known as the *granulosa lutein cells.*

At the electron microscope level the granulosa lutein cells exhibit a large prominent nucleus, numerous mitochondria, large numbers of scattered ribosomes, a prominent Golgi apparatus, and a supranuclear centrosome. Smooth-surfaced endoplasmic reticulum is also a prominent cytoplasmic organelle (Fig. 19-7).

The cells derived from the theca interna occur in groups located at the periphery of the lutein layer and are known as *theca lutein cells.* Although they also contain lipid granules and are similar in shape to the granulosa cells, they may be distinguished from the latter by their location in the periphery, their smaller size, and their denser appearing nuclei.

The structure in a fresh specimen has a yellow color and is called the corpus luteum. The length of life of the corpus luteum and the size to which it grows depend upon the fate of the ovum that was discharged from the follicle. If the ovum is fertilized and becomes implanted in the uterine wall, the corpus luteum continues to grow and is called a corpus luteum (of pregnancy). If the ovum is not fertilized, the corpus luteum begins to degenerate about 14 days after ovulation. Such corpora lutea are soon replaced by scar tissue (corpus albicans). These relations will be discussed more fully.

Atretic follicles. In the preceding paragraphs we have discussed the normal development of an ovum and its follicle. It often happens, however, that follicles that have developed to the graafian stage degenerate rather than reaching ovulation. The first step in atresia is the death of the ovum itself, which is followed by the degeneration of the follicular cells; the result is a mass of detritus left at the center

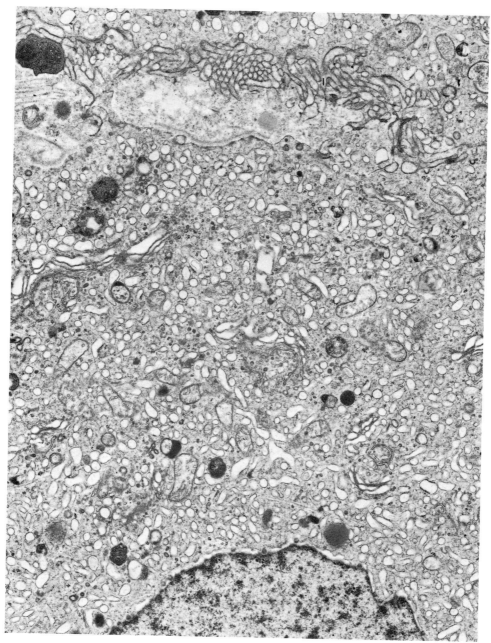

Fig. 19-7. Electron micrograph of a lutein cell from a functional human corpus luteum. Note infolded border of upper cell, *I*, and abundance of agranular endoplasmic reticulum. (×15,600.) (Courtesy Dr. Enders, St. Louis, Mo.)

of the follicle. The cells of the theca interna undergo a hypertrophy similar at first to that occurring in corpus luteum formation. It is, however, carried further, so that the striking characteristic of an atretic follicle is the ring of enlarged theca cells surrounding it (Fig. 19-2). At this stage these cells have some resemblance to the cells of the corpus luteum but are smaller, less eosinophilic, and not conspicuously vacuolated.

The theca cells gradually fill the space left by the degenerating ovum and follicular cells, thus forming a solid mass. In this condition they may remain in the stroma of the ovary for some time.

It has now been established that the ovaries elaborate hormones, estrogens and progestins. Estrogen is formed mainly by the growing follicles. This hormone is concerned with the growth and development of the female reproductive tract and also the mammary glands. Progesterone, derived from the corpus luteum, is responsible for the secretion of the uterine glands and also conditions the uterine mucosa for the reception of the fertilized ovum. The formation of these hormones is cyclic in nature and corresponds to changes that occur in the reproductive tract and uterine mucosa. These events are activated to a large extent by the gonadotropins secreted by the anterior pituitary gland.

• • •

Summary. In addition to the connective tissue stroma, one may find in the ovary the following elements: (1) germinal epithelium, (2) interstitial cells, (3) primary follicles, (4) growing follicles, (5) graafian follicles, (6) blood clots, (7) corpora lutea, (8) scars, and (9) atretic follicles.

FALLOPIAN TUBE (OVIDUCT)

When the ova are extruded from the ovary, they pass into the open end of the oviduct. The oviducts consist of a mucosa lined with a mixture of ciliated and nonciliated secretory cells, an underlying highly vascular lamina propria, and a subjacent muscularis consisting of an inner circular and an outer longitudinal layer of smooth muscle. There is no muscularis mucosa or submucosa. The tube is covered on the outside by a sleeve of peritoneum, a *serosa,* consisting of a thin sheet of squamous epithelium and a stroma of collagenous fibers.

Functionally and structurally the tube can be divided into four segments that differ in (1) the complexity of folding of the lining mucosa, (2) the proportion of ciliated to nonciliated cells in the mucosa, and (3) the thickness of the muscle coat. These four segments are named the infundibulum, ampulla, isthmus, and intramural zones. The *infundibulum* (funnel) with its fringed ends (fimbriae) is the opening or mouth (ostium) of the oviduct near the ovary. Near the time of ovulation, the fimbriae, which contain a tissue resembling erectile tissue, become turgid and motile. These thin-walled fringes hug the ovary and serve as an "egg catcher." The wall of the infundibulum is extremely thin and consists of a sheet of connective tissue interlaced with smooth muscle covered by a ciliated mucosa. The *ampulla* occupies the distal part of the tube, and it is here that fertilization takes place. The mucosa is covered in the main by ciliated cells. Also present is a thin muscle coat and a loose lamina propria that undergoes swelling at the time of ovulation.

A longer segment of the oviduct called the *isthmus* occurs between the ampulla and the uterus. This part of the tube is smaller and firmer and exhibits a larger lumen with a less complicated mucosa. Grossly, it is rather difficult to distinguish the isthmus from the broad ligament. Ciliated cells become less frequent and are confined to the crypts in the mucosa as the tube approaches the uterus. The muscular coat is thick and prominent. The movement of the mucosal cilia and the peristaltic waves set up in the smooth muscle moves the egg slowly toward the uterus. It is not known how the oviduct can simultaneously transport an egg toward the uterus and sperm toward the ampulla. The muscular activity and ciliary beat are influenced by estrogens and by prostaglandins.

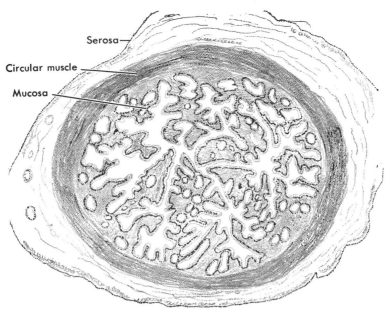

Fig. 19-8. Fimbriated end of oviduct of cat. Note extremely irregular outline of mucosa.

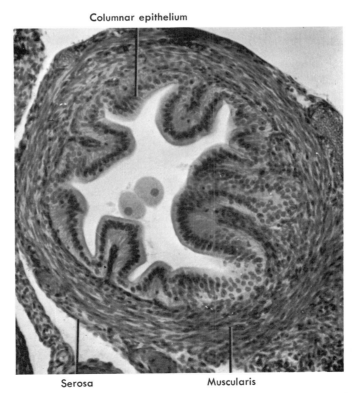

Fig 19-9. Section of fallopian tube of mouse showing two fertilized eggs in the lumen. (×200.) (Courtesy Dr. H. Browning, Houston, Tex.)

The junction of the oviduct with the wall of the uterus is called the *pars interstitialis* or *intramural zone*. This channel is very short in humans, less than 1 mm at the most. An egg cannot pass through this narrow slit until it has been stripped of its halo of granulosa cells (corona radiata), a process that usually takes place as it travels down the oviduct. If fertilization takes place, the developing embryo is still within the confines of the zona pellucida at the time of its passage into the uterus, perhaps ensuring that it will not expand in size and block its own passage. Changes in the size of the slit of the intramural zone during the reproductive cycle can control entry of sperm into the oviducts.

UTERUS

The human uterus is a pear-shaped muscular organ having two parts, a body and a neck, or cervix. At its upper, broader end it receives the oviducts; its lower end opens into the vagina.

Its wall consists of three layers: (1) the endometrium, which corresponds to the mucosa and submucosa; (2) the myometrium, or muscularis; and (3) the perimetrium, a typical serous membrane. The myometrium is a very thick layer of interwoven bundles of smooth muscle, forming three fourths of the uterine wall. At the lower end or cervix of the uterus the fibers are arranged in three fairly distinct layers; the middle layer is circular, and the outer and inner layers are longitudinal (Fig. 19-10).

Endometrium

The endometrium is lined by columnar epithelium that contains scattered groups of ciliated cells. It contains numerous tubular glands that open at the surface (Figs. 19-10 to 19-12). The mucosa undergoes cyclic variations, which are related to changes occurring during the ovulatory or menstrual cycle. Although the changes that occur in the endometrium are not abrupt, structural differences occur that have resulted in the classification of four morphologically distinct stages: (1) the proliferative, also known as the estrogenic stage, (2) the progravid or secretory stage, (3) the premenstrual stage, and (4) the menstrual stage.

Proliferative stage. The proliferative phase of the cycle begins at the termination

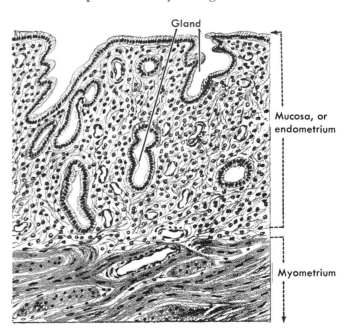

Gland

Mucosa, or endometrium

Myometrium

Fig. 19-10. Mucosa and part of muscularis of human uterus.

Epithelium

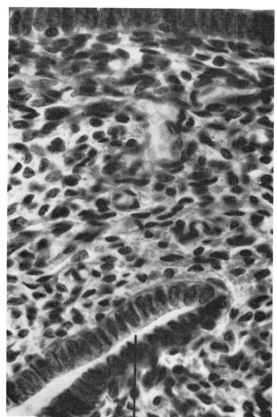

Gland

Fig. 19-11. Section of endometrial wall of human uterus. (×640.)

of the menstrual phase and continues until the thirteenth or fourteenth day of the cycle. It is characterized by the rapid regeneration of the endometrial wall and a replacement of epithelial cells to cover the surface of the mucosa (Fig. 19-13). Also the gland cells increase in number and the glands themselves increase in length. Vascularity of the tissue becomes more pronounced, and indications of edema are also evident.

Secretory (progravid) stage. The secretory stage is characterized by a marked increase in the hypertrophy of the endometrium, which is the result of proliferation of the glandular tissue, and a marked increase in edema and vascularity of the mucosa (Fig. 19-14). This stage begins on the thirteenth or fourteenth day of the cycle and continues until the twenty-sixth or twenty-seventh day.

Premenstrual stage. In the premenstrual part of the cycle changes occur in the vascular components, which result in a loss of the superficial portion of the mucosa. During this time fragmentation of the glands and the extrusion of blood and tissue debris into the lumen of the uterus occur. The premenstrual stage is confined to 1 or 2 days and is said to terminate at the first external signs of bleeding.

Menstrual stage. The menstrual stage usually occupies 3 to 5 days of the cycle and is characterized by a considerable

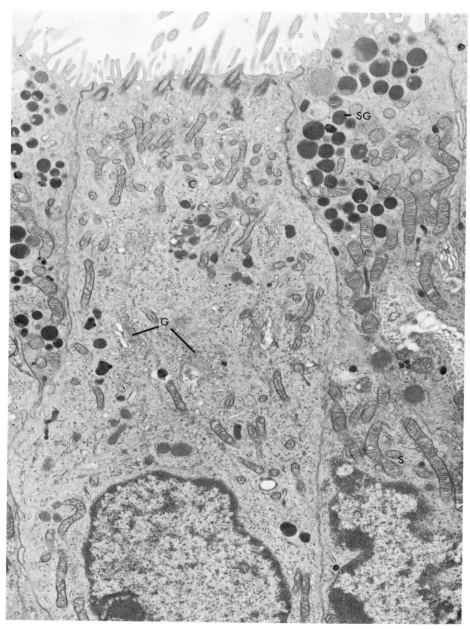

Fig. 19-12. Electron micrograph of endometrial cells from the uterus simplex of an armadillo, showing parts of two secretory cells, *S,* and a ciliated cell, *C. SG,* Secretory granules; *G,* Golgi apparatus. (×11,400.) (Courtesy Dr. Enders, St. Louis, Mo.)

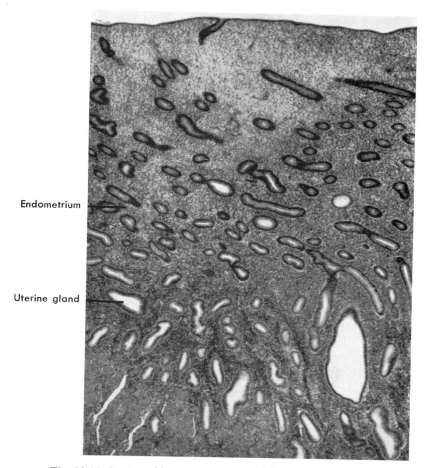

Endometrium

Uterine gland

Fig. 19-13. Section of human uterus in proliferative stage. (×40.)

amount of endometrial destruction, which consists essentially in the sloughing off of the upper three fourths of the endometrium. It involves the destruction of the epithelium and connective tissue and the rupture of blood vessels.

Pregnancy. During pregnancy the structure of the endometrium undergoes marked hypertrophy to provide for the nutrition of the embryo. For a full description of the placenta the student should consult a textbook of embryology. We shall consider here only as much as will explain the place of pregnancy in the female sexual cycle. The changes that take place in the secretory stage are preparations for the implantation of a fertilized ovum. The endometrium is full of large irregular pockets, and in one of these the fertilized ovum becomes embedded. The surrounding tissues enclose it in a sac, from the walls of which the placenta develops. At first, while the embryo is small, the sac surrounding it is smaller than the cavity of the uterus. Later, the embryo and its membranes increase in size so as to completely occlude the uterine cavity. The part of the endometrium that first covered the ovum fuses with the wall of the opposite side, and the only space in the uterus is that immediately surrounding the fetus.

At the end of pregnancy (parturition) the muscles of the uterus contract and the fetus is expelled. Shortly after this another

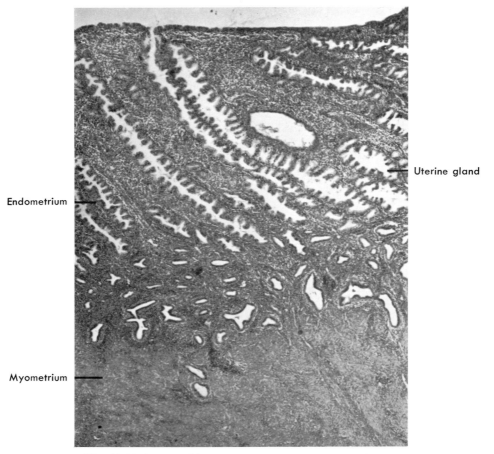

Fig. 19-14. Section of human uterus in secretory stage. (×40.)

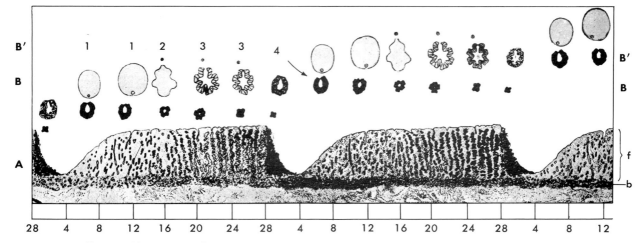

Fig. 19-15. Diagram illustrating relation of menstruation to ovulation. *A,* Cyclic changes in uterine mucosa; *B, B',* ovarian cycles; *b,* basal layer of mucosa; *f,* functional layer of mucosa; *1,* maturing follicle; *2,* rupture of follicle and discharge of ovum (ovulation); *3,* corpus luteum in full function; *4* and remaining figures, degenerating corpus luteum. Numbers at base indicate days of menstrual cycle. (After Schroeder.)

series of contractions empty the organ of the so-called afterbirth. This includes the placenta and the upper layers of the endometrium. After parturition the uterus is in a condition such as that which follows each menstruation, and it enters a period of repair similar to that of the postmenstrual period. From this stage it continues to the proliferative stage and to a renewal of the menstrual cycle. In Fig. 19-15 are shown the probable relations between the uterine cycle and the changes that occur in the ovary (ovulation and the formation of corpora lutea). The cycle represented is one in which there is no coitus and consequently no fertilization of the ovum. Ovulation occurs about the middle of the latter part of the interval between menstrual periods (12 to 14 days before the beginning of the next menstrual flow). The unfertilized ovum travels slowly down the fallopian tube, reaching the uterus in from 5 to 8 days. In the meantime, the ruptured follicle is being transformed into a corpus luteum, and the endometrium is undergoing the progravid hyperplasia. The ovum reaches the uterus when the latter is ready to receive a fertilized egg. But in the cycle under consideration the ovum is dead, and the endometrium enters the menstrual period, during which a part of its mucosa is sloughed off. The ovum also is expelled with the menstrual flow, and the corpus luteum begins to degenerate. If the ovum has been fertilized, it reaches the uterus, as before, when the latter is in the progravid condition. The endometrium provides a suitable place for the embedding of the ovum, which remains in the uterus for the 9 months of the gestation period. If pregnancy occurs, the corpus luteum does not undergo involution but grows larger and persists throughout pregnancy.

The foregoing account is supported by a considerable body of evidence, though it is not definitely proved to be accurate. It appears quite certain that the regulating mechanism of the cycle is in the ovary, not in the uterus, and that it is of endocrine nature. The time of ovulation varies from one cycle to the next. It is now believed that ovulation is triggered by increased estrogen secretion, which in turn stimulates the pituitary to release FSH and LH.

CERVIX

The most inferior and the narrowest portion of the uterus, differing in structure from the rest of the organ, is the cervix. The cervix is a dense tube of connective tissue containing some smooth muscle. The cervix serves two main functions: (1) to secrete mucus, which plays an important role in fertility (since it is the first secretion met by a sperm entering the female tract), and (2) to change from a narrow constricted channel to a dilated, soft tube at the time of parturition. This softening and dilation require considerable change in the matrix. The smooth muscle present may help to contract the cervix again after childbirth until the matrix has had time to reorganize.

The cervical canal is flattened anteroposteriorly with longitudinal ridges on the walls (the *plicae palmatae*, Fig. 19-16). The ridges are composed of long narrow folds of mucosa that make up cryptlike shelves in the wall. Over 100 such crypts are present and they produce 20 to 60 mg. of mucus per day, increasing to over 700 mg. per day at the time of ovulation. The crypts are lined with secretory cells interrupted by an occasional ciliated cell whose beat helps to convey the mucus into the vagina. Occasionally the mouths of the crypts become occluded, leading to the development of cysts, often of considerable size. Beneath the mucosa there is a cellular lamina propria that is less dense than the stroma of the uterine endometrium. It contains elongate fibroblast-like nuclei and a large amount of matrix.

The canal itself is lined with simple columnar epithelium, but near the external opening of the canal (Fig. 19-16) the epithelium changes abruptly to a stratified squamous epithelium that covers the vaginal wall as well. In humans, the cervix undergoes changes in morphology during the menstrual cycle. Cyclic changes can be noted in the length and diameter of the

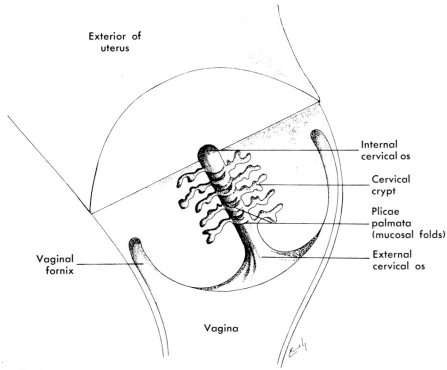

Fig. 19-16. Schematic drawing of human cervix showing mucosal folds. (Drawing by Emily Craig.)

cervical canal and isthmus and the appearance of the mouth (os). No striking histologic changes have been reported.

VAGINA

The wall of the vagina includes a mucosa, submucosa, and muscularis. As in the oviduct and uterus, the mucosa and submucosa are blended. The epithelium is of the stratified squamous variety (Figs. 19-17 and 19-18); the muscularis is of interlacing fibers of smooth muscle that form somewhat indefinite circular (inner) and longitudinal coats.

The epithelium of the human vagina undergoes changes during the menstrual cycle, although these are less marked than those of the uterine mucosa. During the premenstrual period, a zone of keratinized cells is formed in the middle layers of the epithelium. At the menstrual period the cells above this zone are sloughed off and the keratinized cells are thus brought to the surface. In some mammals the changes are more marked, so that vaginal smears furnish an indication of the stage of the estrus cycle of the animal from which they are made.

MAMMARY GLAND

The mammary gland is a compound alveolar gland that develops from the lower layers of the epidermis. It consists of from fifteen to twenty lobes separated by broad bands of dense connective tissue. The lobes are divided into lobules by connective tissue septa, from which strands extend into secreting units. The intralobular connective tissue is fine areolar. The alveoli of each lobule open into small intralobular ducts that unite to form interlobular ducts, and these, in turn, lead to the main excretory

Stratified squamous
epithelium

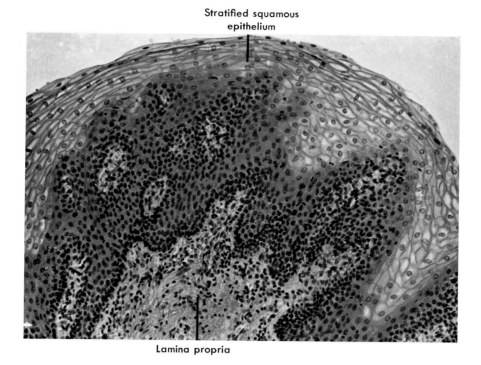

Lamina propria

Fig. 19-17. Section of mucosa of human vagina. (×160.)

(lactiferous) ducts (Fig. 19-19). The inactive and active phases of the gland are marked by difference in appearance.

Resting gland. A section of the mammary gland during a period of inactivity hardly resembles a gland at all on first inspection. The secreting tissue is represented by scattered ducts, around the terminal portions of which one may see a few collapsed or very small follicles and a few solid cords of epithelial cells (Fig. 19-20). Such groups of intralobular epithelial tissue lie in a thin investment of loose connective tissue, and this is surrounded by a dense mass of collagenous fibers. The connective tissue occupies by far the greater portion of the section. Examined under high power, the ducts are seen to be lined with two or three layers of cuboidal cells, whereas such follicles as may be found are composed of simple cuboidal epithelium.

Active gland. During pregnancy the epithelial portions of the mammary gland undergo a pronounced hypertrophy, so that by the fifth month of the period of gestation the organ presents a histologic picture very different from that of the resting gland. Alveoli have developed from the cords of tissue that were to be seen before. The small areas of intralobular connective tissue have expanded, and the lobules appear as relatively large areas filled with alveoli and ducts. The amount of interlobular connective tissue is correspondingly reduced.

During the latter part of the gestation period the development of alveoli and ducts continues, so that at childbirth they occupy the greater part of the organ. They are lined with an epithelium that varies from tall columnar in actively secreting units to low cuboidal in those that have been drained of milk (Fig. 19-21). The cells in active alveoli are filled with fat droplets, which distend them at the free surface and give an irregular outline to

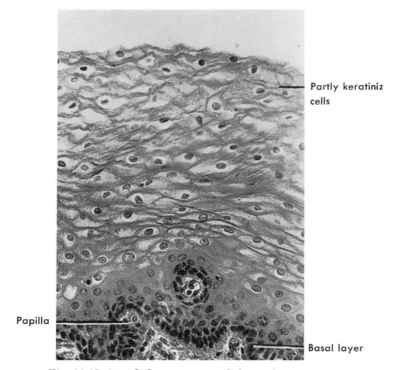

Partly keratiniz
cells

Papilla

Basal layer

Fig. 19-18. Stratified squamous epithelium of vagina.

Excretory duct   Adipose tissue

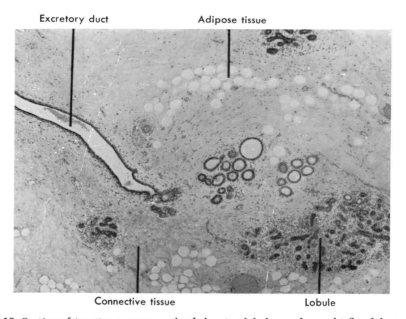

Connective tissue   Lobule

Fig. 19-19. Section of inactive mammary gland showing lobules made up chiefly of ducts. (×40.)

Duct

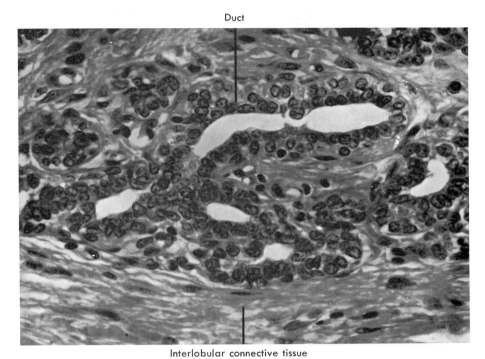

Interlobular connective tissue

Fig. 19-20. Lobule of resting (inactive) mammary gland of cat. (×160.)

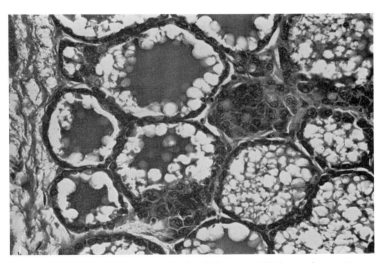

Fig. 19-21. Lactating mammary gland showing follicles and secretion.

the lumen. The ducts leading from the alveoli are lined with low columnar cells, which are replaced by pseudostratified epithelium in the excretory ducts. Near the nipple the epithelium changes to stratified squamous, which is continuous with the skin.

Hormonal control of secretion. The mammary glands are under the control or influence of several hormones. Although the glands undergo some development in the preadolescent state, this process is accentuated during adolescence and is under the influence of two ovarian hormones, estrogen and progesterone, the secretions of which are, in turn, regulated by hormones derived from the anterior pituitary gland. During gestation, production of female hormones is at a high level. At term, active lactation occurs. This process is maintained by the action of prolactin derived from the anterior pituitary and probably secretions derived from other glands, such as the adrenal gland, as well.

The mammary gland remains in the active condition for a variable period after childbirth and then returns to the resting stage. After the menopause it undergoes involution in which the alveoli and parts of the ducts degenerate and their places are taken by connective tissue.

The mammary gland in the male. The early development of the mammary glands in males and females is similar, consisting of the formation of a bandlike thickening of epidermis, the *mammary line* or ridge, which is evident in the 7-week embryo. Along this ridge there is a proliferation of epithelium, which sinks into the underlying mesenchyme and spreads radially to form a *mammary bud.* Androgens cause the mammary buds in males to separate from the surface to which they were previously attached by means of lactiferous ducts (galactophores). In females these duct connections remain intact. In males, the secretory tissue becomes isolated in separate cords. The development of this tissue reaches a maximum in males during adolescence and by age 30 the glands begin to regress. The first tissue to regress in males is the glandular (parenchymal) tissue followed later by the stroma. At the beginning of the fifth decade of life some regrowth of parenchyma and connective tissue may occur. Under conditions of abnormal hormonal stimulation, the duct tissue can increase in males *(gynecomastia)* and in rare cases some milk may actually be secreted *(galactorrhea).*

Blood vessels, lymphatics, and nerves. Blood is brought to the mammary gland by the intercostal, internal mammary, and thoracic branches of the axillary artery. The terminal branches of these vessels lie among the alveoli. Lymph vessels, which are numerous, drain chiefly toward the axilla. Nerves from the cerebrospinal and sympathetic systems supply the epithelial tissue and the blood vessels.

20

Endocrine organs

ENDOCRINE GLANDS

Secretory cells may be divided roughly into two categories, those that release their secretory products into a duct connected to a body or organ cavity (such as the salivary glands) and those that release their products directly into body fluids, via the capillaries or the lymphatics. Glands whose secretions are transported by ducts are called exocrine glands (Chapter 11); those without ducts are known as endocrine glands. Both the endocrine glands (ductless glands, glands of internal secretion) and the exocrine glands arise from epithelial linings. The endocrine glands eventually lose contact with the surface and become isolated islands of epithelium embedded in a connective tissue matrix. The parenchymal cells of these glands secrete *hormones,* chemical regulators of specific tissue metabolism occurring elsewhere in the body.

Endocrine cells may occur singly or in groups making up separate glands. Single endocrine cells may be distinguished from unicellular exocrine glands by the fact that their secretory pole (the portion of the cell containing mature secretory products) is directed toward the capillary bed beneath an epithelium rather than toward the lumen of the organ lined by that epithelium (compare mucous cells and argentaffin cells in the gut wall) (Figs. 14-7 and 14-11). Typical endocrine glands consist of a collection of secretory cells arranged in sheets, cords, or small irregular nests of cells infiltrated by a complex capillary or sinusoidal blood vessel network located in

a thin connective tissue framework. The secretions of the cells of endocrine glands are released into the perivascular spaces and then enter the capillary bed. The term *endocrine gland* is usually reserved for glands that secrete hormones into the bloodstream, although in a functional sense an organ such as the liver that also secretes substances (glucose, blood proteins, and the like) that enter the blood indirectly might be considered in this category.

The cells of endocrine glands exhibit to some degree ultrastructural specializations correlated with the chemical composition of the hormones they secrete. Steroid hormone–secreting cells (Leydig cells of the testis, follicle wall and corpus luteum of the ovary, adrenal cortical cells) have large round nuclei, a prominent Golgi apparatus, extensive smooth endoplasmic reticulum with a sparse rough endoplasmic reticulum, numerous mitochondria often containing unusually shaped cristae, and many lipid and lipofuscin droplets in the cytoplasm. At the light microscope level, the presence of abundant lipid material removed by routine tissue preparation produces a vacuolated appearance of the cytoplasm. Cells that produce polypeptide or protein hormones (such as the cells of the anterior pituitary, thyroid, and so on) resemble the classic acinar cell of the exocrine pancreas except for the fact that the secretory products accumulate near the vascular (basal) rather than at the apex of the cell. Numerous mitochondria are present, usually of a classic rod shape with transverse cristae. At the light microscope

293

level the cytoplasm of these cells is usually basophilic and granular.

A general problem in endocrinology has been to isolate and identify hormonal substances and then to trace these hormones to their cells of origin. Until recently, only two methods of experimentation were in general usage: the biologic effects of (1) removal of a suspected endocrine structure and (2) injection of substances derived from tissue extracts of that structure.

The first of these methods is not always practical. The second method may be questioned on the ground that extracts from organs do not necessarily represent the secretion elaborated by them. The use of the two methods may be illustrated by the work on the thyroid, which has yielded fairly clear-cut results. If this gland is removed from a laboratory animal, a marked retardation of the metabolic rate follows, but this becomes normal again when thyroid extract is administered. The extract also raises the metabolic rate of normal (unoperated) animals. Clinical and postmortem evidence also supports the belief that the thyroid contains a substance that influences, directly or indirectly, the rate of metabolism of the body. This effect is not produced by extracts of other glands. Moreover, the thyroid is a ductless organ composed of secreting epithelial cells, so that its morphology supports the conclusion derived from experimental and clinical work that it secretes a hormone.

In recent years, new techniques have been utilized. These methods are based upon (1) correlation of histologic and ultrastructural changes with functional states in which hormone secretion can be shown to be elevated or depressed, (2) histochemical localization of enzymes responsible for the synthesis of a hormone (restricted to those hormones whose pathways of synthesis have been worked out fairly well, such as the catecholamines and steroids), and (3) identification of hormone storage sites by means of immunofluorescent techniques in which an antibody to a proteinaceous hormone is tagged with a fluorescent compound and then made to react with a tissue containing the hormone antigen.

In some suspected endocrine glands, the results of physiologic experiments are contradictory; in others they are unsupported by morphologic evidence of secretion. One may group in the following way the organs that have been thought to have an endocrine function.

Thyroid gland, parathyroid glands, hypophysis, adrenal glands, and islands of Langerhans. These five organs are composed of cells that have the appearance of glandular tissue. Clinical and experimental evidence is preponderantly in favor of the view that each secretes one or more hormones.

Gonads. There is ample experimental evidence that the testis and ovary produce hormones that control the development and maintenance of secondary sexual characteristics and that the ovarian secretion influences the estrus cycle.

Thymus and pineal glands. Evidence of the endocrine-like function of the thymus has only recently been established. By the activity of a hormone called thymosin, the thymus influences the development of host resistance in a number of species, primarily by affecting the maturation and proliferation of lymphoid cells.

The pineal gland is the source of several monoamines and other substances that can influence the activity of other endocrine glands. It has been called a "regulator of regulating systems," that is, it affects other endocrine control systems in the body although the details of these interlocking relationships are just beginning to be ascertained.

Organs from which hormones are isolated. A fourth group may be made of organs from which, at various times, investigators have claimed they have isolated hormones. For instance, a substance called secretin has been extracted from the wall of the duodenum, and it has been shown that this substance stimulates the alveoli of the pancreas. Which mucosal cells produce secretin? The current view is that epithelial cells of the villus may do so.

· · ·

The grouping of organs just described

indicates a part, at least, of the confusion existing in this field. The complications of the physiologic side of the science are great, since all members of the endocrine group are closely interrelated, and disturbance of one may be expected to affect some or all of the others. Fortunately the histology is less complicated than the physiology. We shall now discuss the thyroid, parathyroid, hypophysis, adrenal, and pineal glands. The islands of Langerhans and the gonads, also in good standing as endocrines, have already been described (see discussion on pancreas, testis, and ovary).

THYROID GLAND

The thyroid gland consists of two lobes and a connecting isthmus. It lies in the neck in contact with the upper part of the trachea and the lower part of the pharynx. The thyroid is enclosed in a connective tissue sheath derived from the cervical fascia. Inside this loose capsule is a second glandular capsule of fibroelastic connective tissue firmly attached to the gland. Trabeculae from the inner capsule penetrate into the gland to provide internal support. These partitions divide the gland into lobules and provide a pathway for the vascular and nerve supply of the gland.

The connective tissue within the gland is largely reticular and is extremely rich in nerve and vascular plexuses although these are not very evident at the optic level.

The functional unit of the thyroid is the follicle, which consists of a simple epithelium enclosing a cavity (the follicular cavity) containing a colloid secretion (Fig. 20-1). Follicles average about 200 μ in diameter but may vary considerably in size. Twenty to forty follicles bound together by a sheet of connective tissue supplied by a single lobular artery make up a thyroid lobule. It is thought that a lobule may give rise to thyroid nodules, local enlargements of a follicle cluster observed in certain thyroid diseases.

The shape of the follicles, the appearance of the cells, and the amount and consistency of the colloid vary with different functional states of the thyroid. In the inactive state, the follicles are round or oval and have regular outlines. In the hyperactive state, the follicles are more folded and irregular in shape. The thyroid may contain as many as 3 million follicles in various stages of activity. In the newborn, most of the follicles are active and are made up of tall follicular cells, exhibiting a slightly basophilic colloid and vacuo-

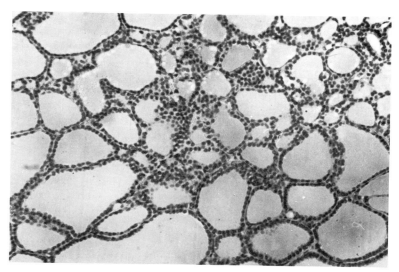

Fig. 20-1. Section of human thyroid gland showing variation in size of follicles. (×40.)

Colloid

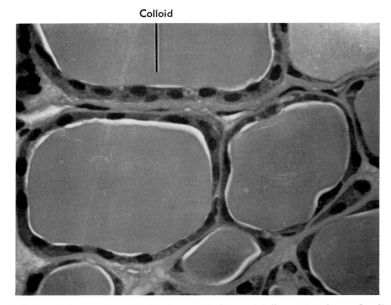

Fig. 20-2. Follicles of human thyroid showing epithelium of different heights and colloid secretion in follicles. (×640.)

lated surfaces between the follicle cells and the colloid. This vacuolation has been shown to be an artifact of fixation. In the adult, most of the follicles are in the storage or inactive phase. In this state the follicle cells are cuboidal or flattened, the colloid is pink and viscous. The central zones of the gland tend to contain more active follicles while the peripheral follicles are larger and inactive. In some mammals, the cells of the follicles are uniform in size, while in humans, the cells are variable in height.

Fine structure of the thyroid follicular cells

The thyroid epithelium consists of two cell types: follicular cells and parafollicular cells (light cells, C cells). The follicular cells are the predominant cell type. They are polarized structurally with their apices directed toward the lumen of the follicle, and their bases rest upon a basement membrane that encloses the follicle wall. The prominent nucleus is usually located in the basal part of the cell. Rarely is a cell observed in mitosis; however, when stimulated by TSH, the cells are capable of division. Marked proliferation may occur following partial removal of the thyroid, in dietary iodine deficiency, or after treatment with antithyroid drugs.

The apical border of the cell exhibits microvilli whose height and number increase with cellular activity. The cell membranes of adjoining cells interdigitate. The cytoplasm contains ribonucleoprotein. The endoplasmic reticulum, which consists of numerous dilated cisternae studded with ribosomes, is usually extensive, especially in active cells. Under the electron microscope, the most characteristic features of the cell are the numerous dilated cisternae (Fig. 20-3). Mitochondria are scattered throughout the cytoplasm but are most numerous in the apical region. The Golgi apparatus is usually located in the supranuclear region and presents no special features. A centrosome is also present in the apical part of the cell. Several inclusions, which vary in number and size during different states of cell activity, are also present. They may be observed as colloid droplets, clear vacuoles, basal colloid vacuoles, and fine granules (Fig. 20-2).

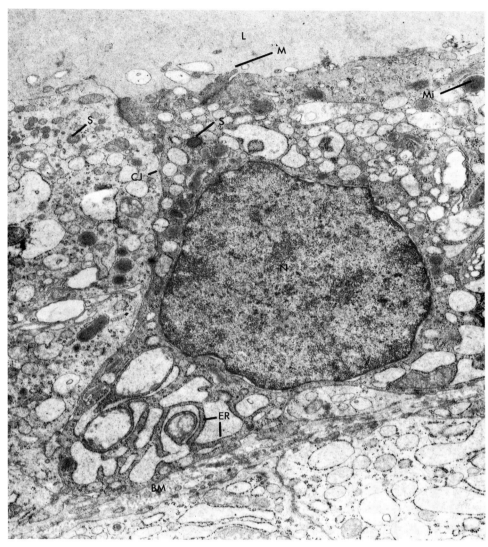

Fig. 20-3. Electron micrography showing parts of two follicle cells of the thyroid of a cat. *BM*, Basement membrane; *CJ*, cell junction; *ER*, cisterna of endoplasmic reticulum; *L*, lumen of follicle; *M*, microvillus; *Mi*, mitochondrion; *N*, nucleus; *S*, secretory granules. (×18,000.)

Parafollicular cells

Most of the cells making up the epithelial wall of the thyroid follicles are derived from the floor of the pharyngeal gut and are concerned with the elaboration and secretion of thyroid hormones (thyroxine and triiodothyronine). A small percentage of cells (2% to 5%) are of different embryologic origin, arising from the

fifth pharyngeal pouch of the embryo. These cells, called parafollicular cells, are derived from the ultimobranchial body, which is later incorporated into the thyroid gland. The parafollicular cells (C cells, light cells) are separated from the lumen of the follicle by slender cell processes derived from the neighboring epithelial cells. They are larger than epithelial cells and have a watery eosinophilic cytoplasm, a prominent Golgi apparatus, and many secretory granules. They have been shown to be the source of the hormone *calcitonin,* a polypeptide that depresses blood calcium levels. It apparently serves to regulate the concentration of calcium in body fluids in combination with the parathyroid hormone of the parathyroid glands and vitamin D, both of which elevate blood calcium. The parafollicular cells have been conclusively demonstrated in the human thyroid, where they are most abundant in the middle third of the gland. They are thought to give rise to medullary carcinomas that produce excess calcitonin.

The colloid, which appears structureless when stained with hematoxylin and eosin, is produced by the cells making up the follicle wall and is usually rich in iodine. It also contains thyroid hormones, thyroxine and triiodothyronine. In this respect, the thyroid is different from other endocrine glands in that it stores an appreciable amount of hormone in an extracellular depot (the colloid). The function of the thyroid gland is controlled by the thyroid-stimulating hormone (TSH), a glycoprotein produced by the anterior pituitary gland. TSH stimulation causes first an increase in the release of thyroid hormone by the gland, then growth of the glandular tissue. The thyroid is very labile in size and structure. Decrease in thyroid activity is associated with high temperatures, fasting, and aging, while increased activity occurs in cold temperatures, during pregnancy, and in periods of emotional stress.

Increase in the activity of the thyroid is associated with a decrease in follicle size and a reduction in the amount of colloid present. The cells become taller and the nuclei, which normally are centrally located in inactive follicles, migrate to the base of the cell. The amount of rough endoplasmic

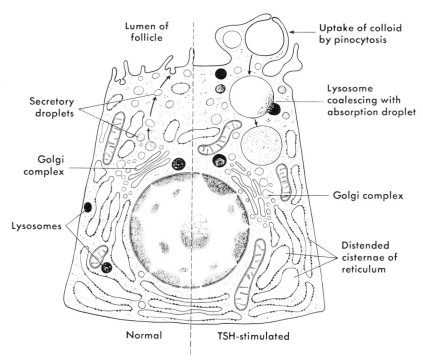

Fig. 20-4. Diagrammatic representation of ultrastructural changes produced in TSH-stimulated thyroid follicle cells. (From Fawcett: Rec. Progr. Horm. Res. **25**:315, 1969.)

reticulum and free ribosomes increases, the Golgi apparatus hypertrophies, the height of the surface microvilli increases, and the number of intracytoplasmic colloid droplets increases (Fig. 20-4). Decreased activity is associated with an enlargement of the follicle, a flattening of the follicle epithelium, and storage of excess colloid. Prolonged stimulation by TSH may cause enlargement of the thyroid gland (goiter). A deficiency of iodine in the diet or the consumption of large amounts of goitrogenic foods, which inhibit utilization of iodine (cabbage, for example, contains thiocyanate, which inhibits iodine uptake by the gland), prevents formation of thyroid hormone. As a result, TSH secretion rises and a simple goiter results, consisting of a diffuse, nonnodular enlargement of the thyroid with signs of overactivity in the follicles. Such stimulation may also occur temporarily at puberty or during pregnancy.

PARATHYROID GLANDS

The parathyroid glands are paired and in man are usually four in number. The glands are surrounded by a framework of reticular tissue, which divides the gland into poorly defined lobules (Fig. 20-5). The lobules are subdivided into sheets or cords by fine extensions of the trabeculae

Capsule

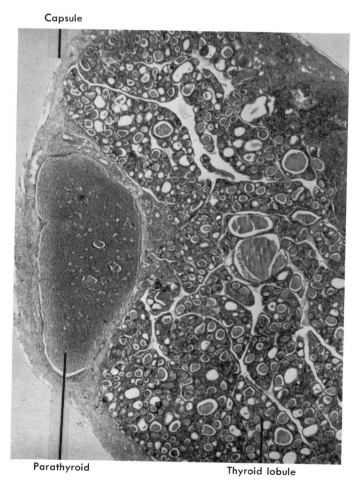

Parathyroid Thyroid lobule

Fig. 20-5. Section of thyroid and parathyroid of cat. (×40.)

Capillary

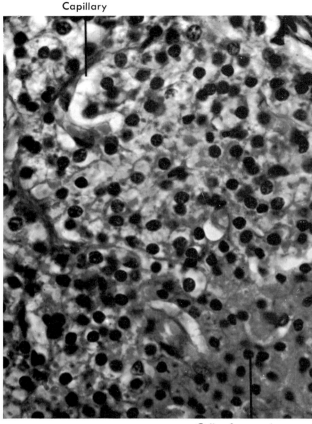

Cells of parenchyma

Fig. 20-6. Human parathyroid. (×640.)

(Fig. 20-6). The connective tissue of the gland contains blood vessels, nerves, lymphatics, and adipose tissue. The cells of the gland are enclosed by a network of reticular fibers in which is found a dense network of capillaries.

The parenchyma of the parathyroid is made up of two kinds of cells in the adult human, chief cells and oxyphil cells, the former being most numerous. The chief cells are polyhedral in shape and exhibit a round, centrally located nucleus and well-defined cell membranes. Chief cells are of two kinds, light and dark. The light cell is most numerous, is slightly larger, and exhibits a clear cytoplasm; both kinds contain glycogen and secretory granules. Evidence appears to indicate that the light cells may be an inactive form of the dark cells.

Oxyphil cells are larger and less numerous than chief cells. They exhibit small, dense nuclei and acidophilic cytoplasm. They can be found by scanning the gland for places where the nuclei appear widely separated, especially near the periphery of the gland. They have been observed only in humans, monkeys, and cattle; in man, they do not appear until the fourth or fifth year of life.

Oxyphil cells interdigitate in a manner that differs from that observed in chief cells. They contain many mitochondria with densely packed cristae. The mem-

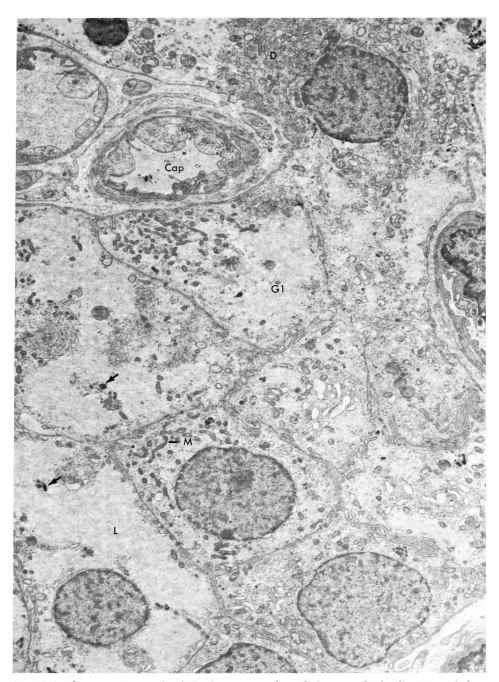

Fig. 20-7. Electron micrograph of the human parathyroid showing chief cells. Most of these cells are the "dark" variety, *D*. The light cells, *L*, show large lakes of glycogen, *Gl*, and relatively few organelles. *Cap*, Capillary; *M*, mitochondrion. Arrows indicate secretory granules. (×4,200.) (Courtesy Dr. B. Munger, Hershey, Pa.)

brane systems of the cells are reduced and the Golgi complex occurs near the cell boundary.

Fatty infiltration of the gland is common in older individuals and at low magnification might be mistaken for bone marrow because of the increase in the amount of adipose tissue, which may come to occupy 50% to 80% of the gland volume.

Fine structure of parathyroid

Active chief cells, the dark cells of light microscopy, contain secretory granules, glycogen, a prominent perinuclear Golgi apparatus, numerous rod-shaped mitochondria, and occasional cilia (Fig. 20-7).

The endoplasmic reticulum is a prominent feature of the dark cells. Lipid granules are present in both dark and light cells (Fig. 20-7).

In the light cells, secretory granules are few in number and glycogen is abundant. These cells generally do not exhibit a Golgi apparatus or endoplasmic reticulum. The cell membranes of all parenchymal cells are smooth, although in some instances examples of interdigitation are observed. Specializations of the membranes, desmosomes, occur in some areas.

Functions of the parathyroids

The parathyroid glands secrete a large amount of hormone per day (about 1 mg.)

and, unlike the thyroid, these glands store very little hormone. Parathyroid hormone (PTH) causes an elevation of blood calcium whenever the plasma level decreases. The plasma level of calcium in the normal mammal is remarkably stable, usually in the vicinity of 10 mg. per 100 ml. Removal of the parathyroids results in a decrease in blood calcium, followed by tetany and death in many mammals. The means by which PTH produces an elevation in calcium is complicated and poorly understood. The best known effect of PTH is on bone. PTH inhibits collagen synthesis in active osteoblasts, enhances resorption of bone by osteoclasts, and probably hastens the maturation of precursor cells into osteoblasts and osteoclasts. The result is to stimulate bone resorption and to release bone salts into the blood. The second major target is the kidney. PTH increases tubular reabsorption of calcium and magnesium, enhances potassium and phosphate excretion, and reduces the loss of hydrogen ions. The phosphate loss (phosphaturia) is the most striking effect of parathyroid hormone. Parathyroid hormone has been purified and is known to be a peptide of low molecular weight (8,500) containing eighty to eight-five amino acids, the number depending upon the species. Commercial preparations of PTH have not been used extensively for clinical treatment,

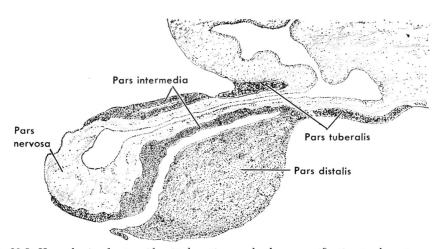

Fig. 20-8. Hypophysis of cat, midsagittal section, under low magnification to show topography.

since vitamin D and its related compounds are usually effective in treating hypoparathyroidism. The actual interaction of PTH, vitamin D and its derivatives, and calcitonin in controlling body calcium balance is an area of active research at the present time. The concept is developing that vitamin D (by way of its active metabolites) may be extremely important for the day-to-day control of calcium homeostasis.

HYPOPHYSIS

The hypophysis or pituitary gland consists of two lobes, each of which is again subdivided (Fig. 20-8). These parts, unlike the lobes of a secretory gland such as the parotid, are composed of tissues that differ from each other in function and (partially) in origin. The gland is actually two organs intimately associated. One part of it, the glandular or *adenohypophysis*, develops from the roof of the oral cavity of the embryo; the other part, the *neurohypophysis*, develops as an outgrowth of the floor of the brain. The hypophysis is located in a fossa of the sphenoid bone, the *sella turcica*, and is invested by an extension of the dura mater. The buccal portion loses its connection with the oral cavity and becomes a solid mass of cells. In some animals the nervous portion retains a cavity in its center.

The adenohypophysis is divided by a lumen in two unequal parts. The *pars distalis* lies anterior to the lumen, and the *pars tuberalis*, an extension of the pars distalis, envelops the neural stalk. The third component, the *pars intermedia*, consists of a thin cellular portion located posterior to the lumen. The anterior lobe refers to the pars distalis and the pars tuberalis; the posterior lobe refers to the pars intermedia and the pars nervosa (the infundibular stalk and median eminence).

The pars distalis of the anterior pituitary gland is composed of glandular cells that are arranged in irregular clumps and cords that are in intimate relation to vascular sinusoids. The anterior lobe is enveloped in a dense connective tissue capsule. In-

Connective tissue capsule   Basophil

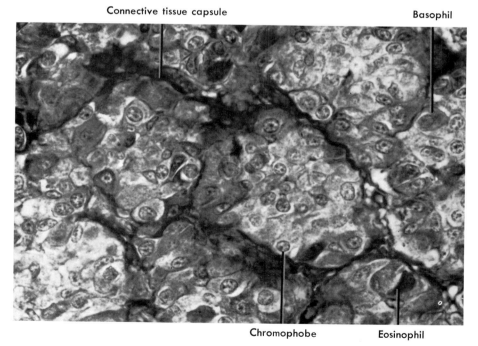

Chromophobe   Eosinophil

Fig. 20-9. Section of anterior pituitary of monkey showing several follicles. (Mallory-azan; ×640.)

ternally, fine reticular fibers arising from the capsule surround the cords of the parenchymal cells and serve to support them and the vascular elements.

The glandular cells are classified as *chromophilic* or *chromophobic* on the basis of their affinity or lack of affinity for routine dyes. The chromophil cells may be divided into two main categories, acidophils and basophils, on the basis of staining reactions following the use of hematoxylin and eosin (Fig. 20-9). Since the anterior pituitary gland secretes at least six different hormones, the classification of these cells as chromophobe, acidophil, and basophil is obviously rather nonspecific. The recent development of more discriminating dyes and the use of ultrastructural analysis have now permitted the identification of a cell type for each hormone known to be secreted by the anterior pituitary. In some cases it appears that the same cell may secrete two related hormones.

Chromophil cells

The acidophils are round or ovoid and measure from 15 to 19 μ in diameter. They possess a prominent Golgi apparatus, numerous rod-shaped mitochondria, and refractile granules that can be seen with the light microscope. The acidophils are of two types: somatotrophs and mammotrophs. The *somatotrophs* secrete growth hormone and the *mammotrophs* secrete prolactin. Together these two cell types account for approximately 35% of the cells of a normal anterior pituitary gland (*pars anterior*). The somatotrophs have dense spherical granules measuring as much as 350 mμ in diameter and are arranged in clusters in the posterolateral region of the gland. They stain specifically with orange G. The mammotrophs can easily be distinguished from somatotrophs by the presence of large irregularly shaped secretory granules 600 to 900 mμ in diameter (Fig. 20-10). In some species the two classes of acidophils cannot be distinguished by staining methods. In man, the mammotrophs stain with erythrosin or azocarmine. In the normal gland, mammotrophs tend to be sparse and poorly granulated. Mammotrophs be-

come predominant in the gland of pregnant or lactating females. In males and in nonpregnant females the acidophils in the human anterior pituitary are somatotrophs and the gland contains a large amount of growth hormone (milligram quantities in comparison to microgram amounts of other hormones). The majority of cells undergoing mitosis in the pituitary are somatotrophs.

The basophils represent 10% to 15% of the cell population of the anterior pituitary. They secrete the following glycoproteins: follicle-stimulating hormone (FSH), luteinizing hormone (LH), and thyrotrophin (TSH). The different types of basophils are more difficult to distinguish histologically than are the acidophil populations. In the human pituitary stained with aldehyde thionine PAS and orange G, the FSH-secreting cells take on a brick red color, the TSH-secreting cells (*thyrotrophs*) stain with aldehyde-thionine only, and the LH-secreting cells exhibit a pale pink color by reacting with both orange G and aldehyde thionine. The LH-secreting cells contain fine granules and occasional lipid inclusions. There is still some doubt as to whether FSH and LH are secreted by separate cells. Some authors have identified two gonadotrophs ultrastructurally. FSH-secreting cells are said to be located along the periphery of the gland and have small (200 mμ) granules. LH-secreting cells are relatively large, angular in shape, and more uniformly distributed. Both *gonadotrophs* (FSH- and LH-secreting cells) have granules of about the same size. The cell that produces TSH contains smaller granules (150 mμ) and is located peripherally. The thyrotroph cells are large, irregular, and polygonal in shape.

In general, basophils occur along the midline and anterior margins of the pituitary while the acidophils are more centrally and posteriorly located.

Chromophobes

In general, chromophobes have less cytoplasm than chromophils and are often located in small clumps between sinusoids. In such clusters, the nuclei appear close to-

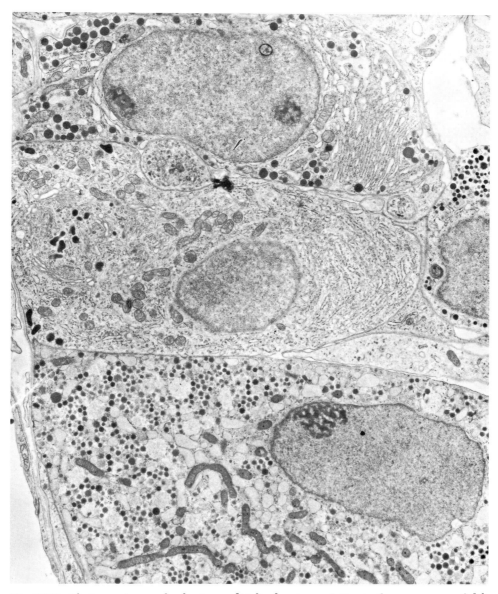

Fig. 20-10. Electron micrograph of rat pars distalis showing variation in the appearance of different cell types. The cells at the top and middle are acidophils; the cell in the lower part is a basophil. At the electron microscope level the size of the granules is the most important diagnostic criterion for the identification of different cell types. (×7,000.) (Courtesy Dr. M. Farquhar, New York, N. Y.)

gether because of the diminished amount of cytoplasm present. It is been suggested that the chromophobes represent a class of differentiating cells that give rise to the various chromophil cell types, but recent evidence fails to support this. On the other hand, it now seems well established that one type of chromophobe, a large cell with 200 mμ granules arranged around its periphery together with irregular long processes insinuating between other cells to reach a sinusoidal bed, may be the source of adrenocorticotrophic hormone (ACTH). These cells are weakly PAS positive (stain for 1,2 glycol groups in carbohydrate-containing substances, with periodic acid–Schiff base reaction) and strongly positive to aldehyde fuchsin. They can be found both in the anterior pituitary and the pars intermedia.

Hormones produced by the pars distalis

The pars distalis is known to produce six hormones, which consist of proteins or polypeptides.

Somatotrophic hormone (STH). One of the earliest hormones to be recognized was the growth or somatotrophic hormone (STH), which stimulates body growth, particularly that of the epiphyses of long bones. Hypophysectomy in growing animals results in a cessation of growth, which can be overcome by the administration of the hormone. Underproduction of the hormone results in dwarfism, overproduction in gigantism. If overproduction occurs when the epiphyseal plate has calcified, a thickening of the bones of the face, skull, hands, and feet occurs. This condition is known as *acromegaly.*

Thyrotropic hormone (TSH). The thyroid-stimulating hormone maintains the integrity of the thyroid epithelium and is responsible for stimulating thyroid secretion. Hypophysectomy results in the atrophy of the thyroid, which, in turn, may be restored by administration of the hormone.

Adrenocorticotrophic hormone (ACTH). The adrenocorticotrophic hormone controls the growth and secretion of the adrenal cortex. Hypophysectomy results in atrophy of the cortex, which can be alleviated by administration of ACTH.

Follicle-stimulating hormone (FSH). The follicle-stimulating hormone stimulates growth of the follicles in the ovary and spermatogenesis in the seminiferous tubules of the testis. Atrophy of the gonads following hypophysectomy can be partially alleviated and the gonads restored to their normal state by the administration of FSH, but complete restoration also requires some luteinizing hormone.

Luteinizing hormone (LH); interstitial cell-stimulating hormone (ICSH). After stimulation by FSH, the luteinizing hormone contributes to the maturation of the ovarian follicle and also to ovulation. In the male, ICSH stimulates the interstitial cells of Leydig in the testes to produce testosterone, which is responsible for the maintenance of the secondary sexual characteristics.

Prolactin (lactogenic hormone) (LTH). Prolactin initiates secretion of milk after hypertrophy of the mammary gland in response to stimulation of ovarian hormones during pregnancy. It also has been shown in the rat that LTH initiates and maintains the secretion of progesterone; hence the synonym, luteotropic hormone (LTH).

Pars tuberalis

The pars tuberalis consists of a thin band of cells enveloping the infundibular stalk. The main cells are cuboidal or polyhedral; the cytoplasm is faintly basophilic and contains small granules. The cells arranged in cords or clusters are in intimate association with a rich supply of blood vessels. Occasional small, colloid-laden vesicles occur among the cells. There are, in addition, undifferentiated cells and also small acidophils and basophils. The function of the pars tuberalis is not known.

Pars intermedia

In man the pars intermedia is rudimentary. It occupies a position adjacent to the residual lumen and is composed of cells and scattered follicles containing colloid. The cells are basophilic and blend with those of the pars distalis. The cells lining the colloid vesicles are frequently ciliated, and some secrete mucus. The colloid does not accumulate iodine.

The only known function of this part of the gland is the secretion of *melanin-stimulating hormone* (MSH), but ACTH may also be produced here, possibly in the same cell.

Neurohypophysis

The neurohypophysis is composed of the infundibular process—the infundibulum and the median eminence of the tuber cinereum. The infundibulum and median eminence of the tuber cinereum have in common the same type of cell, nerve, and blood supply and elaborate similar active substances. The cells of the neurohypophysis are small, have numerous processes, and are known as *pituicytes*. Unlike neuroglia, which they resemble, their cytoplasm contains fat and pigment granules. The nuclei of the pituicytes are round, and the cytoplasmic processes often extend to capillary walls or the septa of the gland.

The nerve cells in the supraoptic and paraventricular nuclei of the hypothalamus elaborate secretory products, which are transmitted by nerve fibers and are stored in the neural lobe and in nerve fiber terminations known as *Herring bodies*.

Two active fractions have been isolated from the neurohypophysis. They have been identified as polypeptides. One of these, *oxytocin*, stimulates uterine contraction during late pregnancy and also activates the myoepithelial cells of the mammary gland, resulting in the flow of milk. The second fraction, *vasopressin*, is an antidiuretic (ADH) hormone. When administered in excessive amounts it also has the ability to raise blood pressure.

ADRENAL GLAND

The adrenal (suprarenal) gland is like the hypophysis in that it is in reality two glands having different functions and arising from different sources. One of these is the cortex, which is derived from mesodermal tissue. The other is the medulla of the

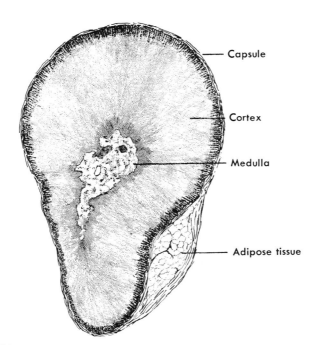

Fig. 20-11. Section through adrenal gland of rabbit showing relation of its parts.

organ, which comes from the same group of cells as those that form the sympathetic ganglia (Fig. 20-11).

The entire gland is surrounded by a capsule of connective tissue (Fig. 20-11). From the capsule delicate connective tissue fibers pass into the cortex at the hilus. They continue into the stroma of the gland as reticular fibers supporting the arterioles and capillaries of the cortex and the sinusoidal vessels of the medulla. The capsule also gives rise to cells that replace the cells of the cortex.

Cortex

The cortex is composed of cords of cells, between which lie capillaries in a fine network of reticular tissue. Three zones are distinguishable, though they are not sharply delimited one from another. They are the zona glomerulosa, zona fasciculata, and zona reticularis.

In the zona glomerulosa the cells are pale and columnar (Fig. 20-12); they are arranged in oval groups separated from each other by fine vascular connective tissue. The nuclei stain intensely, and the cytoplasm is faintly basophilic.

The zona fasciculata is the widest zone of the cortex and is composed of polygonal cells, in the cytoplasm of which fat (lipoid) droplets are present; cells in the zone are arranged in cords that radiate from the center of the gland (Fig. 20-14); the cords are usually two cells in width, being cuboidal and often binucleate. In the outer portion of the fasciculata the cells contain droplets of cholesterol and fatty acids. In

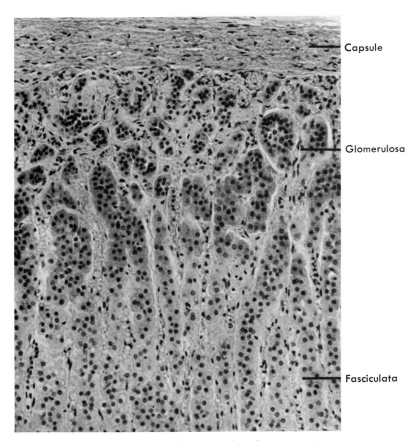

Fig. 20-12. Section of human adrenal cortex. (×160.)

Capsule

Glomerulosa

Fasciculata

the usual preparations these areas appear as vacuoles, giving the cell a spongy appearance. They are sometimes called spongiocytes.

In the zona reticularis, the innermost zone of the cortex, the cords of cells, rather than running in a radial direction, break up into a network. The capillaries are to be found in the spaces of this network. The cells of the reticular zone are somewhat smaller and darker than those of the fascicular zone (Figs. 20-13 and 20-14). Many cells have pyknotic nuclei and contain pigment granules.

Fine structure of cortical cells. Electron microscopy shows that the adrenocortical cells, like other steroid hormone–producing tissues, contain an abundance of smooth endoplasmic reticulum lying between the densely packed mitochondria (Fig. 20-15). Also present are scattered ribosomes, various dense granules, lipid droplets, and multivesicular bodies. The Golgi apparatus is not usually prominent and is often widely distributed throughout the cytoplasm.

Medulla

The medulla consists of irregularly arranged groups of cells that have a granular cytoplasm and polygonal outlines (Figs. 20-13 and 20-14). With hematoxylin and eosin, their color is faintly purple. They react strongly to chromium salts and are therefore called chromaffin cells. Even without this specific stain, they are readily distinguished from the cortical cells by their basophilic reaction, their larger size, and their arrangement. Among the cords is a network of capillaries such as is characteristic of endocrine organs.

Fine structure of the medulla. The chromaffin cells of the medulla have a relatively large nucleus, few scattered mitochondria, ribosomes, and a well-developed Golgi apparatus (Fig. 20-16). A prominent cytoplasmic feature of these cells is the presence of numerous dense granules. These granules apparently arise from the Golgi vesicles and are of two kinds: those containing (1) norepinephrine (dark granules) and (2) epinephrine (light granules). The Golgi vesicles containing the

Reticularis

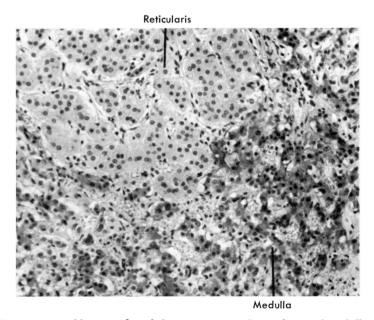

Medulla

Fig. 20-13. Section of human adrenal showing portion of reticularis and medulla. (×160.)

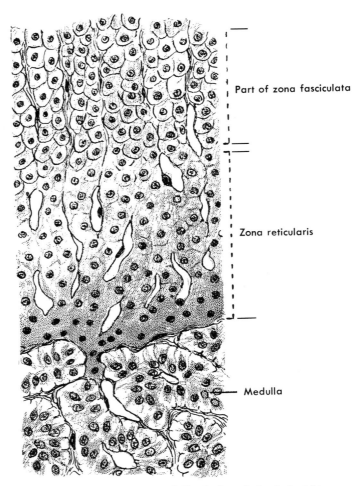

Part of zona fasciculata

Zona reticularis

Medulla

Fig. 20-14. Inner portion of cortex and part of medulla of adrenal gland of rabbit.

formed granules enlarge and migrate to the apical surface of the cell where they are eventually released. In man, the two granule types appear to be contained in the same cell. In most other species they are in separate cells.

Functions of the adrenal gland

The cortex is essential to life, and destruction or removal of the cortex results in Addison's disease, which is fatal. It regulates electrolyte balance and maintains carbohydrate balance, affecting glycogen stores in the liver and muscles; glycogen, in turn, is associated with normal fat and protein metabolism. Another important function of the cortex is the maintenance of connective tissue throughout the body. Connective tissue diseases are often dramatically arrested by the administration of cortisone, an active steroid principle present in the cortex. Deficiency of the hormone is believed to affect adversely other functions such as blood pressure, sexual libido, and vascular permeability. The activity of the adrenal cortex is controlled in part by the adrenocorticotrophic hormone (ACTH) derived from the adenohypophysis whose effect is chiefly on the cells of the zona fasciculata.

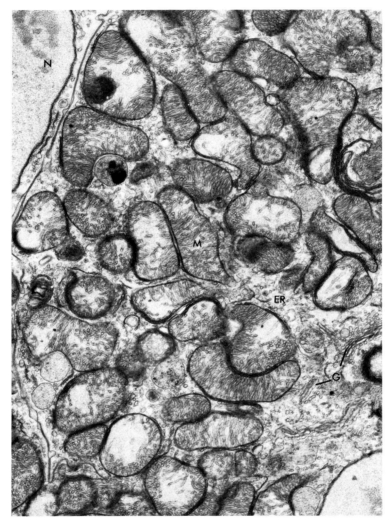

Fig. 20-15. Electron micrograph of a fasciculata cell from the cortex of the adrenal gland of the hamster. These cells have a prominent nucleus, *N*, and the cytoplasm is packed with large mitochondria, *M*. Between the mitochondria are numerous profiles of smooth endoplasmic reticulum, *ER*. Also shown are the laminar portions of the Golgi apparatus, *G*, and granules of various kinds. (×17,880.) (Courtesy Dr. R. Yates, New Orleans, La.)

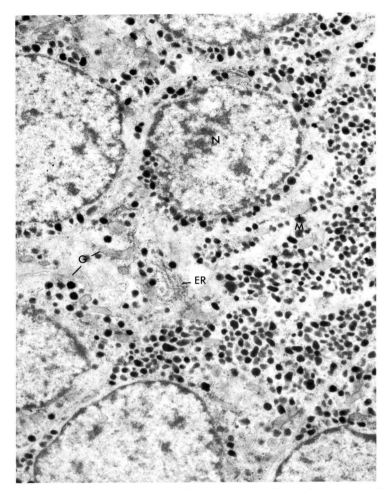

Fig. 20-16. Electron micrograph of part of the adrenal medulla of the hamster. These cells, known as chromaffin cells, have large nuclei, *N*, and numerous dark granules scattered throughout the cytoplasm. The granules of chromaffin cells contain both norepinephrine and epinephrine. The mitochondria, *M*, the endoplasmic reticulum, *ER*, and the Golgi apparatus, *G*, are also shown. (×11,232.) (Courtesy Dr. R. Yates, New Orleans, La.)

Unlike the cortex, the medulla is not essential to life. It elaborates two substances, *epinephrine* and *norepinephrine,* which are catecholamines located in the chromaffin granules of the cells. Epinephrine increases oxygen consumption and the mobilization of glucose from glycogen that is stored in the liver. It also causes contraction of smooth muscle in some vascular beds and relaxation of others, increases cardiac output, and is active in situations of stress or emergency. Epinephrine will also stimulate the secretion of ACTH by the adenohypophysis under experimental conditions. Norepinephrine, a precursor of epinephrine, serves as a transmitting agent of adrenergic nerves regulating blood pressure of the heart and blood vessels. The human adrenal medulla secretes *both* epinephrine (E) and norepinephrine (N). The rate of conversion of N to E depends upon glucocorticoids.

PINEAL BODY

The pineal body, also known as the *epiphysis cerebri,* is a small, flattened, conical body attached to the roof of the third ventricle by a slender stalk. It is divided into lobules by connective tissue septa derived from the capsule in which it is enclosed. When stained with hematoxylin and eosin, the pineal body appears to consist of cords of epithelial cells, which are irregular in shape and have a large nucleus and pale-staining cytoplasm. These are the most numerous cells that occur in this organ and are known as *pinealocytes.* When stained with silver, they are shown to have long radiating processes that terminate in the supporting connective tissue in bulbous processes. Also present are neuroglial cells (interstitial cells), which are believed to serve as supporting elements. At the sixth or seventh year in the human, the pineal body attains its maximum development, and from this time on it undergoes retrogressive changes. The human pineal body often contains concretions, *acervuli* (brain sand), which are extracellular in location and are composed of a mineralized organic matrix having a lamellate appearance.

The function of the pineal gland is not well understood. The pineal in man has been shown to contain *serotonin* and *melatonin.* It is believed to exert a neuroendocrine function and to participate in hormonelike mediation. The details of these processes still await clarification.

21
Brain and special sense organs

BRAIN
Cerebrum

The cerebrum consists of two large symmetrically arranged lobes or hemispheres that are connected by a bridge of white matter, the corpus callosum. Each hemisphere contains a central mass of white matter, the medulla, in which are to be found aggregations of cells known as the internal nuclei and a covering of gray substance known as the cortex.

The cortex is thrown into many folds that are marked by convolutions separated by intervening fissures and sulci. The cells located within the cortex are arranged in layers that are parallel to the surface of the convolutions. Different areas of the cortex vary in the number of cell layers. Some areas contain as few as four whereas others contain as many as eight cell layers. The neurons of the cerebral cortex are believed to consist of two main physiologic types: (1) neurons whose axons enter projection pathways that connect the cortex with the spinal cord and other lower centers; (2) neurons whose axons enter association pathways that connect different areas of the same or opposite hemisphere. These cells make up the majority of the neuron population.

Inasmuch as the arrangement of cells differs slightly in different areas of the cortex, a general description will be presented (Figs. 21-1 and 21-2).

The outer molecular layer consists of a network of fine fibers that is composed chiefly of dendrites derived from cells in the deep layers. These fibers are arranged in tangential meshes below the pia. Small polymorphous cells are sometimes observed among the fibers. They are believed to be displaced from the deeper layers.

The most prominent cell found in the cerebral cortex is the so-called pyramidal cell (Fig. 21-3). Pyramidal cells are distributed in two strata. The stratum located below the molecular layer contains small pyramidal cells, which are about 10 to 12 μ in width; the second stratum is adjacent to that containing small pyramidal cells, on the one hand, and to the white matter on the other. The neurons in this stratum, which is known as the layer of large pyramidal cells, vary in both size and form. The smaller cells in this layer are approximately 20 μ in width, whereas the largest, which are located in the motor cortex, attain a size of from 60 to 80 μ. In the motor cortex, they are known as the cells of Betz. The shape of the cell body is also variable and has been described as pyramidal, triangular, or piriform.

The pyramidal cells are so arranged in the cortex that their pointed apices are directed toward the surface. The pyramidal cells usually exhibit two sets of dendrites. The largest set leaves the cell at the apex and passes to the outer molecular layer. The second set leaves the cell at the sides of the basal part. These dendrites are distributed in the same plane as that in which the cell bodies are located. The axon of the pyramidal cell usually originates at the base of the cell and, after giving off several collateral branches, enters the white matter.

314

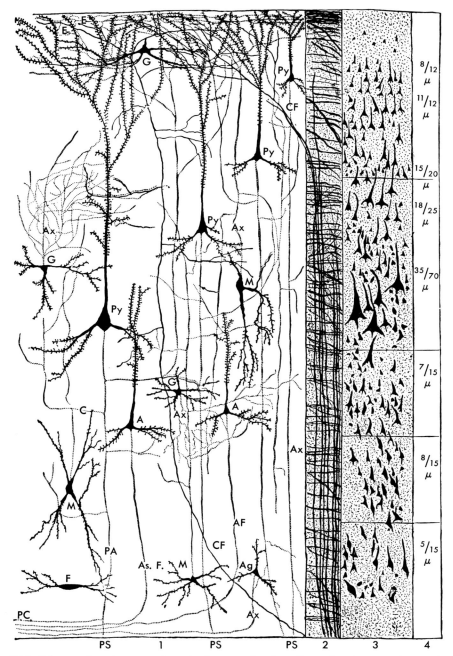

Fig. 21-1. Scheme of motor area of cerebral cortex showing effect of various staining methods. *1*, Golgi's stain; *2*, Weigert's stain; *3*, hematoxylin and eosin; *4*, relative depth of each layer. *A*, Association neurons; *Ag*, angular cells of polymorphous layer; *AF*, association fibers; *Ax*, axons; *C*, collateral; *CF*, centripetal fibers; *E*, terminal fibers; *F*, fusiform cell of polymorphous layer; *G*, Golgi cells, type II; *M*, cells of Martinotti; *PC*, collateral of pyramidal cell; *Py*, pyramidal cells; *PA*, axon of pyramidal cell; *PS*, pyramidal axons passing to cerebral medulla. (After Berkley; from Jordan: Textbook of histology, Philadelphia, D. Appleton-Century Co., Inc.)

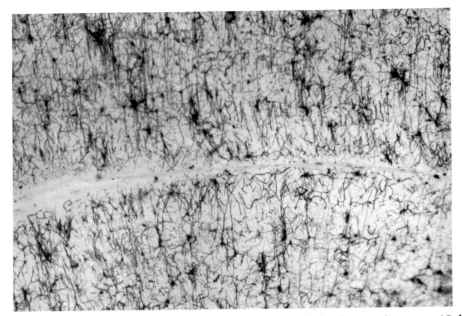

Fig. 21-2. Section of cerebral cortex showing arrangement and distribution of neurons. (Golgi method; ×140.)

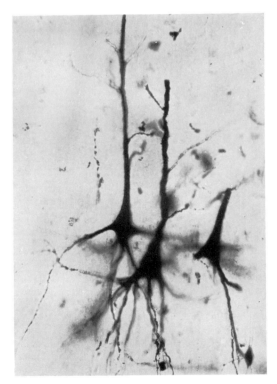

Fig. 21-3. Pyramidal cells from cerebral cortex. (Golgi method.)

The polymorphous layer, sometimes referred to as the inner polymorphous layer, is somewhat thicker than the layer of large pyramidal neurons and consists of cells that may appear stellate, fusiform, or granular. The cells in this layer are less densely distributed than in the other layers and are somewhat smaller than the small pyramidal cells. The axons of these cells pass for the most part to the white matter of the medulla, some reaching the neighboring convolutions. Some of the dendrites are distributed within the layer in which they arise, but most of them pass to the outer pyramidal layers. The granule cells located within this layer are extremely small.

In general, it has been observed that the dendrites of cells in all the layers of the cerebral cortex are either distributed in the same plane as the cell body or pass to the surface of the convolutions. The axons, on the other hand, are directed toward the white matter of the medulla where they continue as association or projection fibers to distant parts of the nervous system.

Cerebellum

The cerebellum is made up of two main lobes or hemispheres, which are connected by a third lobe known as the vermis. Each lobe consists of several subdivisions, the lobules, which are thrown into several transverse convolutions or folia. Like the cerebrum, the cerebellum consists of a central core of white matter, the medulla, and a thick external covering of gray matter, the cortex.

The cerebellar cortex is comprised of an inner granular layer and an outer molecular layer. Between these two zones is a single layer of large conspicuous cells known as Purkinje cells (Figs. 21-4 and 21-5).

The molecular layer contains mostly a dendritic arbor consisting of densely

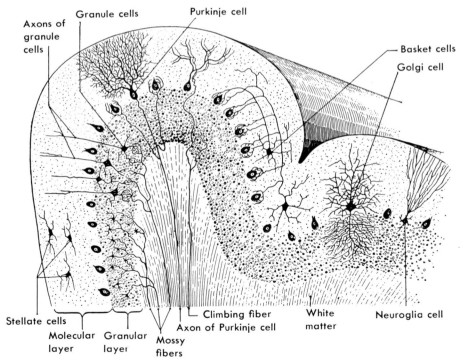

Fig. 21-4. Diagrammatic drawing of cell forms and fiber arrangement of cerebellum. (After Cajal; from Globus: Practical neuroanatomy, Baltimore, The Williams & Wilkins Co.)

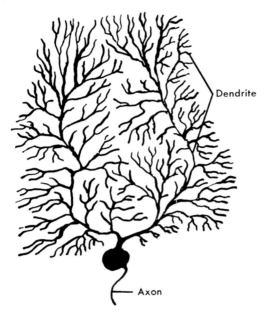

Fig. 21-5. Purkinje cell. (Redrawn from Bremer and Weatherford.)

packed thin axons running parallel to the long axis of the folia and two types of neurons, the large cortical or basket cells and the small stellate cells.

The basket cells are relatively large multipolar cells with short, thick, branching dendrites and a long axon, which passes horizontally in the same plane as that occupied by the dendrites of the Purkinje cells. In its course it gives off five or six collaterals, which pass centrally to end in basketlike arborizations around the Purkinje cells. The basket cells are confined for the most part to the middle and outer part of the molecular layer. They are believed to be association neurons.

The small stellate cells are also multipolar neurons but are smaller than those just described; in addition they are more variable in size. They send out from two to five dendrites that are distributed mainly in the same plane as the Purkinje cells. A single, short, slender axon, which is horizontally placed, is characteristically looped and usually sends out several collaterals. These cells are found to be distributed throughout the molecular layer; they are, however, most numerous in the outer half of this part of the cortex.

The Purkinje cells form a single layer of conspicuous neurons, which is interposed between the molecular and granular layers. These cells are histologically the most distinctive neurons that occur in the cerebellar cortex (Fig. 21-4). They are large, flask-shaped, multipolar cells that possess a thick dendrite directed toward the surface of the convolution (Fig. 21-5). Immediately on leaving the cell body the dendrite divides into two thick branches, each of which undergoes many successive dichotomous branchings. They appear at the surface as a dense profusion of fine fibrils. When viewed in its entirety, the dendrite appears fan shaped, and its characteristic expansions are placed at right angles to the long axis of the convolution. When these dendrites are examined in sections of the convolutions cut lengthwise, they are relatively much less extensive. The single axon arises from the deep surface of the cell and passes through the granular layer to the medulla. Before reaching the medulla the axons send out several collaterals that turn back into the molecular layer and end in association with adjacent Purkinje cells.

The granular or nuclear layer contains three types of cells: (1) granule cells, (2) large stellate cells, and (3) solitary cells that are extremely small and fusiform in shape.

In ordinary stains, the granular layer presents itself as a field of closely packed nuclei looking rather like lymphocytes, with occasional clear spaces or "cerebellar islands" in which resides a complex synaptic tangle called a glomerulus. This structure involves the terminals and dendrites of granule cells and Golgi cells that make contact with incoming fibers (mossy fibers).

Granule cells are small multipolar nerve cells, which are distributed throughout the granular layer in great numbers. These cells have from two to four short dendrites, which pass toward the surface and terminate in peculiar clawlike processes that are in intimate association with small granular spheroidal masses known as eosin bodies. On reaching the surface the axon divides into a T-shaped process, the fibers of which pass parallel to the long axis of the convolutions.

The large stellate cells are also multipolar neurons with profuse dendritic processes that contribute to the molecular layer. The axons and collaterals of these cells are also profuse and contribute to the granular layer, where they end in association with the granule cells.

The medulla contains three main types of fibers: (1) the axons of the Purkinje cells, which are the main efferent fibers from the cortex; (2) the climbing fibers, which are afferent and end in association with the Purkinje cells; and (3) mossy fibers, which are afferent fibers ending in mossy terminations with the granular layer.

Meninges

The brain and spinal cord are enclosed by connective tissue coverings known as the meninges. The meninges (Fig. 21-6) consist of three membranes: the dura mater, the arachnoid, and the pia mater. In the spinal cord the dura is separated from the periosteum of the vertebrae by a space occupied by a loose fibrous and adipose tissue. This region is known as the epidural space.

The dura of the spinal cord is a single-layered structure made up of fibrous tissue containing a few elastic fibers. The fibers in this part of the dura are longitudinally disposed. The cranial dura consists of two layers: an outer vascular portion, serving as the periosteum, and an inner layer, the dura proper. The cranial dura forms reduplications, which extend between the cerebral hemispheres and between the hemispheres and the cerebellum. The two layers of the dura separate along the lines of attachment to form the venous dural sinuses, which receive blood from veins of the brain.

In the cord where the outer surface of

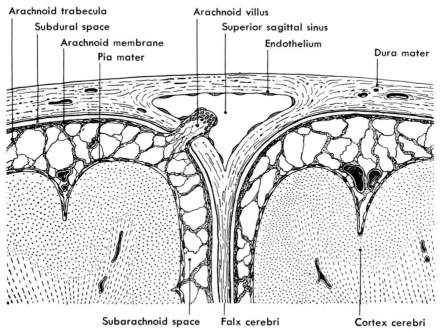

Fig. 21-6. Diagram of arachnoid and subdural spaces. (After Weed; from Bremer and Weatherford: A text-book of histology, New York, 1948, The Blakiston Co.)

the dura is not attached to the adjacent bone, the covering consists of a layer of thin mesenchymal epithelium, which serves as the lining of the epidural space. The inner surface is also lined with a layer of mesenchymal epithelium. This forms the outer wall of the subdural space.

The arachnoid is a loose netlike membrane that intervenes between the dura and the pia. The outer surface consists of a thin fibrous sheath, which is covered by a layer of epithelium. Numerous delicate strands of this membrane pass to the outer surface of the pia.

In the cranial part of the arachnoid, numerous fingerlike structures that project into the venous sinuses are to be found. They are known as the arachnoid villi.

The pia mater is a delicate, vascular, fibrous layer that is closely adherent to the brain and spinal cord. In the region of the roof of the third and fourth ventricles, the vascular membranes that cover them are in some areas invaginated to form the choroid plexuses. Similar invaginations also occur in the lateral ventricles. The vessels of the plexuses are enclosed in connective tissue, which, in turn, is covered by a granular cuboidal epithelium. The entire complex is known as the tela choroidea. The choroid plexuses are one of the main sources of the cerebrospinal fluid.

EYE

On cutting the eye in a meridional horizontal plane, one may readily see the following features.

The eye is a hollow globular structure with a thick, fairly elastic wall, the inner lining of which appears darker than the remainder. It is divided into two unequal parts by a transversely placed structure, the iris. The portion between the iris and the cornea is the anterior chamber; the remainder is divided by the lens and its capsule into the small posterior chamber and the large vitreal space (Fig. 21-7).

The curvature of the outer coat as it

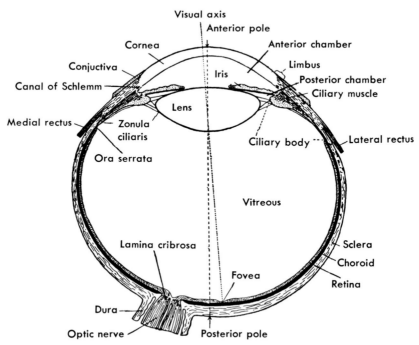

Fig. 21-7. Schematic horizontal meridional section of right eye. (×3.) (Redrawn and modified from Salzmann.)

passes over the anterior chamber is sharper than that around the posterior part of the eye, so that the eyeball is not a perfect sphere. The coat is modified in structure also in its anterior portion, forming the transparent cornea. The anterior chamber contains a fluid, the aqueous humor.

The iris does not lie flat in the transverse plane. Its center is slightly anterior to its periphery so that it has the form of a low truncated cone. It is pierced at the center by the pupil, which is a round aperture of varying dimensions.

The posterior part of the eye contains the lens and the vitreous body or humor. The latter is a jellylike mass, the former a smaller and more solid body lying just posterior to the iris. The lens is suspended in this position by a group of fine fibers, the suspensory ligament. The fibers of the ligament are attached at one end to the lens capsule and at the other to the ciliary body. This is macroscopically visible as a thickening of tissue posterior to the periphery of the iris.

The optic nerve is seen as a stalk leaving the eye at a point slightly medial to the posterior pole. The thick covering of the eye extends over this stalk, and, in a complete dissection of the eye, the optic nerve, and the brain, one would find that the

sheath of the eye extends to and is continuous with the dura mater of the brain.

Coats of the eye

On microscopic examination it is apparent that the coating of the eye has three parts as follows. (1) The fibrous coat includes the sclera covering the vitreal cavity and the transparent cornea of the anterior chamber. (2) The vascular layer extends around the posterior chamber inside the sclera and turns inward to form the iris. The choroid is thickened to form the ciliary body. (3) The retina lines the vitreal cavity. A part of the retina extends over the ciliary body and the posterior surface of the iris.

Fibrous coat. The fibrous coat consists of the sclera and cornea.

Sclera. The sclera surrounds the vitreal cavity and extends a short distance anterior to the margin of the iris. It consists mainly of closely packed fibers and fibroblasts. At its inner margin exists a layer of looser connective tissue containing pigment cells (lamina fusca). Elastic fibers are abundant in the sclera, especially at the points of insertion of the muscles that move the eye.

Cornea. The corneal portion also consists mainly of fibers arranged in flat lamellae parallel to the surface. It has, in addition, two epithelial layers. The outer one is a thin stratified squamous epithelium (from four to six layers of cells), which rests on a relatively thick basement membrane called the anterior basal membrane (of Bowman) (Fig. 21-8). The posterior surface of the cornea is covered with a mesenchymal epithelium, which consists of one layer of flattened cells and rests on an exceptionally transparent membrane called the posterior basal or Descemet's membrane.

Vascular layer. The vascular layer corresponds to the pia mater of the brain and is fundamentally a layer of loose connective tissue containing blood vessels. The part surrounding the posterior chamber is called the choroid. The anterior part forms two structures, the ciliary body and the iris.

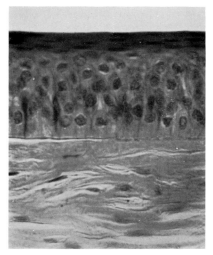

Fig. 21-8. Cornea showing stratified epithelium.

Choroid coat. Blood vessels and connective tissue are not evenly distributed throughout the choroid. Nearest to the sclera is a layer of connective tissue with few, if any, blood vessels. The next layer contains the largest arteries and veins; the innermost layer, a plexus of capillaries. The choroid is bounded on the inside (next to the retina) by the hyaline membrane of Bruch, part of which is said to be a cuticular formation of the cells of the retina.

Ciliary body. The ciliary body is a thickening of the vascular layer to which the suspensory ligament of the lens is attached. It extends into the posterior chamber in a series of from seventy to eighty radially arranged ridges, the ciliary processes. It contains all the elements of the choroid coat except the capillary layer. In addition, there are smooth muscle fibers in it, the contraction of which alters the shape of the lens. The muscles form three groups: meridional, radial, and circular. The ciliary body is covered by a forward extension of the retina, and fibers extend from it to the capsule of the lens. These two elements will be discussed with the retina and the lens, respectively.

Iris. Anterior to the ciliary body the vascular layer forms the iris, which acts as a diaphragm to control the amount of light falling on the retina. The anterior surface of the iris is covered by flattened mesenchymal epithelium similar to the innermost layer of the cornea. The epithelium is interrupted by irregular crypts, which extend into the underlying stroma. The connective tissue of the anterior part of the stroma is a loose network of stellate cells and fine fibers. Some of the stellate cells are pigmented. Fibers are more numerous in the posterior layers of the stroma, and the cells may or may not contain pigment. In this part there are a few elastic fibers, radially arranged, and two groups of muscle fibers. One group of muscle forms the dilator, the other the sphincter, by which the size of the pupil is altered. A part of the retinal layer extends over the posterior surface of the iris.

Retina. The structures described thus far are concerned with the protection of the

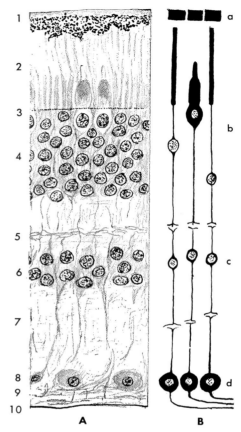

Fig. 21-9. Human retina: A, section of retina; B, isolated cells, diagrammatically presented. Numbers to left of illustration and letters to right correspond to numbers and letters in outline on opposite page.

retina or with focusing light upon it. The retina is the nervous mechanism for the reception and transmission of light stimuli.

The retina arises embryologically as a vesicular outgrowth from the forebrain. As development proceeds, the distal surface of the optic vesicle is invaginated, resulting in a two-layered, cup-shaped structure. The outer layer forms the pigmented epithelium; the invaginated portion gives rise to the remaining layers of the retina, which are, in most of its extent, nine in number.

Three main regions of the retina may be distinguished histologically and topographically: (1) pars optica, lining most of the vitreal space; (2) pars cilaris, covering the ciliary body; and (3) pars iridica, covering the posterior surface of the iris.

Pars optica (Figs. 21-9 and 21-10). In the pars optica, the largest part of the retina, ten layers have been distinguished and named as follows:

1. Pigmented epithelium   a
2. Rods and cones
3. External limiting membrane
4. Outer nuclear (granular) layer   b
5. Outer plexiform (molecular) layer
6. Inner nuclear (granular) layer
7. Inner plexiform (molecular) layer   c
8. Ganglion cell layer
9. Nerve fiber layer   d
10. Internal limiting membrane

The pars optica is, however, more easily understood if we consider that it is composed of a layer of pigmented epithelium and three layers of nervous elements with intervening strata between the perikarya of the latter, which are occupied by axons

and dendrites. This division into four kinds of elements is indicated by a, b, c, and d in the list. Among the nervous elements are found supporting cells, which form the fibers composing the two limiting membranes (3 and 10 in accompanying list). Since cells of this group are scattered throughout all layers of the retina except the first and tenth, they cannot well be included in the list.

The pigmented epithelium is a single layer of cuboidal cells, the cytoplasm of which contains melanin in the form of rod-shaped granules. The cells are said to send out processes among the subjacent rods and cones. In some of the lower vertebrates variations in the extent of such processes can be observed and correlated with differences in the amount of light falling on the retina, but such morphologic variations have not been established as occurring in the mammalian eye.

Immediately next to the pigmented

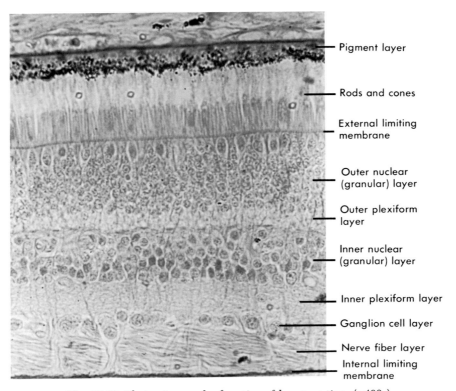

Fig. 21-10. Photomicrograph of section of human retina. (×400.)

Pigment layer

Rods and cones

External limiting membrane

Outer nuclear (granular) layer

Outer plexiform layer

Inner nuclear (granular) layer

Inner plexiform layer

Ganglion cell layer

Nerve fiber layer

Internal limiting membrane

epithelium lie the rods and cones, which are the light receptors. They are part of the first nervous elements involved in the transmission of stimuli. The nuclei of the rod and cone cells form the outer nuclear layer of the retina. Between this layer and the pigmented epithelium, the cytoplasm of the cell assumes one of two forms. In the rod cells the outer segment of the cell is an elongated cylinder 60 μ in length and 2 μ in width. This portion, the rod, is homogenous in appearance. It rests upon an inner segment that contains fine cytoplasmic granules. As it passes through the outer limiting membrane, the cytoplasm of the cell narrows to a thin strand, which traverses part of the outer granular layer until it reaches the nucleus and expands again to form a thin perinuclear film. The nucleus is characterized by the presence in it of from one to three definite bands of chromatin. Beyond the perikaryon the cytoplasm of the rod cells form a fiber that extends into the outer plexiform layer, ending there in a club-shaped enlargement.

The cone cells are less numerous than the rods in most parts of the retina. Their outer segments are relatively short and thick, tapering to a blunted point. The inner segment is broader than that of a rod cell and passes to the perinuclear portion without any marked constriction. The inner process or fiber of the cone cell ends in a pyramidal base in the outer plexiform layer.

The cells of the second layer are bipolar. Each has a dendrite located in the outer plexiform layer, a perikaryon in the inner nuclear layer, and an axon that extends to the inner plexiform layer. Among the perikarya of these cells one may find association neurons, which lie entirely within the inner nuclear layer and serve as horizontal lines of communication between different parts of the retina.

The ganglion cells are typical multipolar nerve cells. Their dendrites synapse with the axons of the bipolar cells, whereas their axons run in a plane parallel to the surface of the retina to the optic disk. This part of the axon is nonmedullated.

Throughout the retina, as in other parts of the nervous system, there is a network of supporting tissue. Concentrations of the fibers elaborated (Müller's fibers) from the external and internal limiting membranes.

The structure of the pars optica is modified in two regions: the optic disk and the macula lutea. The former is the point at which the axons of the ganglion cells meet and turn at right angles to their previous course to leave the eye and form the optic nerve. In the optic disk the outer layers of the retina are interrupted, and the area does not receive stimuli ("blind spot").

The macula lutea is an area near the posterior pole of the eye that appears yellow in the fresh specimen and has the shape of a shallow funnel. The center where the retina is thinnest, is the fovea centralis. From the periphery of the macula to its center there is a gradual reduction of all the retinal elements except the cones, and at the fovea the retina consist of a layer of small cone cells and a few scattered ganglion cells. The fovea is the spot of most acute vision.

The foregoing account of the structure of the retina is based on facts to be observed in special preparations. The ordinary section shows differentiation into ten layers, but the forms and connections of many of the cells are difficult to see.

It is of interest to note that light entering the eye does not fall directly upon the rods and cones. It must first pass through the thickness of the greater part of the retina to the pigmented epithelium. The pigment absorbs the light in the rods and cones.

Pars ciliaris. The pars optica of the retina ends at a point slightly posterior to the ciliary body in a thick irregular margin called the ora serrata. As it approaches this point, the retina undergoes a gradual loss of visual elements, and beyond the margin these disappear entirely. The pars ciliaris of the retina consists of two layers: the pigmented epithelium continues unchanged, and beneath it lies a layer of sustentacular cells arranged in the form of a columnar epithelium. The sustentacular cells produce fibers, some of which are gathered in a hyaline membrane bordering the cavity of the posterior chamber. Other fibers enter into the formation of the ligament of the lens.

Pars iridica. The pigmented epithelium is the only part of the retina that continues beyond the ciliary body to cover the posterior surface of the iris (pars iridica). It becomes somewhat thicker in this region, and the amount of pigment contained in the cells is so great that nuclei and cell boundaries are obscured.

Contents of the eye

The anterior chamber and the small posterior chamber are filled with a fluid, the aqueous humor, whereas the large vitreal cavity encloses the vitreous body. Between the posterior chamber and the vitreal cavity lie the lens and its capsule.

Aqueous humor. The aqueous humor is a colorless fluid that is probably derived partly by transudation from the blood vessels of the region and partly from secretion of the cells covering the anterior surface of the iris and the ciliary body.

Vitreous body or humor. The vitreous body or humor is a mass of jellylike connective tissue that resembles the mucous connective tissue of the umbilical cord. It consists of fine fibers and fibroblasts in a semisolid matrix. The periphery of the vitreous body is covered by a thin membrane of fibers (hyaline membrane), which some authors consider as merely a surface condensation. Others believe it to be a definite membrane uniting the vitreous body to the retina in the posterior part of the eye, turning inward at the ciliary body to contribute part of the suspensory ligament of the lens.

Lens. The lens is an ectodermal structure that was originally cut off as a hollow vesicle from the epithelium. The space within the lens vesicle is filled, as development proceeds, by the growth of the cells on its posterior aspect. These cells elongate until they are fibrous in shape, then lose their nuclei and undego cornification. The anterior surface of the lens is covered by a layer of cuboidal cells. The whole lens is enclosed in a hyaline capsule, which is a specialized basement membrane, and to the capsule are attached the fibers of the suspensory ligament. The fibers of the ligament are supposed to be derived from the basal (sustentacular) cells of the retina and perhaps also from the hyaloid membrane of the vitreous body.

Optic nerve or stalk. The optic nerve is enclosed in extensions of the pia mater and dura mater of the brain, which join the fibrous coat of the eye. The optic nerve consists of the axons of the cells of the ganglionic layer of the retina. These fibers have neither myelin nor neurilemma as long as they remain in the retina. At the optic disk they turn and leave the eyeball, and at this point they acquire a myelin sheath but not a neurilemma. The optic nerve is, in fact, an extension of the substance of the central nervous system rather than a true sensory nerve, and it is more correct to call it the optic stalk.

Circulation and innervation of the eye

The retina and the optic nerve are supplied by the central artery, which passes in the optic stalk. The remainder of the eye receives blood from the opthalmic artery, which forms three ciliary vessels. The latter enter the wall at different levels, supplying the choroid, sclera, iris, and ciliary bodies. Motor nerves form a plexus in the region of the ciliary body, from which are innervated the smooth muscles of the ciliary body and the iris.

EAR

The ear develops from three sources embryologically and retains throughout life its division into three parts: external ear, middle ear, and inner ear. The last-named part develops early in the course of embryonic life as a vesicle that is cut off from the ectodermal covering of the head region and lies in the mesenchyme between the surface and the wall of the developing hindbrain. In this situation, it becomes surrounded by bony tissue as the latter develops from the mesenchyme of the region. The middle ear develops from a diverticulum of the pharynx (first pharyngeal pouch), its ossicles being formed in the surrounding mesenchyme. The external ear is a secondary ingrowth of ectoderm from the surface plus a projection on the surface that forms the pinna.

External ear

The pinna is an irregularly shaped flap of elastic cartilage covered by skin, which is set on the side of the head around the opening of the external auditory meatus. The latter is a tubular channel leading to the eardrum or tympanic membrane. Its outer part is surrounded by elastic cartilage continuous with that of the pinna. Its inner portion penetrates the outer layers of the temporal bone. It is lined with skin that contains sebaceous and ceruminous (wax-forming) glands. Stiff hairs are present at the junction of the cartilaginous and bony parts.

Middle ear

The middle ear is a cavity in the substance of the temporal bone completely separated from the external ear by the tympanic membrane. It is in communication with the pharynx by way of the eustachian tube and separated from the inner ear by a plate of bone containing two apertures, the oval window and the round window. The former is closed by the end of one of the ossicles, the latter by a membrane, so that there is no communication between middle and inner ear. The cavity of the middle ear is crossed by a chain of three small bones, the ossicles.

The tympanic membrane is a fibrous membrane held in a grove of the temporal bone by a ring of fibrocartilage. It is covered on the outside by skin like that lining the meatus and on the inside by a layer of flattened epithelium.

The ossicles are called the malleus (hammer), the incus (anvil), and the stapes (stirrup), the names being descriptive of their respective forms. The handle of the hammer is firmly attached to the inner surface of the tympanic membrane, while its head rests on the anvil. The anvil is articulated also with the upper end of the stirrup, while the foot of the latter is inserted into the oval window. It is by means of

this chain of bones that the vibrations of the tympanic membrane are transmitted across the cavity of the middle ear to the vestibule of the inner ear.

The cavity of the middle ear is lined with flattended epithelium, which rests on the periosteum of the surrounding bone. Epithelium also covers the periosteum of the ossicles.

Inner ear

Osseous labyrinth. The cavity of the inner ear forms a series of irregular spaces in the temporal bone, the whole system being known as the osseous labyrinth. The labyrinth is bordered by layer of compact bone, which may be separated by careful dissection from the spongy bone with which it blends. The bone is covered by periosteum, and the cavity is lined throughout by flattened epithelial tissue. It contains, besides the membranous labyrinth, a fluid called the perilymph. The labyrinth consists of a vestibular portion, semicircular canals, and a cone-shaped cochlear part. It has, in addition, a narrow outlet to the subarachnoid space, the vestibular aqueduct.

Vestibule and semicircular canals. The osseous vestibule is an irregularly rounded cavity from which the semicircular canals, the cavity of the cochlea, and the vestibular aqueduct diverge.

The semicircular canals are three in number. Two of these (the superior and posterior) are set vertically and at right angles to each other. The third canal (lateral) lies in a horizontal plane. Each is a horseshoe-shaped channel in the temporal bone, connecting at both ends with the cavity of the vestibule. One limb of each is enlarged near its connection with the vestibule to form the ampulla. The opposite ends of the superior and posterior canals join and re-enter the vestibule through a common opening; the lateral canal returns to it separately, so that there are five openings from the vestibule to the system of semicircular canals.

Cochlea. The canal of the cochlea pursues a spiral course from the vestibule to the apex of a flattened cone. It surrounds a central mass of spongy bone, the modiolus, which contains the spiral ganglion. A shelf of bone projects into the canal from the modiolus, following the course of the former to its apex. This is called the osseous spiral lamina.

Membranous labyrinth. The membranous labyrinth, which lies within the osseous labyrinth, is separated from it by the perilymph and is divided functionally into two parts: the portion lying in the vestibule and the semicircular canals mediates the sense of equilibrium, while that in the cochlea is the organ of hearing. Fundamentally the structure of the membranous labyrinth is that of a closed system consisting of a sheath of connective tissue lined with flattened epithelium and containing a fluid, the endolymph. The epithelium is modified in various parts of the system to form receptors for the stimuli involved.

Utricle and saccule. The utricle and saccule are rounded sacs that lie in the perilymph of the vestibule and are held in place by trabeculae of connective tissue extending from the periosteum of the surrounding bone. They are united by a narrow duct, which has the form of an inverted V. From the apex of this duct the endolymphatic duct leads away through the vestibular aqueduct to terminate in the endolymphatic sac. Another fine duct joins the saccule with the cochlear duct.

Semicircular canals. The semicircular ducts arise from the utricle. They lie within the osseous semicircular canals, and each is attached along part of its periphery to the periosteum of the bone and is further anchored by connective tissue trabeculae.

The epithelial lining of the vestibular portion of the labyrinth contains patches of neuroepithelium. There is one of these in the utricle, another in the saccule, and one in each ampulla of the semicircular ducts. The neuroepithelium contains hair cells and tall sustentacular cells.

Cochlear duct. One border of the membranous part of the cochlea is attached to the bony shelf of the modiolus, the lamina spiralis. The opposite border forms a wider attachment to the outer edge of the canal, thus dividing the latter into two parts, which are in communication at the apex of the spiral but not elsewhere. The upper part of the osseous canal leads from the vestibule and is known as the scala vestibuli. The lower part ends at the membrane close to the round window (secondary tympanic membrane) and is called the scala tympani. The intervening space, enclosed by the cochlear duct, is the scala media (Figs. 21-11 and 21-12). The scala vestibuli and the scala tympani are lined, as are other parts of the osseous labyrinth, by flattened epithelium resting on the periosteum of the surrounding bone. The epithelium extends, also, over the outer surfaces of the cochlear duct, where the latter is not in contact with the modiolus on the one hand or the outer wall of the osseous labyrinth on the other.

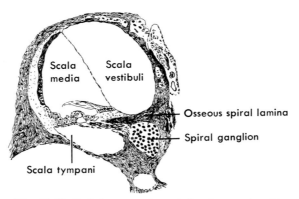

Fig. 21-11. Radial section through basal turn of cochlea.

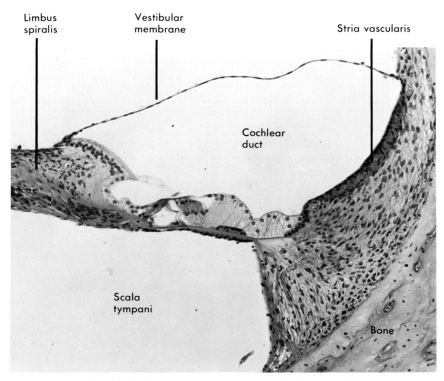

Limbus spiralis   Vestibular membrane   Stria vascularis

Cochlear duct

Scala tympani

Bone

Fig. 21-12. Photomicrograph of organ of Corti. (×100.)

The scala media is separated from the scala vestibuli by a thin membrane, the vestibular membrane, which extends from the modiolus to the outer wall of the cochlear canal. Along this part of the wall the periosteum is thickened, forming a ligament, the lower edge of which projects toward the bony spiral lamina of the modiolus. The gap between the ligament (spiral ligament) and the lamina is closed by the basal membrane. The scala media is, therefore, separated from the scala tympani by three structures: the spiral ligament, the basal membrane, and the osseous spiral lamina. Between the latter and the vestibular membrane a thickening of connective tissue called the limbus spiralis projects outward from the modiolus into the space of the scala media. The vestibular membrane is attached to the upper surface of the limbus. Its lower surface is concave, forming, with the spiral lamina, a groove

known as the spiral sulcus. The space enclosed by the structures just enumerated has, in section, the form of a right-angled triangle of which the vestibular membrane forms the hypotenuse.

Histologically the different portions of the cochlear duct present striking variations from the structure of the remainder of the membranous labyrinth (Fig. 21-13). The vestibular membrane consists of a very thin layer of connective tissue. It is covered on the outside by an extension of the mesothelium lining the remainder of the vestibule; its inner surface is also lined with flattened epithelium of ectodermal origin.

The epithelial lining of the scala media continues unchanged around the outer edge of the triangle where the duct is in contact with the border of the osseous canal. The connective tissue of this portion is much thickened, forming a relatively

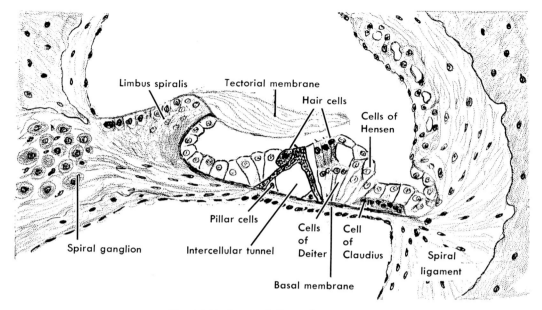

Fig. 21-13. Organ of Corti of guinea pig.

wide band between the epithelium and the bone. A part of this layer is very vascular, and its lower portion is extended toward the modiolus as the spiral ligament. At the angle between the base and the outer side of the scala media, the lining epithelium changes from flattened to cuboidal or low columnar cells.

The basal membrane running from the tip of the spiral ligament to the tip of the osseous lamina is a connective tissue membrane considerably thicker than that forming the vestibular membrane. Like the latter, it has an outer covering of mesothelium that is, in this case, part of the lining of the scala tympani. The epithelium on the side toward the scala media, which is the ectodermal lining of the cochlear duct, is modified for the reception of sound waves and forms the organ of Corti. Starting at the outer edge and tracing the organ toward the modiolus, we may distinguish the following parts:

1. The cells of Claudius, which are small cuboidal cells with dark, granular cytoplasm, lie along the membrana basilaris between the latter and the cells of Hensen in that region.

2. The cells of Hensen lie next to those of Claudius, are columnar, and increase in height as they continue toward the modiolus.

3. Outer hair cells and sustentacular cells (of Deiter), as their name implies, are provided with hairlike projections from their surfaces and are the actual receptors of the organ. They form a band three or four cells wide at the surface of the epithelium but do not reach to the basement membrane. Deiter's cells rest on the basement membrane and have narrow distal ends extending to the surface between the hair cells. They have stiff cuticular borders that give a firm support to the hair cells.

4. Two rows of pillar cells run through the length of the organ of Corti. They are tall columnar cells in which the cuticular substance forms a stiff rod. One row of these rods is inclined toward the modiolus, the other away from it, so that while their distal ends meet, there is a considerable space between their bases. They thus enclose two sides of a tunnel, which is triangular in cross section, the base of the triangle being formed by the membrana basilaris of the scala media. The enclosed

space is called the inner tunnel. It is crossed by naked dendrites of the cells of the spiral ganglion.

5. One row of inner hair cells lies next to the inner pillar cells. These cells are usually of the low columnar type and do not reach the basement membrane. They are supported by tall columnar cells much like the cells of Hensen in appearance.

6. The spiral sulcus is lined with cuboidal epithelium. There is, however, no sharp line of demarcation between the border cells and those lining the spiral sulcus.

At the inner angle of the scala media are the osseous spiral lamina and the spiral limbus, which partially enclose the internal spiral sulcus. The periosteum of the osseous lamina extends outward from the bony shelf to meet the basal membrane. The

spiral limbus is composed of connective tissue and projects into the space enclosed by the scala media. Its apical convex surface is covered by columnar cells that have a thick cuticular border. Its lower surface is covered by cuboidal cells. From the border between these two surfaces projects the tectorial membrane, which extends into the scala media and rests upon the portion of the organ of Corti that contains the hair cells. The tectorial membrane is a noncellular structure composed of fine fibers in an adhesive matrix. It is supposed to be attached, in life, to the organ of Corti, although the two are almost always separated in fixed preparations.

The spiral ganglion, situated in the osseous lamina, is composed of bipolar nerve cells. The dendrites of these cells pass to-

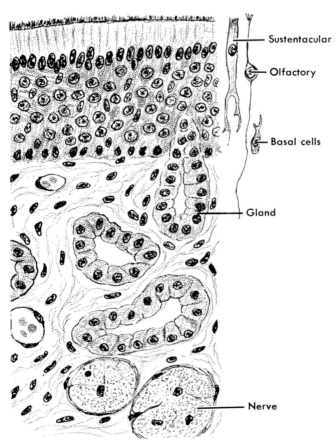

Fig. 21-14. Olfactory mucosa of rabbit. (After Jordan.)

ward the organ of Corti, forming a conspicuous band of myelinated fibers in the lamina. As they leave the latter, they lose their myelin sheaths. Some of them cross the inner tunnel, other pass below it, and both groups end in arborizations among the hair cells. The axons of the cells of the spiral ganglion carry impulses to the appropriate region of the brain.

The exact mechanism of the transmission of sound waves to the organ of Corti is a subject of controversy. It is clear, however, that sound waves cause vibrations of the tympanic membrane and that such vibrations are transmitted to the perilymph of the vestibule by the movement of the ossicles of the middle ear. The movement of the perilymph causes movement of the basal membrane of the organ of Corti,

and the consequent alteration of position of the hair cells in relation to the tectorial membrane is the stimulus that is transmitted to the brain as sound.

OLFACTORY ORGAN

The receptors for olfactory stimuli, or sensations of smell, are located in the nose. This organ also functions as a part of the respiratory system, since air passes through it into the trachea by way of the nasopharynx. The nose consists of two passageways separated by the nasal septum. Each passage may be divided into a vestibule lined with skin and a nasal cavity that opens into the nasopharynx through an aperture known as the choana. The outline of the nasal cavity is irregular, its lateral margin having three longitudinal elevations

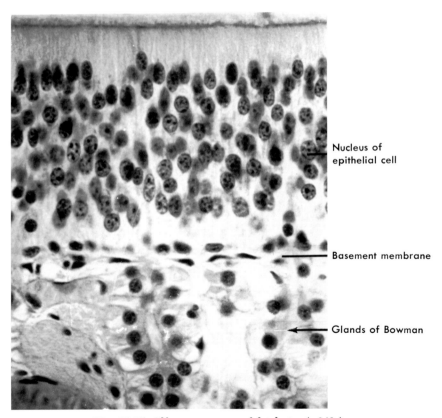

Nucleus of epithelial cell

Basement membrane

Glands of Bowman

Fig. 21-15. Olfactory mucosa of fetal pig. (×640.)

of the surrounding tissue. These are the conchae or the turbinate bones. The lining of the cavity is, for the most part, columnar or pseudostratified epithelium but may contain some patches of stratified squamous epithelium.

The olfactory part of the nose is an area of neuroepithelium extending from the superior concha across the roof of the nasal cavity and part way down the septum. The epithelium in this region appears as stratified columns and contains sustentacular cells, olfactory cells, and basal cells (Figs. 21-14 and 21-15).

Sustentacular cells

Sustentacular cells are tall columnar cells that form the superficial layer. Their basal portions are extended in irregular branching processes among the olfactory and basal cells. Their apical ends contain pigment granules, are ciliated, and have a distinct cuticular border. The nuclei of the sustentacular cells are oval and lie for the most part in a zone between the surface of the epithelium and the nuclei of the olfactory cells. Some oval nuclei may be found scattered among the deeper layers.

Olfactory cells

The olfactory cells are true nerve cells, bipolar in form. Their dendrites extend to the surface of the epithelium, passing through minute openings in the cuticle and ending in a tuft of cilia. The perikarya are small rounded elements with spherical nuclei. They form a broad band below the zone of oval nuclei called the zone of round nuclei. The axons of the olfactory cells pass inward through the lamina propria where they may be seen as large groups of nonmyelinated fibers. They terminate in the olfactory bulb.

Basal cells

The basal cells are thought to be reserve sustentacular cells. They are short, irregularly shaped cells, which form a layer next to the lamina propria. Like the sustentacular cells, they have oval nuclei. Their distal ends form short processes that extend among the branched ends of the sustentacular cells.

The lamina propria of the olfactory mucosa contains glands that open into the surface through wide ducts. The epithelium lining the glands (of Bowman) has the appearance of serous-secreting tissue but sometimes contains mucus.

The olfactory mucosa has a rich blood supply, the veins of which drain into the superior longitudinal sinus.

Index